Instruments for Clinical Nursing Research

Instruments for Clinical Nursing Research

Editor

Marilyn Frank-Stromborg, R.N., Ed.D.
Professor
School of Nursing
Northern Illinois University
DeKalb, Illinois

With a Foreword by
Nola J. Pender, R.N., Ph.D., FAAN

JONES AND BARTLETT PUBLISHERS
BOSTON   **LONDON**

Editorial, Sales, and Customer Service Offices

Jones and Bartlett Publishers
One Exeter Plaza
Boston, MA 02116

Jones and Bartlett Publishers International
PO Box 1498
London W6 7RS
England

Library of Congress Cataloging-in-Publication Data

Instruments for clinical nursing research / editor, Marilyn Frank
-Stromborg ; with a foreword by Nola J. Pender.
      p.   cm.
   Originally published: Norwalk, Conn : Appleton & Lange, c1988.
   Includes bibliographical references and index.
   ISBN 0-86720-340-4
   1. Nursing--Research. 2. Clinical medicine--Research. I. Frank
-Stromborg, Marilyn.
   [DNLM: 1. Clinical Nursing Research--instrumentation.   2. Clinical
Nursing Research--methods.   WY 20.5 I59 1988a]
RT81.5.I157 1991
610.73'072--dc20
DNLM/DLC
for Library of Congress   91-35377
ISBN   0-86720-340-4   CIP

Printed in the United States of America
95 94 93   10 9 8 7 6 5 4 3

To Nels and Danny—my joy
To Paul—my support
To my parents—my inspiration

Contributors

Susan Larsen Beck, R.N., M.N.
Doctoral Candidate, University of Utah, College of Nursing, Oncology Nurse
Specialist, University of Utah, Health Sciences Center, Salt Lake City, Utah

Nancy Bergstrom, R.N., Ph.D.
Associate Professor, Graduate Nursing Program, College of Nursing, University of
Nebraska Medical Center, Omaha, Nebraska

Barbara J. Braden, R.N., M.S.
Doctoral Candidate, University of Texas at Austin, Associate Professor, Creighton
University School of Nursing, Omaha, Nebraska

Mary L. Brown, R.N., M.S., C.A.N.P., O.C.N.
Clinical Nursing Coordinator, Compromised Host–Bone Marrow Transplant Unit
C020, Stanford University Hospital, Stanford, California

Caroline Bagley-Burnett, R.N., M.S.N.
Doctoral Candidate, The Johns Hopkins University, School of Hygiene and Public
Health, Arlington, Virginia. Formerly with the Medical Breast Cancer Section,
National Cancer Institute, Bethesda, Maryland

Nancy Burns, R.N., Ph.D.
Professor of Nursing, University of Texas at Arlington, School of Nursing,
Arlington, Texas

Rebecca F. Cohen, R.N., Ed.D., C.P.Q.A.
Associate Administrator–Quality Assurance, Sycamore Hospital, Sycamore, Illinois,
Instructor, School of Allied Health, Northern Illinois University, DeKalb, Illinois

Patricia H. Cotanch, R.N., Ph.D.
Associate Professor–Nursing, Assistant Professor–Psychiatry, Duke University
Medical Center, Durham, North Carolina

Sue B. Davidson, R.N., M.S.
Doctoral Student, Oregon State University, Corvallis, Oregon, Associate Professor,
School of Nursing, Oregon Health Science University, Portland, Oregon

Hannah Dean, R.N.C., Ph.D.
Associate Dean for Administration, School of Nursing, University of California,
Los Angeles, California

Judy M. Diekmann, R.N., Ed.D., O.C.N.
Associate Professor, University of Wisconsin–Milwaukee, School of Nursing,
Department of Health Restoration, Milwaukee, Wisconsin

Marylin J. Dodd, R.N., Ph.D.
Associate Professor and American Cancer Society Professor of Oncology Nursing,
University of California, San Francisco, Department of Physiological Nursing,
San Francisco, California

Linda Bartkowski-Dodds, R.N., M.S.
Oncology Clinical Nurse Specialist/Senior Clinical Research Associate, XOMA
Corporation, Berkeley, California

Susan Gross Fisher, R.N., M.S.
Doctoral Candidate, School of Public Health, University of Illinois, Biostatistician,
Veterans Administration Cooperative Studies Program Coordinating Center,
Hines, Illinois

Mary C. Fraser, R.N., M.A.
Clinical Nurse Specialist/Epidemiology Research Nurse, Cancer Nursing Service and
Environmental Epidemiology Branch, National Cancer Institute, National Institute of
Health, Bethesda, Maryland

Marcia M. Grant, R.N., D.N.Sc.
Director, Nursing Research and Education, City of Hope National Medical Center,
Duarte, California

Sharol F. Jacobson, R.N., Ph.D.
Professor and Director of Nursing Research, University of Oklahoma, College of
Nursing, Oklahoma City, Oklahoma

Suzanne Hearne Kaempfer, R.N., M.N.
Doctoral Student, Department of Physiological Nursing, Earle C. Anthony Graduate
Dean's Fellow, University of California, San Francisco, California

Ada M. Lindsey, R.N., Ph.D.
Professor and Dean, School of Nursing, University of California,
Los Angeles, California

Ruth McCorkle, R.N., Ph.D., FAAN
Professor and American Cancer Society Professor of Oncology Nursing, School of
Nursing, University of Pennsylvania, Philadelphia, Pennsylvania

Deborah B. McGuire, R.N., Ph.D.
Assistant Professor, The Johns Hopkins University School of Nursing, Coordinator,
Nursing Research, The Johns Hopkins Oncology Center Nursing Department,
Baltimore, Maryland

Carol McMillen Moinpour, Ph.D.
National Research Service Award Fellow (NIMH/DHHS-MH08949-02),
Postdoctorate Fellow, Department of Biostatistics, University of Washington,
Seattle, Washington; Staff Scientist, Fred Hutchinson Cancer Research Center,
Seattle, Washington

Sharon Rothenberger, R.N., M.S.
Research Nurse, Department of Infectious Diseases, Veterans Administration
Medical Center, Buffalo, New York

Jan M. Ellerhorst-Ryan, R.N., M.S.N., C.S.
Surgical Oncology Clinical Nurse Specialist, Department of Nursing Consultation,
University of Cincinnati Medical Center, Cincinnati, Ohio

Judith Saunders, R.N., D.N.Sc.
Project Director, Improving Cancer Patient's Hospital–Home Transition, Department
of Nursing Research and Education, City of Hope National Medical Center,
Duarte, California

Martha H. Stoner, R.N.-C., Ph.D., A.N.P.
Assistant Professor, School of Nursing and Assistant Director of Nursing for
Research, University Hospital, University of Colorado Health Sciences Center,
Denver, Colorado

Roberta A. Strohl, R.N., M.N.
Clinical Nurse Specialist, Radiation Oncology, University of Maryland at Baltimore,
Baltimore, Maryland

Marilyn Frank-Stromborg, R.N., Ed.D.
Professor, School of Nursing, Northern Illinois University, DeKalb, Illinois

Jo Ann Wegmann, R.N., Ph.D.
Assistant Administrator, Nursing Services, Pomerado Hospital, Poway, California

Reviewers

Jean Brown, R.N., M.S.
Associate Professor, School of Nursing, University of Rochester,
Rochester, New York

Mary C. Corley, R.N., Ph.D.
Director of Nursing Research, Veterans Administration Medical Center,
Seattle, Washington

Alice J. Dan, R.N., Ph.D.
Associate Professor, The University of Illinois, College of Nursing, Chicago, Illinois

Mary Maxwell, R.N., Ph.D.
Clinical Specialist, Oncology, Director, Nursing Research Program, Veterans
Administration Medical Center, Portland, Oregon

Contents

Foreword

Nursing research generates knowledge about human responses directed toward optimizing health, preventing disease, and coping with acute or chronic illness throughout the lifespan. The processes of "care" rather than "cure" are the primary focii of nursing investigations. Because nursing is an evolving science, the repertoire of research tools and instruments available for measuring holistic dimensions of human functioning and client status as a basis for care decisions is limited. Yet, the development and use of valid and reliable instrumentation in research is critical to the advancement of nursing science and ultimately to the quality of practice within the profession. Rigorous development of instrumentation and precise use of measurement tools already available are critical to promote quality inquiry as the nursing profession assumes an increasingly important role in formulating and addressing the national and international health research agendas.

This book provides a timely overview of instruments for use in clinical nursing research. Not only is attention given to the criteria for evaluating instruments prior to use in clinical research, but compilations of tools for assessing health and function as well as clinical problems in more than 25 areas are provided. These areas range from quality of life, spirituality, and self-care, to dyspnea and alterations in taste and smell. The editor is to be commended for bringing together the respective expertise of over 25 nurse researchers who describe and critique the instruments presented. The instruments included have been developed by both nurses and non-nurses. The contributors provide an excellent review of the various tools available to measure the target phenomena of scientific interest to nursing. Thus, highly practical assistance is offered to nurses seeking instrumentation for their own investigative work or for that of their students.

The perspective of the book has special relevance for persons who are currently involved in the arduous task of instrument development. It provides direction and prototypes for instrument construction and evaluation. This book is not only a valuable resource for nurses in research, education, and practice, but in addition, should stimulate further development of instrumentation which can profoundly enhance the future of nursing science and practice.

Nola J. Pender, R.N., Ph.D., FAAN
Professor
Community Health Nursing
School of Nursing
Northern Illinois University
DeKalb, Illinois

Preface

A clearly identified priority in nursing research is the need to develop instruments to be used by nurses to conduct clinical research. Barriers to accomplishing this goal have been multiple and are of long standing duration. Some of these barriers include:
1. a tendency for nurses to develop a new tool for each research endeavor, to use small samples when instruments are developed, to conduct minimal validity/reliability testing, and to discard the tool after the study has been completed.
2. repeated investigations of certain variables because of the lack of psychometrically refined instruments, while other variables remain unstudied because appropriate instruments are not available.
3. the inaccessibility of instruments developed by other researchers.

In 1981, in response to the barriers listed above, several national groups (the Division of Nursing, the U.S. Department of Health and Human Services, and the Western Interstate Commission for Higher Education) compiled and published two books that were designed to aid researchers in selecting appropriate measurement tools. While these publications (*Instruments for Measuring Nursing Practice and Other Health Care Variables* and *Instruments for Use in Nursing Education Research*) were initially excellent sources for meeting the needs of nurse researchers for greater access to psychometrically refined instruments, there is clearly a need for additional publications in this area. Furthermore, because of the increasing emphasis on the importance of research-based practice, there remains a need for additional information about instruments designed for *clinical research.*

Background Information: *Instruments for Clinical Nursing Research* is an outgrowth of a project undertaken by the Oncology Nursing Society. The Oncology Nursing Society (ONS) is a professional nursing organization of 12,000 nurses that was founded eleven years ago. In 1984, the research committee wrote a series of scholarly articles for the *Oncology Nursing Forum,* the official journal of the ONS. Each article focused on one concept and described the available instruments that could be used to measure that concept. The major impetus for undertaking this project was: 1. the need to increase clinical research activity among the members of the Oncology Nursing Society, and 2. the realization that a major barrier to nurses conducting clinical research revolved around their lack of knowledge about the availability and suitability of instruments.

Feedback on the articles was overwhelmingly positive and requests for reprints were received from across the country. It became obvious to the members of the ONS Research Committee that there was high interest in the articles from nurses outside of the organization and that the information on the tools had stimulated multiple nursing research efforts by students and clinicians alike. One difficulty identified by the committee was that the address-ing of a concept with an article prevented in-depth discussion and inclusion of many essential instruments because of page limitations.

The decision was made to develop a book which would: 1. review the tools that are presently available to measure a selected phenomena, 2. describe the psychometric proper-ties of each tool, 3. detail the samples or studies that have utilized the tool, 4. identify the strengths and weaknesses of the instrument, and 5. discuss the instruments in relationship to use in all areas of nursing, *not* limiting it to oncology nursing. The ONS Research Committee, which was composed of researchers in both academic and clinical settings, next identified clinical phenomena for which instruments had been developed for assessing health, function, and/or clinical problems. These became the individual chapters that make up the book. The committee also felt that in addition to the chapters devoted to discussions of instruments, one other chapter was needed to assist the reader. The Overview section reviews the important characteristics of tools (reliability, validity) that need to be addressed in instrument develop-ment. For the beginning researcher, the Overview section is designed to provide a review of key concepts related to psychometric properties of research tools. Also included are the legal/ethical considerations that attend instrument use.

As with any book it becomes the task of the editor to set limits on what can and cannot be included. Obviously this endeavor could not include every variable nor every instrument available to measure that variable. Therefore, the decision was made to include only those variables associated with the most commonly occurring clinical problems, and to include those related to measuring holistic dimensions of human functioning and client status. The intent of this book is to provide nurses desiring to conduct research with one resource that identifies clinical nursing research instruments, that specifies references to locate each instrument, and that describes sample questions from each instrument. The intended audience of this book are nurses in education, practice, and research settings who are interested in conducting clinical research. It is anticipated that the nurse who has had a beginning level research course would have no difficulty understanding the material in this book.

There are several ways that this book can be used. One way is to select a concept and read the related chapter. Another way is to find a specific instrument in the Index and find the chapter(s) where it is discussed. Some of the instruments (e.g., Sickness Impact Profile-SIP) are discussed in multiple chapters because they measure more than one concept. It is anticipated that most readers will select specific chapters that describe the concepts they are interested in researching.

Organization of the Text: The 25 chapters are subdivided into three parts. In Part I the reader will find information related to evaluating research instruments.

Part II contains 16 chapters devoted to instruments that can be used to assess health and function. This section begins with the chapter devoted to instruments for measuring func-tional status, by Moinpour, McCorkle, and Saunders. Fraser's chapter on selecting instru-ments to measure mental status and level of consciousness includes in-depth discussions of the components of mental status, general issues in measuring this area, specific instruments that can be used to measure level of consciousness/mental status, and applications for the clinical setting, including AIDS. Quality of life instruments are detailed in the next two chapters from two different frameworks. Stromborg presents multiple quality of life defini-tions including health as a dimension of quality of life, as well as other dimensions which are hypothesized to constitute quality of life. In this chapter, there is a discussion of the issues which should be considered when selecting a quality of life tool and the single instruments which measure quality of life. In contrast, Dean conceptualizes quality of life as a multidimensional, complex concept that is best measured by multiple instruments. Lindsey, Wegmann, and Stoner in each of their respective chapters detail the concepts of social support, coping, and hope, and the related instruments available to measure these concepts.

Instruments to measure spiritual needs, spiritual well-being, spiritual coping, and the spiritual needs of nurses and patients are found in Ryan's chapter. Bagley details information-seeking activities reported in consumer and health care literature and the instruments that can be used to measure information-seeking behavior. Dodd's chapter gives a comprehensive discussion on the concept of self-care and health-deviation self-care, and the universal self-care instruments that can be used to measure this concept. Diekmann's chapter includes the issues that must be considered when measuring the body image concept. Included are scales and questionnaires to measure body image, means for direct measurement of perceived body size, and methods for using distortion techniques and videotape recordings.

Kaempfer and Fisher have compiled an extensive listing of instruments that can be used to measure multiple aspects of sexuality. The initial part of their chapter includes a thorough review of the clinical and research perspectives of human sexuality. Bergstrom's chapter analyzes the multiple methods for measuring the outcomes of dietary intake including clinical examination, biochemical analysis of blood, serum, and urine, and anthropometric measures. The current state of the science of sleep measurement is detailed in Beck's chapter including a discussion of the present conceptualization of sleep. The last two chapters in this part deal with measurement of attitudes—attitudes toward chronic illness and attitudes toward cancer. Cohen provides a comprehensive review of the tools that are designed to measure a patient's attitudes toward chronic disease and traces the development of these instruments that are utilized to measure the many dimensions of attitudes toward chronic illness. Burn's chapter includes an overview discussion of the differences between beliefs, attitudes, and values, the selection of a belief or attitude tool, and the tools that can be used to measure attitudes toward cancer.

Part III contains the instruments that can be used for the most commonly occurring clinical problems encountered by nurses. The phenomenon identified range from nausea and vomiting to skin integrity. The measurement instruments that are included in this part are both paper and pencil, and laboratory and physiological procedures. Cotanch presents a review of the issues that must be considered when measuring nausea and vomiting, the treatment advances that are being made in this area, and the instruments that can be used. The researcher who desires to measure bowel elimination has many choices to make including whether to use scale, radiologic, colorimetric, particulate, chemical, isotopic, or gastrointestinal motility measures. These methods are detailed in the chapter by Bartkowski-Dodds. McGuire's extensive review of tools which can be used to measure pain includes introductory pages that discuss the multiple definitions of pain, the different types of pain, the problems in measuring pain, and the perception and experience of pain. Strohl points out that disturbances in taste and/or smell are difficult to measure but offers concrete information that will help the nurse researcher desiring to conduct research in this area. The chapter describes the normal taste and smell response, the changes in taste and smell that result from disease states (i.e., cancer, diabetes, renal disease), and the tools that can be used to measure these alterations. Brown presents the instruments that can be used to measure dyspnea and the problems that are encountered in clinical research investigating this symptom.

Many instruments are available to measure skin integrity. Braden discusses the instruments that permit direct measurement or estimation of skin integrity. Mucocutaneous alterations of the oral cavity and the vaginal vault are covered in the last two chapters in this section. Rothenberger points out that stomatitis is a treatment-associated side effect and describes the tools and methods that are available to assess this condition. The definition, occurrence, and parameters used to describe vaginitis are covered in the chapter by Grant and Davidson, along with a discussion of assessment of subjective and objective symptoms and available assessment tools.

Acknowledgments

The editor wishes to acknowledge the excellent contributions of the many authors and their willingness to contribute to the project and meet the deadlines. Many of the authors of this book are the original members of the ONS Research Committee who participated in the decision to produce the series of research articles, as well as later members of the committee who participated in the decision to produce a book. A substantial number of the chapters were done by authors who have concentrated their research efforts on the concept they wrote about. The input of the multiple reviewers of the manuscript was appreciated and each suggestion contributed to strengthening the final product. The support of the Oncology Nursing Society Board of Directors and Pearl Moore, R.N., M.S.N., Executive Director of the Oncology Nursing Society, contributed greatly to the ease in producing this book. I would also like to thank Claudette Varricchio, R.N., D.S.N., Vickie Beck, R.N., M.S.N., and Kerry VanSloten Harwood, R.N., M.S.N., for their contributions to this book.

All royalties are being donated to the Oncology Nursing Foundation and will be used to support oncology-related nursing research activities. It is our sincere hope that this compilation will help foster and promote more clinical research among nurses.

Marilyn Frank-Stromborg, R.N., Ed.D.
Editor

PART I

Overview

CHAPTER 1

Evaluating Instruments for Use in Clinical Nursing Research

Sharol F. Jacobson, R.N., Ph.D.

Historically, nurse researchers who wished to measure clinical phenomena had little choice but to develop their own instruments. Fortunately, this situation is changing. In response to recent reviews of the state of measurement in nursing,[1,2] the development of more and better instruments for nursing research has become a high priority. As this book attests, compilations of instruments are appearing to help researchers locate useful measures.

The purpose of this chapter is to provide a brief review of key concepts in measurement and a summary of current recommendations for the selection, use, and continued development of existing instruments in clinical nursing research. Major topics include assessing the conceptual basis and measurement framework of a tool, a review of the nature of the major psychometric properties of tools and common item analysis procedures, a description of the state-of-the-art of measurement in nursing, and a summary of the ethical and legal considerations in using existing tools. The emphasis is on practical information for decision making. The chapter is aimed at nurses who have had at least one course in research methods and statistics but whose background in measurement and research may be neither extensive nor recent. It is not the purpose of the chapter to serve as a comprehensive research or measurement text. Readers who need fuller or more theoretical explanations should consult the References; those with asterisks are particularly useful, comprehensive, or recent.

In this chapter, the terms "measure," "tool," "test," and "instrument" are used interchangeably for the measurement device. The terms "trait," "concept," and "attribute" refer to what is being measured.

ASSESSING THE CONCEPTUAL BASIS OF INSTRUMENTS

Instrument development, like other research, can be based on a conceptual or a theoretical model. Developers may select concepts and models from other disciplines that are compatible with nursing perspectives,[3,4] or they may design instruments to operationalize nursing perspectives. For example, the author based her tools for assessing stress and coping on

Lazarus' model because this mediated, transactional view seemed more compatible with nursing perspectives than Selye's more biochemical mechanistic approach. Kearney and Fleischer developed an instrument to measure the exercise of self-care agency based on Orem's model of nursing.[5]

Even when instruments are not based on an identifiable model, some assumptions, biases, and values can be detected in them. For example, one must be cautious with older instruments. A tool developed in 1954 to assess female sex role adjustment may be based on now untenable assumptions about the female destiny. Tool users should ascertain that the tool's basis is at least compatible with, if not identical to, their individual and professional perspectives on the problem. Failure to do so is more than a mere philosophical matter. It may create a validity problem in that the findings obtained with a particular tool cannot be interpreted adequately.[6]

MEASUREMENT FRAMEWORKS

There are two major frameworks for measurement.[6] The norm-referenced framework is used when the aim is to evaluate an individual's performance in relation to other individuals in a specified comparison or norm group. Norm-referenced measures promote variability, that is, they seek to spread people out over a possible range of scores. The ideal distribution of scores will look like the normal curve, with most scores in the midrange. The Graduate Record Examination is an example of a norm-referenced measure. A student's scores are interpreted in relation to the scores of other students seeking admission to graduate school who took the same test.

The criterion-referenced framework is used when the aim is to determine what a person knows or can do in relation to a fixed performance standard. How a person compares to others is irrelevant when this framework is used. Criterion-referenced measures (CRMs) produce classifications on judgments, such as satisfactory/unsatisfactory or met/not met. Scores from a CRM have a narrower range than those from a norm-referenced measure and are skewed (clustered) toward one end of the scale. Criterion-referenced measures are often useful in clinical research requiring measurement of process or attainment of outcome variables.[6] For example, the Denver Developmental Screening Test, adjustment or nonadjustment to the parental role, and the National Cancer Institute's criteria for the proper performance of breast self-examination are useful CRMs.

CHOOSING A METHOD OF DATA COLLECTION

Every instrument uses one or more methods of data collection to operationalize the variables of interest. Each method has its own advantages and disadvantages for certain purposes and populations and its special reliability and validity problems. For example, because semantic differentials are rapid to complete, many items can be used. Q sorts are time consuming and are best suited to intensive analysis of individuals or to small samples.[7] Tools whose items use identical response formats, such as Likert or numerical rating scales, are prone to response sets, in which subjects respond to items in characteristic ways regardless of the item content; such tendencies are threats to validity.[8]

Although it is beyond the scope of this chapter to describe the features of each data collection method, tool users need this knowledge. Comprehensive research and measurement tests[6-9] provide basic information. There are also specialized texts that focus on one method, such as Osgood, Suci, and Tannenbaum's *The Measurement of Meaning*[10] (semantic differentials) and Stephenson's *The Study of Behavior*[11] (Q methodology). Current research literature comments on data collection methods, problems, and strengths. Unfortunately, if methodology is not the focus of the article and is not reflected in the title or abstract, this very useful information can be difficult to locate.

OTHER CONSIDERATIONS

A common error in choosing an instrument is to assume that it is sound if it is widely used. This is not necessarily so and must be determined on a case-by-case basis.[12] For example, the Holmes and Rahe Schedule of Recent Experiences is still widely used despite a decade of profound criticisms of its psychometric properties and sex bias and the subsequent development of superior instruments.[13] Often researchers could avoid this error by continuing to review the literature after reading a report of a promising instrument.

Assessing the apparent qualifications of the author may be a helpful, minor strategy in appraising a tool. Most journals give a statement about an author's education and institutional affiliation. An advanced degree is desirable. If the measured concept is clinical, a clinical position held by the author may be significant. The text of the article may describe the kind of experiences on which a tool is based, information that will help users decide whether the tool is appropriate for their circumstances.

PSYCHOMETRIC CHARACTERISTICS OF INSTRUMENTS

Theory of Measurement Error

In classic measurement theory, an observed score on any measure is seen as a combination of a true score (what the subject would get if the instrument were perfect) and random and systematic error. Random error results from chance variations in the test (the directions may not be clear), the subject (he or she may have a headache today), or the conditions of test administration (the room may be very hot, or not all administrators may use the same instructions). By sometimes raising and sometimes lowering the observed score, random error reduces the consistency of measurements and, indirectly, makes it difficult to know what exactly is being measured.

Systematic error results from the presence of some extraneous factor that affects all measurements made with the tool in the same way. For example, a scale that reads 3 pounds high is systematically upwardly biased. Systematic bias compromises validity, the extent to which an instrument measures what it is intended to measure. The aim of all reliability and validity measures is to minimize the portion of the observed score that is due to error and to maximize the portion that is true. The larger the portion of random error in a score, the lower the reliability coefficient of the tool. The lower the reliability coefficient, the lower the confidence that can be placed in any subsequent judgments or relationships using that tool.[14]

Reliability

The first characteristic that any instrument must possess is reliability. Concerns about reliability involve the consistency or repeatability of measurements made with the instrument.

Reliability can be conceptualized in terms of stability, equivalence, or internal consistency. It is often possible and desirable to use more than one approach.[8,15] All reliability assessments are reported as correlation coefficients. Theoretically, correlation coefficients may range between -1.00 and $+1.00$, but in reliability assessment, they usually fall between 0.0 and 1.0. The closer the correlation coefficient is to 1.00, the more reliable is the tool.[8]

Reliability as Stability. Reliability as stability takes two forms. Test–retest reliability is the correlation between scores from the same subjects tested at two different times. The interval between testings should not be so short that subjects' recall of items can spuriously inflate the reliability coefficient[16] nor so long that one is studying the stability of the characteristic over time rather than the performance of the instrument.[17] Test–retest reliability is more useful for measures of enduring traits than for changeable states and for affective rather than cognitive measures.[6] For example, a test–retest correlation is more suited to a measure of introversion/extroversion (an enduring affective trait) than to a measure of knowledge of the warning signals of cancer (a changeable cognitive state).

The second form of reliability as stability is intrarater reliability, the consistency with which one rater assigns scores to a single event on two different occasions. The correlation is calculated from the scores of the same observer at time 1 and time 2.[6]

Reliability as Equivalence. Reliability as equivalence has two forms. Parallel forms reliability requires the development of two different tests that measure the same trait in the same way. The correlation coefficient is based on the scores of the same individuals taking test A and test B sequentially. This procedure overcomes the problem of specific recall associated with the administration of a single test twice. Thus, parallel forms are useful for studies using repeated measures. The disadvantage is that parallel tests are very difficult to construct.[16] The chief application of parallel forms reliability has been with standardized tests in education. Occasionally, one finds parallel forms for a psychologic construct, such as self-esteem.[8]

The second form of reliability as equivalence, much more common in nursing research than parallel forms, is interrater (or interobserver) reliability. Here, two or more trained observers watch an event simultaneously and score it independently, using established scoring criteria.[6] Various correlation coefficients are available for assessing agreement among two or more raters.[8]

Reliability as Internal Consistency. The third approach to reliability, internal consistency, is perhaps the most widely used today. It is based on the assumption that several items (indicators) relevant to the studied trait produce a composite score that is closer to the subject's true errorless score than any single item would be.[18] A tool is said to be internally consistent or homogeneous to the extent that all items measure the same trait.[8]

Historically, the oldest method of assessing internal consistency is the split-half technique. The items of a single test are divided into halves—usually odd and even numbered items—and scored separately. The correlation coefficient is calculated from the scores on each half of the test. Although splitting the test avoids the need to create two tests, it creates another problem. Because reliability is related to test length, a correlation coefficient based on split-halves systematically underestimates the reliability of the entire scale. A statistical correction known as the Spearman-Brown prophecy formula is used to adjust the split-half correlation coefficient for the full-length test.[16] The chief disadvantage of the split-half technique is that different splits (e.g., odd–even, first half–second half) yield different reliability estimates. Because of this problem, psychometricians have developed reliability coefficients that do not require the repeating of items or the splitting of tests.[19]

The preferred measure of internal consistency is the Cronbach coefficient alpha. Coefficient alpha—not to be confused with alpha, the level of significance—measures the extent to which performance on any one item in an instrument indicates performance on any other item in that instrument. If an instrument has internal consistency, the items should have similar and relatively high intercorrelations; items that do not fit with the others can be isolated and modified or deleted.[18]

The Cronbach alpha is a very general reliability coefficient. It subsumes the Spearman-Brown prophecy formula because it is actually an average of all possible split-halves. It also encompasses two other reliability coefficients, known as Kuder-Richardson (KR) 20 and 21, developed for use with dichotomous data.[19]

Coefficient alpha is not appropriate for criterion-referenced instruments.[15] It also underestimates reliability when the interitem coefficients are not high and when the number of items is small.[19]

Interpretation of Reliability Coefficients. Reliability is a matter of degree rather than an all-or-nothing affair, and it is not a property of an instrument but of an instrument when administered to certain people under certain conditions. For all types of reliability, prospective users must ascertain the characteristics of the group on or for whom the tool was developed. The more similar the original group to the user's target group, the more likely that the tool will perform reliably for the new study. Reliability is increased by longer test length (up to a point), by speeded conditions in which all subjects do not finish, by heterogeneous samples, and by variability of scores on the total test.[15,19]

Other things being equal, the tool with the highest reliability is best.[8] Because reliability coefficients are not automatically generalizable, however, reliability coefficients should be recalculated each time an instrument is used.[6]

"How high is high?" is a common question about reliability coefficients. There is no simple answer. The judgment depends on the nature of the trait being measured and the stage of development of the instrument. The reliability of physiologic measures is often expected to be 0.95 or more, whereas that of attitudinal measures may be acceptable at 0.70.[20] Coefficients for interrater and test–retest reliabilities should be at least 0.80.[18] Coefficients of 0.60 to 0.70 may be acceptable for the exploratory use of tools in the early stages of development or if the reliability of other available tools is even lower.[21] If a test is composed of several subtests, the reliability of each subtest must be assessed, as well as that of the total test. Because reliability is a function of test length, the reliability of subtests will be lower than that of the total test.[14]

Reliability of Criterion-Referenced Measures. The forms of reliability assessments most relevant to CRMs are test–retest, parallel forms, and intrarater and interrater agreement procedures.[6] (Internal consistency is virtually assured in the well-constructed CRM.[14]) Although the meanings of these terms are the same in both the norm-referenced and criterion-referenced frameworks, the calculations are different. Traditional reliability methods require a degree of variability usually not found in the results from CRMs; their use with scores from CRMs will produce a lower correlation coefficient that is a conservative estimate, or underestimate, of the actual reliability. Several special procedures for estimating the reliability of CRMs are available. Popham[22] suggested some informal procedures based on testing subjects twice. One could assess the variability of individual scores by determining the percentage of scores that differed by a specified percentage, say ±5 percent, or one could assess the consistency of test-based decisions by determining the percentage of respondents for whom the same decision was made both times. Livingston's formula[23] computes a traditional reliability coefficient and adjusts it for the criterion or cutoff score of the CRM. Two statistics that are useful regardless of the number of categories established by the measure are P_o, the proportion of subjects classified the same way on two occasions, and kappa (K), the proportion of subjects classified the same way on two occasions beyond that expected by chance. P_o and K can also be used to estimate the reliability of parallel forms and intrarater and interrater agreement.[6] Details of the conceptualization and interpretation of these statistics can be found in the References.

Validity

The second characteristic of a measuring instrument is validity, that is, if a tool measures what it claims to measure. Validity is dependent on reliability in that a tool must measure something consistently (be reliable) before one can determine what that something is. An instrument can be reliable without being valid, but an unreliable instrument cannot possibly be valid.[24]

Establishing validity is more difficult than establishing reliability because many validity assessments are subjective and logical rather than data-based.[8] Although the literature contains many typologies of validity, this discussion covers face, content, criterion-related, and construct validity.

Face Validity. Face validity is the weakest form of validity.[24] It is a judgment of what the tool appears to measure, based on a cursory inspection by the layman. If a test appears irrelevant to the stated purpose, subjects may respond carelessly or not at all.[15,16] Face validity is the public relations aspect of a tool; it provides no evidence of what the tool really measures.[25]

Content Validity. Content validity is concerned with whether or not the test items adequately sample the content area: Are the items representative and comprehensive?[18] Judgments on content validity usually are based on consensus among a group of subject matter experts. An Index of Content Validity showing the proportion of agreement among judges can be calculated.[6] Content validity is also aided by consensus in the literature. Although used historically for developing tests of classroom knowledge, content validity is necessary for all measures.[6] There is, however, a great need in nursing research to establish other forms of validity for tools as well.[2]

Criterion-Related Validity. Criterion-related validity is the correlation between a measure and some outsider indicator. It is most pertinent when a tool will be used for decision making.[6] Two types of criterion-related validity commonly are distinguished, depending on when the criterion data are collected. For concurrent validity, data about the measure and the indicator are collected at the same time. For example, a measure of patients' perceived readiness for discharge could be correlated with caregivers' perceptions of their readiness. A high correlation between the scores of the two samples would support concurrent validity.

For predictive validity, data on the criterion variable are collected from the same subjects at a future date. Patients' scores on the perceived readiness for discharge measure could be correlated with the number of days until a subsequent hospital admission. The correlation between the scores of the single sample at two times would estimate predictive validity.[8] Clinical nursing may be an excellent field for determining predictive validity because of the frequency with which behavioral cycles occur, for example, admission–discharge, crisis, patient teaching, and the availability of multiple respondents. Fox believes that tool users should demand evidence of predictive validity in clinical tools.[24]

In principle, criterion-related validity is a strong form of validity. In practice, several factors must be considered when planning or interpreting criterion-related studies. Very often, identification of an adequate criterion is not possible.[8] What would be an appropriate criterion for an abstract concept such as self-actualization? Even if a criterion can be identified, reliable, valid measures of it may not be available. Validity coefficients based on a criterion measure with low reliability will underestimate the true strength of the predictor–criterion relationship.[24] Underestimates of validity will also occur if the procedures used to sample the target population do not ensure a representative or random sample or if attrition is high.[6] The validity coefficient may be falsely high if criterion contamination occurs, that is, if raters or judges know how members of the sample performed on the predictor.[24] In addition, a coefficient from a single criterion-related study will tend to inflate the predictor–criterion relationship. Ideally, cross-validation should occur. This is a procedure in which the predictor–criterion relationship is developed on one sample and tested on a second independent sample from the same population. The cross-validation correlation is usually a lower, more accurate estimate of the true predictor–criterion relationship.[6]

Construct Validity. Construct validity is the most theoretical form of validity. The concept being measured is seen as part of a network of associated concepts and meanings (a construct). From this network, theoretical relationships are proposed and tested. This emphasis on meaning makes construct validity the form of validity most directly concerned with the question of what a tool actually measures; the testing of relationships links theory with the empirical world.[8] Construct validity is especially useful for measures of affect and other abstract concepts for which criterion-related validity is unsuitable.[6,19]

Construct validity can be approached in several ways. In the known-groups approach, the instrument is administered to two groups known to be high and low on the measured concept. If the groups' scores differ significantly, construct validity is supported, in that the tool appears to be measuring the attribute. In the experimental manipulation approach, hypotheses about the behavior of people with varying scores on the measure are tested. If the predictions are borne out, construct validity is supported.[8] Internal consistency reliability data also aid construct validity. A high Cronbach coefficient alpha on a unidimensional tool or on subscales of a multidimensional measure reflects positively on what is being measured as well as on the consistency with which it is measured.[16]

The use of two correlational approaches to construct validity is growing rapidly. Although an adequate description is beyond the scope of this chapter, tool users should cultivate at least a conceptual understanding of both. Briefly, factor analysis identifies clusters (factors) of related items. The names (content) and the mathematical weights of the factors are then used to define the concept or to confirm prior theorizing about its nature. Factor analysis also sheds light on whether a concept is unidimensional or multidimensional—on whether one or several factors are needed to describe it. The multitrait–multimethod approach is based on the principles of convergent and discriminant validity. Convergence is the idea that different measures of the same trait should correlate highly with one another. Discriminant validity means that measures of different constructs should have low intercorrelations. Scores from at least two constructs, each measured in at least two different ways, are entered into a correlation matrix. By reading different diagonals of the matrix, the researcher can obtain separate correlations for reliability and for convergent, construct, and discriminant validity. The technique is efficient and informative, but it may be burdensome to respondents if the tools are several or lengthy. A clear, full description of the procedure is found in *Measurement in Nursing Research.*[6]

Interpretation of Validity Evidence. Validity evidence is harder to interpret than is reliability evidence. Reliability is essentially a matter of the correlation of a test with itself; therefore, the relationship should be high. With validity, the test is correlated with external criteria that may be very different measures of the general concept, and the relationship will necessarily be lower.[18] Tool users should ask: What is being correlated (statistically or logically) with what? How strong can the relationship reasonably be expected to be? Is use of the tool an improvement over use of previous tools or of no measurement at all?[21] How similar is the proposed use to conditions under which the available validity evidence was obtained? What use will be made of the scores?

When correlation coefficients are used as evidence of predictive validity, coefficients in the 0.60 to 0.70 range are usually considered adequate for group prediction purposes. Coefficients in the 0.80s are considered minimal for individual predictions.[14]

Evidence for the construct validity of a tool should be viewed as a cumulative pattern. Each positive study results in greater confidence that a tool is a valid measure of a particular construct. On the other hand, despite many previous successes, one strong negative finding can destroy confidence in the construct as measured.[16] Because validity evidence is specific to an application of the instrument rather than to the instrument itself, users should plan to provide additional evidence of validity from their studies.[6]

Validity of Criterion-Referenced Measures. Because CRMs are designed primarily to measure the achievement of some specific objective, content validity is the major concern. In fact, the content validity of a criterion-referenced tool is usually expected to be higher than that of a norm-referenced measure because the domain of relevant behaviors can be defined more precisely. As with traditional measurement procedures, the content validity of a CRM is a matter of expert judgment,[14] and the number and qualifications of the content experts should be provided. Waltz et al.[6] describe some numerical procedures for use in assessing content validity of CRMs at the item level.

Sometimes CRMs are used to predict future performance. For example, nurses might wish to know whether a certain score on a criterion-referenced examination of activities of daily living predicts elderly patients' abilities to function alone at home. As with reliability, the traditional correlational approach to predictive validity may be inappropriate because of reduced score variability with CRMs. A noncorrelational approach to a predictor–criterion relationship is to develop an expectancy table. This is a two-way table that lists predictor categories (pass/fail, high/medium/low) down the left side and criterion scores or categories (no readmission, early readmission, delayed readmission) across the top. Table entries are the number or percentage of persons in each category.[14]

Other Desirable Tool Characteristics

Sensitivity is the ability of an instrument to make discriminations of the fineness needed for the study. Often, scales with categories of "Yes" and "No" will not allow many subjects to respond accurately. Expanding the scale to five categories ranging from "Strongly Approve" to "Strongly Disapprove" will increase its sensitivity.[26] Sensitivity is especially important when physiologic measurements are being monitored, when measurements will be used to make decisions about an individual rather than a group, and when the experimental and control conditions are not drastically different.[6] These are all common conditions in clinical research. Unnecessary sensitivity may be expensive to achieve and burdensome for either the respondent or the investigator.

Appropriateness is the extent to which subjects can meet the requirements of the instrument. Appropriateness often translates into assessment of the reading level of a tool. An inappropriate tool will produce invalid responses.[26]

Objectivity is the extent to which the data obtained reflect what is being measured rather than some outside influence. Common threats to objectivity are the influence of the race or sex of an interviewer on the subject, instructions that suggest what the answers should be, and observation guides that require the researcher to judge behavior. A tool user should expect the tool developer to spell out the steps taken to protect the objectivity of the data.[24]

The feasibility of an instrument is assessed in terms of the time, cost, and skill needed for the study and in terms of the instrument's acceptability to potential subjects. Cost factors include the time and expense of obtaining subjects, the purchase price of the tool, printing, photocopying, postage, clerical help, computer time, and consultation. Other things being equal, a short, machine-scoreable tool would be more feasible than a longer one that must be hand-scored or interpreted by a specialist.[26] Acceptability involves burden—the time and effort involved for the subject—and the fit between the implicit values or sensitivities of the instrument and the subjects. If subjects consider the items irrelevant or offensive, they may answer casually or not at all.[12]

Psychometric Properties of Biophysiologic Measures

Although data obtained from bioinstrumentation and laboratory procedures are generally accurate, sensitive, and objective, several threats to their reliability and validity do exist. Most involve human error (such as improper use or calibration of equipment, failure to follow established procedures, or clerical errors in reporting results) or equipment failure. Users of biophysiologic measures often must employ quality control strategies, such as regular calibrations of equipment and random checks on adherence to procedures. Although biophysical measures are relatively immune to subjects' distortions of readings, the measurement process itself can alter the variable of interest. For example, the presence of a transducer in the bloodstream can reduce the blood flow in the vessel.[6] Other considerations with biophysiologic instruments include direct versus indirect measurement, invasive versus noninvasive measurement, single versus multiple measures, and sensitivity.[27]

Some biophysiologic phenomena (pain, nausea, fatigue) are more subjective than objective and can be assessed by paper-and-pencil instruments. The chief consideration in choosing the instrument is the conceptualization of the phenomenon being studied. If a visual analog scale or short questionnaire captures the variable of interest and adequate psychometric data are available, there is no point in using an expensive, invasive physiologic procedure.[27]

The texts by Polit and Hungler,[8] Waltz et al.,[6] and Wilson[9] all contain helpful chapters on choosing and using biophysiologic measures.

ITEM ANALYSIS

Reports of instrument development should contain some description of how items were refined. This usually involves some form of item analysis, an examination of the pattern of responses to each item in order to assess its effectiveness and provide guidelines for its revision. The results of item analysis affect both reliability and validity by manipulating the variability of scores, eliminating the extraneous effects of very easy or very difficult items, and strengthening the relationship between items and an external criterion.[14]

Item Analysis with Norm-Referenced Tests

The major aspects of item analysis with norm-referenced measures are the determination of item difficulty and the discrimination power of each item.

Item difficulty (ID), also called "item p level," is the percentage of correct responses to the item. Item difficulty can range from 0 to 100. The closer it is to zero, the more difficult the item is.[6] Average item difficulties, around 50 or with a range of 30 to 70, are generally sought to promote variability of scores and, hence, reliability.[14]

The discrimination power or index (D) represents the degree to which an item distinguishes high and low achievers on the test or to which performance on any one item predicts performance on the entire test; D scores can range from -1.00 to $+1.00$. Positive D scores are desirable and indicate that the item is discriminating in the desired direction—those who answered the item correctly tended to do well on the test. D scores near zero mean that the item is not discriminating and serves no useful purpose in the test. Negative D scores mean that respondents who answered the item correctly tended to do poorly on the total test. These items need major revision.[6] D scores of $+0.30$ are generally accepted as adequate.[14]

Item Analysis with Criterion-Referenced Measures

In CRM, the concepts of average item difficulty and of promoting variability of scores have little or no meaning. Also, because of the great emphasis on content validity, items in CRMs are not discarded lightly. Therefore, item analysis of CRMs focuses mainly on the identification of items that need revision if the measure is to distinguish between those who have achieved the desired outcome and those who have not.[6]

There are two general approaches to item analysis in CRM. The pretest–posttest approach involves testing the same group twice, before and after the treatment. The criterion-group approach involves testing two separate groups at the same time. One group is independently known to possess or score high on the desired attribute, and one group is known to score low on it.[6]

Item difficulty (or item p level) in the pretest–posttest approach should be higher on the posttest than on the pretest. (Higher scores indicate that the respondents found the items easier after the treatment.)

In the criterion-groups approach, item difficulty levels should be higher (easier) for the group known to possess more of the attribute than for the group with less of it.

Item discrimination in the pretest–posttest approach can be determined in at least three ways.[6] The pretest–posttest difference index is the proportion (or percentage) of respondents who answered the item correctly on the posttest minus the proportion of those who answered that item correctly on the pretest. The individual gain index is the proportion of respondents who answered the item incorrectly on the pretest and correctly on the posttest. The net gain index is the proportion of respondents who answered the item incorrectly on both occasions subtracted from the individual gain index, thus considering the performance of all persons who answered the item incorrectly on the pretest.[6] The Waltz, Strickland, and Lenz text[6] provides details of how to select, calculate, and interpret these indexes and additional references on CRM.

OTHER HELPFUL PROCEDURES IN INSTRUMENT EVALUATION

Pretesting and Piloting an Instrument

Pretesting (trying out an instrument with a few volunteers) and piloting (trying out the research procedure as a small-scale trial run) can be useful in choosing and using an instrument. The following is only a partial list of the instrumentation issues that can be addressed in a pretest or pilot study[28]:

- Perform reliability and validity checks.
- Reduce random error by assessing subjects' response to the instrument. Are the

instructions clear? Do they understand the questions and answer them correctly? Do some questions cause embarrassment or resistance? Is cheating or unwanted collaboration among subjects a problem?
- Obtain accurate estimates of the time required to complete the instrument and of the cost of data collection.
- Determine that the tool will indeed yield the needed data and eliminate the collection of unnecessary data.
- Gain staff experience and confidence in working with the subjects and the tool.
- Standardize rater, interview, and other measurement techniques.

A pilot can also be performed to compare two or more instruments and aid one's final choice. Sometimes piloting should be conducted in phases to allow successive refinements or to address problems in some logical sequence.

Subjects for a pilot study should be as similar as possible to those in the eventual study group but should not serve in both the pilot and data-producing groups. Nurse researchers too often are content to obtain only the views of fellow head nurses or graduate students or faculty; although their evaluations may be helpful, they are no substitute for representatives of the study populations. For most trial runs, a sample size of 10 to 20 should suffice. More may be needed if the measurement procedure is complex or if the sample is heterogeneous.[8]

For maximum benefit from a pilot study, the investigator should observe subjects as they complete the tool and then interview them about their reactions. The meaning of subjects' nonverbal responses should be explored. Do frowns, fidgets, and many erasures indicate ambiguity in the tool, resistance to the content or circumstances of administration, or genuine involvement?

Because of the small sample size and the relative artificiality of the situation, a pilot study cannot anticipate or solve all problems.[28] Nevertheless, few research procedures are as useful.

Sources of Help with Instrument Evaluation

Several sources of help with instrument selection and use are available if needed. In addition to the references with asterisks at the end of this chapter and the other references in this book, the research teachers at a nearby school of nursing or the nursing research staff of a nearby hospital may be able to help. One can write to the tool developer or to previous users of a tool. The directories of research and clinical organizations often identify members with expertise in instrumentation and willingness to consult on it. For example, Sigma Theta Tau, the Midwest Nursing Research Society, and the Oncology Nursing Society all publish informative membership directories.

THE STATE-OF-THE-ART OF MEASUREMENT IN NURSING RESEARCH

The conduct of research is rapidly becoming an expectation for both faculty and clinicians. With that maturity, attention can turn from quantity to quality. The literature of the 1980s reveals an increasing emphasis on the quality of measurement in nursing research.

Waltz and Strickland[2,29] have done the most extensive appraisals of measurement in nursing research. In two studies they analyzed research articles published in major nursing research journals from 1980 to 1984 to determine the characteristics of tools used to measure nursing research variables and the use of measurement principles and practices in nursing research. A content analysis procedure was used to obtain the data.

Major findings of the second study[29] included the following:

1. The majority of tools used (53 percent) were existing nonnursing tools. Existing nursing measures accounted for 8.8 percent of the total, and 37 percent were developed by the investigators for their studies. Over half (51.7 percent) of tools measured attitudinal or perceptual variables.
2. Although the number of tools used to measure a variable ranged from 1 to 6, 85.1 percent of the variables were measured with one tool.
3. The most frequently used formats for gathering data were questionnaires (33.2 percent) and rating scales (30.7 percent). Physical measures were used in 20.2 percent of the cases.
4. Conceptual frameworks were identified for only 20.2 percent of the measures. For about 56 percent of these, the frameworks for the tool and the study were consistent. In about 40 percent, the consistency of the tool and study frameworks could not be determined; in 4.6 percent, the tool and study frameworks were clearly inconsistent.
5. In over one half of the articles (57.6 percent), reviewers could not determine whether tools were norm-referenced or criterion-referenced. About 22 percent were clearly norm-referenced, and 12.6 percent were criterion-referenced.
6. No reliability data were reported for 38.4 percent of the measures. The most frequently reported forms of reliability assessments were test–retest and internal consistency (each 15.1 percent) and interrater reliability (13.9 percent).
7. No validity data were reported for 58 percent of the measures. The most frequently reported form of validity evidence was criterion-related validity (22.3 percent).
8. Reliability and validity data from both the current study and previous studies were provided in only 1.7 percent and 2.1 percent of the cases, respectively. "In a few instances" (p. 85), authors mislabeled reliability and validity procedures or cited inappropriate evidence.

Strickland and Waltz concluded that the state of measurement in nursing is not high and that there was no improvement in measurement over the 4 years of the two studies. They recommended that researchers, readers, and manuscript reviewers place more emphasis on measurement principles and practices.

There is a relationship between the amount of relevant psychometric information provided by the developer or publisher of a tool and the quality of a tool. Missing data can be assumed to be negative.[14]

Norbeck[30] addressed the issue of what constitutes a publishable report of instrument development. She suggested that the minimal standard for publishing psychometric testing should include at least one type of content validity, test–retest reliability, internal consistency reliability, and at least one type of construct or criterion-related validity. Moreover, results should not be published until the minimal indicators of reliability and validity reach acceptable levels as specified by measurement theory.

The necessary descriptive information about the instrument consists of the conceptual basis for the tool, the methods of item generation and refinement, sociodemographic characteristics of the intended respondents, details of administration, method of scoring, type of data obtained, and any other instrument-specific information. Variable means, standard deviations, and range of scores should be provided so that users may compare their study samples with others. An initial report should also provide examples of the tool format and sample items or a complete copy of the instrument in an appendix. Norbeck recommended that beginning work on instruments be reported through papers or posters at research meetings or research newsletters and that all planned psychometric testing should be included in the initial published report. If heeded, Norbeck's recommendation should improve the quality of articles on instrument development and reduce the need to search for fragmented reports.

The authors in this book have noted that a distressing number of tools have been developed on very small samples.[31] Small samples are, by nature, less representative of the population and more prone to sampling error (the tendency of obtained statistics to fluctuate from one sample to another) than larger samples.[8] Therefore, one cannot be as confident that a tool developed on a small sample will perform that way again. Correlation coefficients obtained from small samples should be tested for statistical significance to be sure that the relationships are not due to chance.[14,18] Factor analysis, used as evidence of construct validity, requires at least five, and preferably ten, subjects per variable (tool item) for a reliable result.[32] A pretest on the intended population is especially desirable before adopting an instrument developed on a small sample.

PUTTING IT ALL TOGETHER

The following list of questions is offered as a guideline for the evaluation of existing instruments:

Author	What are the qualifications of the author for developing this tool?
Purpose	Is the purpose of the tool (description, screening, diagnosis, prediction, or prescription[6]) specified? Is the purpose similar to that of my study?
Measurement framework	Is the measurement framework specified? Is it appropriate for my study?
Conceptual base	Is the conceptual base stated? Implied? Is it at least compatible with my orientation to the problem?
Subjects	Are the intended subjects clearly described? Are they similar to those in my proposed study? If not, how do they differ? Are they more or less heterogeneous than my subjects will be? How many subjects have contributed to the development of this tool?
Data-gathering method	What method is used? Is the method properly used? What are the advantages and disadvantages of this method?
Content	Is the content dated or current? Is a rationale apparent for each item?
	Do the items cover the key elements of the concept? If not, what is missing?
Administration and scoring	Are these clearly described? Will the conditions of administration be similar in my study? Will I need help in scoring or interpreting the results?
Reliability and validity	Can the responses be faked or distorted easily (a threat to validity)?

	Is evidence of both reliability and validity reported? Are the forms of evidence reported appropriate? Are multiple forms of evidence reported? Are reliability and validity coefficients appropriately high for the concept being measured?
Sensitivity	Will this instrument make discriminations of the necessary fineness?
Appropriateness	Is the reading level suited to the intended subjects? Are assumptions made about things like standard of living or cultural backgrounds that do not fit the intended subjects?
Objectivity	Has the developer identified steps taken to insure the objectivity of the data? Are there any unidentified threats to objectivity?
Feasibility	How much time will subjects need to complete this tool? Will subjects be able to do this task under the conditions of my study? Can I afford to use this tool?
	Will this tool need to be modified before I can use it? Do I have the expertise to make these modifications? If not, can I find help to do this?

Because few instruments have model histories, the evaluation of instruments is always a judgment call. If you answered most questions positively and you generally believe that the tool meets your needs, use it. If there are major doubts, look for another tool or conduct a pilot study. A helpful hint: Saving the written assessment of tools will soon result in a useful tool file.[6] Tools not used for one study may suit another.

ETHICAL AND LEGAL ASPECTS OF TOOL USE

The ethical and legal use of instruments places obligations on the investigator to the subjects, the developer or publisher of the tool, and to the professional and scientific communities. Because obligations to subjects are described in most research texts or can be clarified by research review boards, this discussion will focus on obligations to the developer and the larger community.

Ethical considerations are inherent in the measurement considerations just discussed. The thoughtful selection of an appropriate instrument and its proper use are themselves ethical acts. Failure to perform them is at best a waste of time and at worst a hindrance to the advancement of nursing knowledge.

Obligations to the Instrument's Developer

The user's first obligation to the developer is to obtain his or her written permission to use the tool. Doing so may or may not be simple. Because research literature gives very little guidance about this, the following experiential suggestions are offered.

Ideally, the tool's developer will be at the institution named in the source of the tool. If not, an address may sometimes be obtained from a later publication by the developer or from another user of the tool or from a publisher. Membership directories of professional organizations, conference brochures, lists of conference participants, and one's own network may also be helpful.

The letter to the tool's developer should be short and simple. The user should state that he or she wishes to use Instrument X described in Journal Y for Purpose Z. (The name of the tool and the source are important because authors may have published more than one tool or in more than one source.) A short abstract or a three- or four-sentence description of the project should be provided. It is permissible to ask authors if they have more recent information about the tool to share, but they should not be expected to review the literature. The letter should close with an offer to share the findings, an indication of when they may be available, and a statement that full credit will be given to the developer. If 6 weeks pass without a reply, a courteous second letter may be sent, inquiring whether the previous one was received and requesting a prompt reply.

Although most authors are delighted when people wish to use their instruments, the replies are not always favorable. Some authors do not release their tools until they are highly developed or until they have written a certain article or grant proposal. Others grant permission for use but attach a list of conditions. For example, they may charge for the tool's use, limit the number of copies allowed, stipulate that the instrument may not be altered, request a report of the results, or ask that the responses to the tool be shared for the ongoing validation of the tool. Users are obligated to fulfill those conditions unless they can negotiate otherwise.

The user's second obligation to the tool's developer is to report the results of the tool's use to the developer, whether or not such feedback was requested. Information about difficulties encountered, additional determinations of reliability and validity, and suggestions for modifications or future use help the developer improve the tool and aid the accumulation of knowledge about it. [6]

Obligations to a Test Publisher

Some instruments are available from commercial test publishers. The publisher can be identified in the publication describing the tool, by the author, or by the publisher's catalog. In this case, users purchase the manual and copies and may be asked to document their qualifications for using the instrument properly. Acceptable documentation may consist of a graduate degree in a field that emphasizes measurement, the titles and credit hours of measurement courses, membership in professional organizations concerned with measurement, and a brief list of one's research activities. Investigators who cannot provide such documentation must order through a qualified individual who consents to supervise the use of the instrument. Improper use could result in the loss of ordering privileges for the supervisor.

Obligations to the Scientific and Professional Communities

Knowledge about tools and their applications cannot accumulate if the research is never published. The most available and enduring form of publication is a journal article.

The goal of a report on tool use is to provide enough information so that a reader can determine that sound measurement principles were observed and reach justified conclusions about the findings. In these reports, full credit must be given to the original developer. Any modifications in tool content, administration, scoring, or interpretation must be clearly described, along with psychometric data about the changes. Information about extraneous or confounding variables that might have influenced subjects' scores should be provided. Reports of problems and failures with a tool are as useful to other investigators as reports of success. [6]

Copyright Considerations

Copyrights involve both legal and ethical aspects of tool use. According to Dr. Florence Downs, editor of *Nursing Research*, [33] if an entire instrument is published in a journal, it is considered to be in the public domain and may be used without formal permission unless the author has retained the copyright, which will be indicated by a copyright symbol, ©. An example is found in the article by Hymovich. [34] If the author has the copyright, he or she must be contacted; in either case, it is both wise and courteous to do so because further work may have been done on the tool. The journal retains a copyright on the article regardless of who owns the tool, and proper citation of the published source is mandatory. Permission is needed to adapt items or to alter the tool.

The question, "Can I use a tool if I can't find the author after a reasonable effort to do so?" occasionally arises, usually in reference to a situation in which the author published a tool in full and retained the copyright. The wording of the Copyright Revision Act of 1976[35] leaves this author pessimistic that one may do so. Under the old law, copyright protection lasted from 28 to 56 years. Under the revised law, works created on or after January 1, 1978, are protected for the life of the author and for 50 years after the author's death, to be ascertained by mortality records in the Register of Copyrights. Even if this timespan were feasible for the investigator, the tool would probably need major revision to update it. Downs[33] recommends that questions about reasonable access and use of copyrighted works be taken to a copyright lawyer. The legal counsel of a hospital or school of nursing may also give advice on these matters.

SUMMARY

The use of existing instruments for nursing measurement can be a contribution to nursing knowledge. The necessary conditions are that:

> . . . an instrument should be selected only if it is congruent with the intended purpose, conceptually consistent with the theoretical and measurement perspectives being employed, and psychometrically sound. Selection of an existing instrument should be based on careful evaluation of those available in the light of specific needs. Once selected, the instrument should be used according to the criteria and specifications set by the developer, and the results of its use communicated to the nursing community (p. 336).[6]

REFERENCES

1. Batey, M. Conceptualization: Knowledge and logic guiding empirical research. *Nurs Res,* 1977, *26*(5):325.
2. Waltz, C.F., & Strickland, O.L. Measurement of nursing outcomes: State of the art as we enter the eighties. In W.E. Field (Ed.), *Measuring outcomes of nursing practice, education, and administration: Proceedings of the First Annual Southern Council on Collegiate Education for Nursing Research Conference.* Atlanta: Southern Regional Education Board, 1982, p. 47.
3. Ellis, R. Characteristics of significant theories. *Nurs Res,* 1968, *17*(3):217.
4. Fitzpatrick, J., Whall, A., Johnston, R., & Floyd, J. *Nursing models and their psychiatric mental health applications.* Bowie, MD: Brady, 1982.
5. Kearney, B., & Fleischer, B. Development of an instrument to measure exercise of self-care agency. *Res Nurs Health,* 1979, *2*(1):25.
*6. Waltz, C.F., Strickland, O.L., & Lenz, E.R. *Measurement in nursing research.* Philadelphia: F.A. Davis, 1984.
*7. Kerlinger, F.N. *Foundations of behavioral research* (2nd ed.). New York: Holt, Rinehart, and Winston, 1973.

*Recommended readings.

*8. Polit, D., & Hungler, B. *Nursing research: Principles and methods* (2nd ed.). Philadelphia: Lippincott, 1983.
*9. Wilson, H.S. (Ed.) *Research in nursing.* Menlo Park, CA: Addison-Wesley, 1985.
10. Osgood, C., Suci, G., & Tannenbaum, P. *The measurement of meaning.* Urbana, IL: University of Illinois Press, 1957.
11. Stephenson, W. *The study of behavior.* Chicago: University of Chicago Press, 1953.
*12. Norbeck, J.S. Collecting data with psychosocial instruments. In H. S. Wilson (Ed.), *Research in nursing.* Menlo Park, CA: Addison-Wesley, 1985, p. 296.
13. Rabkin, J.S., & Struening, C.B. Life events, stress, and illness. *Science,* 1976, *194*(3269):1013.
*14. Gay, L.R. *Educational evaluation and measurement.* Columbus, OH: Charles E. Merrill, 1980.
15. Waltz, C., & Bausell, R.B. *Nursing research: Design, statistics, and computer analysis.* Philadelphia: F.A. Davis, 1981.
16. Helmstadter, G.C. *Principles of psychological measurement.* New York: Appleton-Century-Crofts, 1964.
17. Knapp, T.R. Validity, reliability, and neither. *Nurs Res,* 1985, *34*(3):189.
18. Krueger, J.C., Nelson, A.H., & Wolanin, M.O. *Nursing research: Development, collaboration, and utilization.* Germantown, MD: Aspen, 1978.
*19. Zeller, R.P., & Carmines, E.G. *Measurement in the social sciences.* Cambridge, England: Cambridge University Press, 1980.
20. Humenick, S.S. *Analysis of current assessment strategies in the health care of young children and childbearing families.* Norwalk, CT: Appleton-Century-Crofts, 1982.
*21. Nunnally, J.C. *Psychometric theory.* New York: McGraw-Hill, 1967.
22. Popham, W.J. *Educational evaluation.* Englewood Cliffs, NJ: Prentice-Hall, 1975.
23. Livingston, S.A. Criterion-referenced applications of classical test theory. *J. Educ Meas,* 1972, *9*(1):13.
24. Fox, D.J. *Fundamentals of research in nursing* (4th ed.). New York: Appleton-Century-Crofts, 1982.
25. Anastasi, A. *Psychological testing* (4th ed.). New York: Macmillan, 1976.
26. Kovacs, A.R. *The research process: Essentials of skill development.* Philadelphia: F.A. Davis, 1985.
*27. Lindsey, A.M., & Stotts, N.A. Collecting data on biophysiologic variables. In H.S. Wilson (Ed.), *Research in nursing.* Menlo Park, CA: Addison-Wesley, 1985, p. 324.
28. Fox, R.N., & Ventura, M. Small scale administration of instruments and procedures. *Nurs. Res* 1983, *32*(2):122.
29. Strickland, O.L., & Waltz, C.F. Measurement of research variables in nursing. In P.L. Chinn (Ed.), *Nursing research methodology: Issues and implementation.* Rockbridge, MD: Aspen, 1986, p. 79.
*30. Norbeck, J.S. What constitutes a publishable report of instrument development? *Nurs Res,* 1986, *34*(6):380.
31. Stromborg, M.A. Personal communication, June 6, 1986.
32. Bentler, P.M. Factor analysis. In *Research issues 13: Data analysis strategies and designs for substance abuse research.* Rockville, Maryland: National Institute on Drug Abuse No. 017-024-00562-2, December, 1976, p. 139.
33. Downs, F.S. Personal communication, May 29, 1985.
34. Hymovich, D. The chronicity impact and coping instrument: Parent questionnaire. *Nurs Res,* 1983, *32*(5):275.
35. *Copyright Revision Act of 1976.* Chicago: Commerce Clearing House, 1976, p. 45.

PART II

Instruments for Assessing Health and Function

CHAPTER 2

Measuring Functional Status

Carol McMillen Moinpour, Ph.D., Ruth McCorkle, R.N., Ph.D., and Judith Saunders, R.N., D.N.S.

Over the past two decades, there has been increasing interest in the measurement of functional status during illness. Some of the reasons for assessing functional status include determination of patients' needs and problems, assessment of the adequacy and composition of staff for institutional settings, and determination of the effectiveness of various modes of treatment and care. The purposes of this chapter are to present an overview of the conceptualization of functional status, to discuss the methodologic issues in measuring functional status, to review specific functional status instruments, and to summarize the critical elements to consider when selecting an instrument.

CONCEPTUALIZATION OF FUNCTIONAL STATUS

The terms "physical functioning" and "functional status" have been used interchangeably and are often equated with other terms, such as health status, level of impairment, and disability. Health status measures reported in the literature have included some or all of the following factors: type of diagnosis, self-assessed health, pain, doctor visits, days in bed, number of therapeutic drugs, and performance of everyday activities. Examples of health status measures are the Sickness Impact Profile (SIP) and the Rand Health Insurance Experiment instruments. Impairment and disability are related, although slightly different, concepts. The American Medical Association has defined *impairment* as the extent of organic pathologic change, determined by a physician. An example of a scale to measure impairments is the Cumulative Illness Rating Scale. *Disability,* on the other hand, refers to how impairment limits activities and functioning. More scales deal with disability than with impairment, and numerous examples can be found, for example, the Barthel Index.

The concept of functional status is important in nursing because nurses are often responsible for assisting patients with maintaining or improving their functional status. In order to do assessments and target interventions at an individual's functional status, the term must be defined. Functional status for purposes of this chapter means any systematic attempt to measure the level at which a person is functioning in any of a variety of areas, such as physical health, quality of self-maintenance, quality of role activity, intellectual status, social activity, attitude toward the world and toward self, and emotional status.[1]

Changes in a person's functional status threaten his or her independence or autonomy. The threat potentially decreases the person's sense of power, control, and self-esteem; only a functional existence is considered meaningful and worthwhile in our society. Associated with chronic illnesses are disabilities that necessitate some degree of functional changes. The extent of the changes may progress to the stage where patients may regress to a situation reminiscent of early childhood, when even the most rudimentary and intimate functions are performed by others. Not only does dependency impinge negatively on the patient's self-esteem,[2] but social relationships may be dramatically altered.[3] Previously unresolved conflicts and new problems arise in relationships with significant others, in addition to challenges in meeting daily life adaptations. Both family and members of the health care system may maladaptively reinforce excessive social dependency.[4]

One of the first steps necessary in defining functional status is the establishment of criteria to judge a person's abilities. Competence is usually judged against an implicit set of collective norms of health care specialists caring for the patient. These levels of competencies represent a certain picture of how people in society should live and do not necessarily reflect the patient's circumstances. For example, it may be important for some groups of people to bathe everyday and for others only once a week. Such variables as the weather and strenuousness of activities may influence how much a person will need to bathe. Therefore, scores on bathing may differ because of individual habits and values and not necessarily because of changes in illness effects.

Another important step in defining functional status is to distinguish between the usual performance of the person versus his or her capacity to perform. Those supporting the use of performance-based items argue that such measures are more objective (i.e., either the observer sees the patient actually functioning at the particular level or the patient indicates that he does function at that level). Proponents for capacity-oriented items argue that circumstances unrelated to the person's health or functional status can determine the response (e.g., the effect of weather or other life demands on "Do you walk on a regular basis?"). Kuriansky and Gurland noted that:

> If a patient is observed and rated as "not eating," it is not known if he just does not want to eat at the time of observation, or if he is physically unable to go through the motions to do so. This distinction is necessary for making a differential diagnosis and for making decisions about treatments (p. 345).[5]

A dilemma occurs when health care providers in different institutions do not make parallel observations. For example, on a follow-up assessment, the focus may be on the patient's usual routine, the information may come from self-report rather than direct observation, and the pre and post measures may result in conflicting information.

Various authors have made distinctions among different types of functional status. There is considerable agreement that self-care and mobility are central to the determination of functional status. Beyond these two categories of function, the domains of measurement included by various authors show little congruence. Many have tried to address the broader World Health Organization (WHO)[6] definition of well-being, which includes physical, emotional, and social aspects of health. The concepts used by authors vary from concrete and discrete categories of self-care to global measures of health, work activities, and socialization with others. It is important to be clear about one's purpose before determining which items are needed to measure functional status. Clearly, some components of functional assessment are well developed, whereas others are not. For example, ideas of activities of daily living and mobility have a solid methodologic base and are applied broadly in similar terms, whereas measures of psychosocial and socioeconomic function are less well developed and are applied in a nonuniform manner.

The assessment of functional status of chronically ill patients is common practice for nurses. What is needed is a common language and standardized tools to compare the assessments of functional status and results of nursing interventions targeted at changing functional status.

DESCRIPTION OF THREE FUNCTIONAL STATUS INSTRUMENTS

There have been three major methods used to measure functional status: clinical assessment of the individual's functional status, questioning the individual about his or her current level of functioning, and standard tests of an individual performance conducted by a trained observer. We thoroughly reviewed the literature for functional status instruments and found many. The next step was to select specific instruments to include in this review. All of the instruments included were judged content appropriate for general assessment of functional status in a chronically ill population or in populations who may have functional impairment. Before an instrument was selected for inclusion, it had to have psychometric properties established in the literature. The reader may refer to the Appendix for an alphabetized listing of the instruments and a concise overview of their properties and uses.

Three specific instruments are presented in more detail. These are the Katz Index of Activities of Daily Living (ADL), the SIP, and the Enforced Social Dependency Scale (ESDS). These instruments were selected because they can be used as both clinical and research tools.

▪ INDEX OF ACTIVITIES OF DAILY LIVING (INDEX OF ADL)

One of the best known and most widely used instruments to measure activities of daily living is the Katz Index of ADL.[7-15] This instrument was developed empirically during the 1950s from observations of a large number of activities performed by patients with fractured hips. The Index of ADL was developed to study results of treatment and prognosis in the elderly and chronically ill adult. Six functional activities are rated: bathing, dressing, toileting, transfer, continence, and feeding. These activities are hierarchical and represent a natural sequence of functions lost as dependency increases. During recovery, the regaining of the activity is reversed. For most patients, the last function where independence was lost was the ability to feed themselves, and this function was usually the first area where independence returned as their condition improved.

The worksheet has the rater judge the amount of human assistance the patient requires. Three levels of independence are used for each function by rating the amount of assistance needed. Assistance is defined as supervision or direction of personal assistance. An example is presented from the worksheet for bathing (p. 47)[12]:

BATHING—either sponge bath, tub bath, or shower

Receives no assistance (gets in and out of tub by self if tub is usual means of bathing)	Receives assistance in bathing only part of the body (such as back or a leg)	Receives assistance in bathing more than one part of the body (or not bathed)

A similar procedure is followed by the rater for completing the worksheet for the other five functional activities. These ratings are then translated into a dichotomous 8-point rating scale, where A equals total independence in all six areas of functioning and G equals dependence in all six areas. Each category is well defined, and instructions for the rating are standardized. For example, bathing is considered independent if assistance is provided only in bathing a single part (as the back or disabled extremity) or if the person bathes self completely. Bathing is considered dependent if bathing is provided on more than one part of the body or if assistance is provided in getting in or out of the tub or if the person does not bathe self. The complete independence index of the ADL is presented below (p. 46)[12]:

A   Independent in feeding, continence, transferring, toileting, dressing, and bathing
B   Independent in all but one of these functions
C   Independent in all but bathing and one additional function
D   Independent in all but bathing, dressing, and one additional function
E   Independent in all but bathing, dressing, toileting, and one additional function
F   Independent in all but bathing, dressing, toileting, transferring, and one additional function
G   Dependent in all six functions
Other Dependent in at least two functions, but not classifiable as C, D, E, or F

Experience in the health care field and a knowledge of the patient are needed to use this instrument. Minimal training is needed because the categories are well defined, behavioral in nature, and require little inference. Each area of functioning is scored by rating it either independent or dependent, as defined on the observation sheet. The scoring then is compiled by noting those areas of independent functioning and locating the correct corresponding letter on the index. It takes only a few minutes to complete both the worksheet and the rating scale.

The Index of ADL has been used in many studies to evaluate care and to develop data about a person's progression through the longitudinal course of an illness. This instrument has been used to assess ADL in patients with many types of chronic illnesses and has not been limited to patients with fractured hips.[7] Although formal reliability analyses have not been reported, differences between observers seem to be infrequent. Mangen and Peterson[15] noted the need for more systematic studies of reliability. Predictive validity of the instrument was established originally through predicting the amount of assistance patients would need. One year after the onset of the illness, an independent measure of the amount of family and nonfamily assistance being provided to the patient was assessed. As predicted, 79 percent of patients who were rated D, E, F, or G were receiving nonfamily attendant care, whereas only 45 percent of those rated B and C were receiving this type of assistance. No patient who had been classified as A had nonfamily attendants.[7]

This instrument can be used in a variety of settings, such as a person's home, a long-term care facility, or an acute care setting. Scores can be artifically lowered in some settings, however, if these settings have practices of providing assistance to patients whether there is a demonstrated need or not. For example, hospitals often assist patients with bathing and dressing even when the person is capable of doing this without assistance.

▪ SICKNESS IMPACT PROFILE (SIP)

The original purpose for developing the SIP was to monitor the functional performance of individual patients in a physician's practice. The SIP has been used with a wide variety of chronic disease populations[16,17,18-27] and the elderly.[28-29] It has been translated into Spanish.[30]

The SIP was developed in 1972 and, after extensive field testing in 1973, 1974, and 1976, consists of 136 items.[31-36] Table 2–1 provides examples of items from each of 12 subscales. The following types of scores can be obtained: total, physical dimension, psychosocial dimension, and scores for each of the 12 categories. Validity and reliability analyses are strongest for SIP total scores. The developers believe that the ability of the SIP to discriminate levels of health status is best when the entire instrument is administered. In addition, there are no data favoring one subscale over another for various populations. However, reliabilities for individual scales are adequate for group and individual comparisons (internal consistency: alpha = 0.94, reproducibility = 0.92). The extensive psychometric evidence does not support eliminating items from a scale.

The SIP has been validated in a number of ways. Examples of convergent validity include the Sugerbaker et al.[19] study in which the SIP, Katz Index of ADL, and a psychosocial adjustment scale all showed more dysfunction for the limb-spared versus the limb-amputated patients. Liang et al.[37] found a high correlation between the AIMS and SIP measures (r = 0.97) and moderate correlations with other arthritis measures (e.g., Functional Status Index,

TABLE 2–1. SICKNESS IMPACT PROFILE (SIP) CATEGORIES AND SELECTED ITEMS

Dimension	Category	Selected Items
Independent categories	Sleep and rest (SR)	I sleep or nap during the day.
	Eating (E)	I am eating special or different foods.
	Work (W)	I am not working at all.
	Home management (HM)	I am not doing heavy work around the house.
	Recreation and pastimes (RP)	I am going out for entertainment less.
I. Physical	Ambulation (A)	I walk shorter distances or stop to rest often.
	Mobility (M)	I stay within one room.
	Body care and movement (BM)	I do not bathe myself at all; I am bathed by someone else.
II. Psychosocial	Social interaction (SI)	I am doing fewer social activities with groups of people.
	Alertness behavior (AB)	I have difficulty reasoning and solving problems, for example, making plans, making decisions, learning new things.
	Emotional behavior (EB)	I laugh or cry suddenly.
	Communication (C)	I do not speak clearly when I am under stress.

From Bergner et al. Med Care, 1981, 19(8): 789.

$r = 0.62$; Index of Well-Being, $r = 0.61$). Evidence of discriminant validity can be seen in higher correlations between the SIP and measures of dysfunction than between the SIP and measures of sickness.[32] This pattern was found both for self-assessments of dysfunction and sickness and for clinician assessments of dysfunction and sickness. The SIP has demonstrated descriptive validity in a number of ways: it has discriminated head injury patients from controls for most scales,[25] discriminated Group Health enrollees from cardiac arrest survivors,[17] and distinguished Nocturnal Oxygen Therapy Trial (NOTT) patients with chronic obstructive pulmonary disease (COPD) from controls with regular scores but not with a 6-month change score.[21] Sickness Impact Profile change scores but not straight scores discriminated two myocardial infarction patient treatment groups.[22]

Clinical validity was obtained by comparing SIP scores with scores on clinical measures used to monitor patients with specific conditions. Three such groups were examined: hip replacement, hyperthyroidism, and rheumatoid arthritis patients. Hypotheses were, in general, accepted (e.g., the SIP physical score correlated more highly with the Harris Analysis of Hip Function score than did the SIP psychosocial scores).

Regarding sensitivity to presence of disability, Liang et al.[37] found that the SIP detected less disability among patients who were clinically similar than did the Index of Well-Being and four other measures of health status developed for arthritis patients. Bloom[38] reported that the SIP (along with the Karnofsky Index and the Index of ADL) does not detect differences among patients with early-stage cancer. Deyo and Inui[24] evaluated rheumatoid arthritis patients with the SIP, a physician-completed American Rheumatism Association (ARA) Functional Classification Scale, a physician-rated change in overall patient status scale (5-point scale), a physician-rated 7-point scale of overall functioning, and a patient-rated 5-point scale of overall change in status. When the measures were compared for patients within ARA classification II (adequate for normal activities despite discomfort or limited motion), the SIP predicted clinical measures (e.g., hemocrit, erythrocyte sedimentation rate, and employment status) better than did the patient self-rating scale. In contrast to the findings of Liang et al.[37] and Bloom,[38] these data demonstrate the SIP's ability to detect meaningful/clinical differences for patients with low-level disability. There is no question that the SIP is an appropriate measure of functional status for most clinical populations.

Regarding sensitivity to change, the SIP detected greater dysfunction at time period two than at periods one, three, and four for hip-replacement patients; during period two, the patients were hospitalized.[32] Both the SIP and a clinical measure Adjusted T-4 (hormonal measure) detected a significant difference between times one and four for hyperthyroid patients.[32] In the Deyo and Inui study,[24] a maximum of six assessments were performed in a 6-month period. Clinical change was defined as both patient and physician perception that change had taken place. A 1 percentage point change on the SIP was equivalent to clinical change for large groups of patients but not for individuals. This difference was due to the wide variation in score changes per categories. Of the four methods used to assess sensitivity to change, the patient self-rating (7-point functional scale) was as good or better than the SIP or the ARA physician ratings. In general, the SIP predictive values were equal to or better than the other measures using a score change of 3 or more points as a criterion. However, the patient self-assessment predicted clinical improvement better than did the other measures. The authors noted that all of the measures were basically insensitive (". . . a functional score change occurs in only a minority of cases for which change is said to have occurred on clinical grounds," p. 283). Deyo and Inui[24] suggested the need for an item measuring transition or change in status on health status measures. Patients could be asked whether they are "better," "worse," or "the same" with regard to all the statements in a category and within some timeframe, such as "since your last visit."

Generally, the SIP takes about 20 to 30 minutes to administer. However, very sick patients (e.g., patients on respirators) have taken much longer, and you should check administration time in a pilot test if your sample includes such people. Another criticism of the SIP is its negative health orientation; some researchers and clinicians prefer more positively worded items (e.g., activities the respondent can or does do). On the other hand, many instruments share this approach to measuring negative performance. Carter and Deyo[39] demonstrated patient acceptance of the SIP and its procedures with Veterans Administration outpatients and with arthritis patients.

The SIP is one of the most carefully developed and tested instruments available. Its psychometric properties and ease of administration make it an excellent candidate for functional status monitoring. The sensitivity of the SIP with less dysfunctional individuals has not been as solidly established as its sensitivity for chronically ill patients. If your study includes a number of less dysfunctional individuals, it might be wise to pilot the SIP with such individuals to make certain that response variation is possible. Existing data on the SIP with less disabled groups certainly support its consideration.

• ENFORCED SOCIAL DEPENDENCY SCALE (ESDS)

Enforced social dependency is defined as the state in which patients require help or assistance from other people that under ordinary circumstances adults can perform by themselves.[4] Under ordinary circumstances in society, adult human beings who are not handicapped by disease or injury are socially independent creatures in the sense that they have considerable choice about entering into a state of dependence on other people. This state of dependence refers to a situationally required state of reliance on other people for help with activities ordinarily carried out by the individual. The ESDS was developed to be used as an outcome measure to assess the impingements of disease and treatment effects on patient responses.

The original scale, developed in 1978, consisted of three components: everyday self-care competence, mobility competence, and social competence. Initial validity and reliability were established on 60 patients with progressive chronic illnesses.[4,40,41] The scale has demonstrated face and content validity for measures of usual daily activities and social roles. The reliability coefficient alpha was 0.90. Subsequently, the scale has been revised and used with other patient groups (e.g., lung cancer and myocardial infarction,[40] melanoma and quality of life in the elderly,[29] amyotrophic lateral sclerosis[27]). McCorkle and Benoliel[40] reported reliability coefficients for the total scale by disease groups (alpha = 0.84 for cancer and alpha = 0.80 for heart disease) and test–retest correlations of 0.62. Increased dependence was associated with fewer social activities, including changes in the role responsibilities at home, work, and social activities with others. In addition, factor analysis confirmed the two unique factors: personal and social competence. Other researchers have studied social dependence as related to such variables as self-esteem, self-concept, morale, satisfaction, intimacy, and physical impairment.[2,3] Fink[27] reported the internal consistency reliability at 0.92 and found a high correlation between the ESDS and the SIP measurements ($r = 0.89$).

The scale has undergone revisions, during which two of the three initial scales, self-care competence and mobility competence, were reduced to the current subscale of personal competence. These subscales were combined because they were highly correlated. The category of personal competency is comprised of six activities judged central to performing as a normal adult: eating, dressing, walking, traveling, bathing, and toileting. Each activity is coded on a 6-point, Likert-type scale. Scores for personal competency are summed, ranging from 6 to 36.

Content areas for social competency have remained the same. Three specific role activities are included: activities in the home, work activities, and social and recreational activities. A fourth behavior related to communication is included. Each role activity is coded on a 4-point, Likert-type scale. The communication competency is coded on a 3-point scale. Scores for social competency are summed, ranging from 4 to 15. The total ESDS ranges from 10 to 51, with higher scores reflecting greater enforced dependency (Table 2–2).

TABLE 2–2. ENFORCED SOCIAL DEPENDENCY SCALE COMPONENTS AND SELECTED ITEMS

Component	Activity	Interview Guide for Items	Coding of Items
Personal competence	Dressing Eating Walking Traveling Bathing Toileting	Do you have problems dressing yourself now that you did not before your illness? Does it take you more time? Do you need help in putting on some of your clothes?	*Dressing* 1. Dresses in street clothes without help 2. Dressing involves minor change since illness 3. Dresses with help of equipment 4. Dresses with help of another person; includes major changes in pattern of dressing 5. Dresses only with help of another person 6. Is not dressed in street clothes
Social competence	Home Work Social and recreation Communication	Can you describe what your primary responsibilities have been in your home? In what ways have these changed since your illness? Who prepares the meals? Who runs the errands?	*Home Activities* 1. Usual activity; no change in quantity or quality of activities characterizing usual household role performance 2. Modified activity; all activities continue as before, but with some limitations in degree 3. Restricted activity; some activities characterizing usual household roles can no longer be performed 4. No activity; major activities defining role are no longer being performed

From McCorkel et al. A manual of data collection instruments, 1981, pp. 3–17. Courtesy of the University of Washington.

The advantages of this scale are threefold. First, it takes a relatively short time for an interviewer to administer the scale, between 10 and 20 minutes. Second, the scale is constructed as a semistructured interview guide and gives the subject an opportunity to share his or her perception of what is happening. The first question for each item is general and open-ended. Often, the subject will give enough information in response to this question that no further questions are necessary for that particular item. If more information is needed, more detailed questions follow the general question. The questions are constructed on the principle that as many questions as necessary should be asked using the standardized form to determine where a patient scores on a particular item. Third, responses are scored on standardized code dimensions so that findings can be compared across groups of patients and over time.

The scale was developed to determine the extent to which the patient's dependence on external sources of support has changed during the course of illness. The scale is sensitive to changes in levels of dependence over time. In addition to its research use, the scale has had applicability to the clinical area. One home health agency in Seattle uses the scale to screen patients to determine homebound status in order to apply for reimbursement of services.[42]

Application
Any of these three instruments could be used by nurses to assess the functional status of patients with chronic illnesses. Nurses make assessments of their patients routinely but often do so from individually established criteria. Use of a standardized instrument is one way nurses can assess their patients more systematically and can identify changes over time. These instruments can assist nurses to assess changes in their patients so they can adjust their nursing care interventions. For example, a change in the functional status of a patient may signal the need for teaching the patient methods of approaching a particular activity. Also, systematic changes in functional status, measured by one of these instruments, may alert nurses to a change in self-care ability. If changes occur, the nurse can adapt interventions to increase or reduce the patient's participation in his or her own care. Many instruments that measure functional status can be useful in assisting nurses to evaluate outcomes of the nursing interventions and can be a valuable supplement to clinical impressions of improvement. This review should help a nurse scientist choose instruments that are appropriate to the research question and the population of interest. Consideration of a broad array of instruments in terms of content and psychometric pluses and minuses can facilitate a better match between research goals and outcomes.

SUMMARY

In this chapter, we have compiled a range of functional status scales for use with various populations. We discussed the conceptual and methodologic issues that need to be taken into account when selecting a functional status instrument. Some critical questions that you must ask yourself when selecting an instrument to measure functional status are listed below. A similar set of questions is presented in Chapter 1 to guide the choice of instruments for clinical research. We considered the following questions particularly important when assessing functional status:

- What is your purpose for measuring functional status? (clinical assessment versus research study)
- Are the individual items on the functional status instrument useful for your needs?
- What population do you want to study? (age, types of illness, setting)

- Who will administer the instrument? (self versus recorder)
- How long does it take to complete the functional status instrument, particularly with respect to the condition of your subjects?
- What standardization procedures are necessary for administering and scoring the functional status instrument? (clear and concise instructions; training sessions for recorders and scorers)
- Is the functional status instrument reliable and valid?
- How is the functional status instrument scored?
- Do you need more than one functional status instrument? If so, how do you combine results?
- Does the discussion of the functional status instrument in the literature match what you want your outcome to be? Does it allow you to describe patients in a manner consistent with your research/clinical goals?

ACKNOWLEDGMENT

Carol McMillen Moinpour, Ph.D. is a National Research Service Award Fellow (NIMH/DHHS-MH08949-02), Department of Biostatistics, University of Washington, Seattle, Washington.

APPENDIX. FUNCTIONAL STATUS MEASURES

Name of instrument	Arthritis Impact Measurement Scale (AIMS)
Dimensions, superordinate categories	Assess physical, psychologic, or social health status. 9 scales: mobility, physical activity, dexterity, household activities, ADL, social activity, anxiety, depression, pain, and general health and health perceptions. Dexterity, pain, and ADL developed by authors; other 6 based on Rand Health Insurance Experiment[43] and Index of Well-Being[44] instruments
Target population	Rheumatoid arthritis patients; extended to other chronic diseases (pulmonary disease, diabetes, hypertension, cancer, cardiac disease)
Number of items	67
Method of administration	Self-administered
Length of administration	15–20 minutes
Scoring	Items summed for each scale and standardized to a 0 to 10 range, with higher values describing worse functional status
Reliability	Internal consistency: (1) >0.7 for all scales, (2) 0.61–0.92 for arthritis patients, (3) 0.40–0.92 for other chronic diseases Test–retest (6 months): r for scales ranged between 0.84 and 0.92
Validity	Convergent and discriminant: High intercorrelations within dimensions and across instruments, e.g., HAQ and AIMS physical scales; lower intercorrelations across dimensions and across instruments, e.g., HAQ physical and AIMS psychologic scales; lower intercorrelations across dimensions and within an instrument, e.g., AIMS physical and psychologic Descriptive: Ranks worse than that of 5 other chronic diseases on physical activity, dexterity, household activities, social activity, and pain Clinical: High r between 9 scales and physician estimates of health Factor analytic support for 3 factors (physical disability, psychologic disability, and pain)
Sensitivity to change	Over 6 months of standard clinical treatment, substantial number of subjects showed minor change; concluded change due not to instrument variability but to intervention, regression to mean, or some other factor 6-month blinded drug protocol; AIMS changes correlated with changes in physician estimates of disease severity and patient estimates of general health
Comments and special limitations	Use with other chronic disease groups; reliabilities need to be rechecked for other chronic disease populations
References	45–49
Name of instrument	Barthel Index—Maryland Disability Index
Dimensions, superordinate categories	Physical disability, ADL, and mobility; ability to feed oneself, groom oneself, bathe, go to the toilet, walk, or propel a wheelchair, climb stairs, control bladder, and control bowels
Target population	Patients with chronic disease
Number of items	16
Method of administration	Other; health care staff
Length of administration	2 minutes
Scoring	100 point scale; points given to each ADL carried out adequately (higher score = less disability)

Reliability	Internal consistency reliabilities (alpha) ranged from 0.943 to 0.965
Validity	Predictive: For scores below 60, the scores were inversely related to subsequent mortality in a sample of CVA patients Clinical: The greater the rise in disability score during hospitalization, the more patients were classified as improved by physicians at time of discharge
Sensitivity to change	Not reported
Comments and special limitations	Has been used clinically; instructions standardized for scoring
References	12, 50

Name of instrument	Cumulative Illness Rating Scale (CIRS)
Dimensions, superordinate categories	Physical impairment in 6 organ systems that covers 13 independent organs: (1) cardiovascular–respiratory, (2) gastrointestinal, (3) genitourinary, (4) musculoskeletal–integumentary, (5) neuropsychiatric, (6) general
Target population	People with current or history of illnesses
Number of items	13
Method of administration	Physician or person skilled in physical assessment
Length of administration	Completing a health history and physical examination is time-consuming; if these data are already available, the rating scale takes only a few minutes to complete
Scoring	Separate scores available for each organ system, then 5 point degree of severity scale (none to extremely severe) summed for an overall score
Reliability	Interrater: Kendall's coefficient of concordance (W) ranged from 0.83 to 0.91
Validity	Predictive: Designated individuals along the lifespan with regard to capacity for survival better than chronologic age measure
Sensitivity to change	Not reported
Comments and special limitations	Ratings are formed from judgments established through health history and physical assessment, therefore, can only be administered by those competent in health histories and physical examinations; authors see this tool as having potential clinically by aiding with prognosis as well as in research
References	12, 51

Name of instrument	Duke-UNC Health Profile (DUHP)
Dimensions, superordinate categories	Dimensions: Symptom status, physical function, emotional function, social function
Target population	Adult health status; primary care setting
Number of items	63
Method of administration	Self-administered
Length of administration	10 minutes
Scoring	Desirability (intuitive, not empirical) of health state basis for score, with least desirable health state = 0 Separate score for each dimension by dividing score by total possible to obtain proportion 0–1.0 (best possible health status) Items were weighted equally No overall score because of complex nature of health
Reliability	Internal consistency: Symptom status (not reported); physical functioning (overall not reported, reproducibility for ambulation

	items = 0.98); emotional functioning (alpha = 0.85); social functioning (reproducibility = 0.93)
	Test–retest (1 to 8 weeks): symptom status ($r = 0.68$); physical functioning ($r = 0.89$); emotional functioning ($r = 0.72$); social functioning ($r = 0.52$)
Validity	Convergent/discriminant: Duke psychologic scale correlates higher with SIP psychologic symptoms than it does with other SIP scales; this correlation is higher than most correlations between the psychologic scale and other scales within either the SIP or the DUHP
	Descriptive: Most predicted associations with demographic characteristics of patients upheld (e.g., younger patients had higher health status scores)
Sensitivity to change	No data
Comments and special limitations	No data on sensitivity to change; clinical applicability not yet documented
Reference	52

Name of instrument	Health Assessment Questionnaire (HAQ) Disability Index
Dimensions, superordinate categories	Health Assessment Questionnaire: death, disability (physical and psychologic), discomfort, drug toxicity, dollar costs
	Disability Index: functional ability measured by 8 components: dressing and grooming, arising, eating, reach, personal hygiene, activities, pain, walking, grip, sex
	Following information pertains to Disability Index only
Target population	Rheumatoid arthritis
Number of items	21
Method of administration	Self-administered
Length of administration	5–8 minutes to administer; 1 minute to score
Scoring	0–3/item; score for component is highest item score; index = average of component scores
Reliability	Internal consistency: Index/component r range from 0.48 to 0.81 (self-administered instrument)
	Test–retest (6 months): $r = 0.98$
	Interrater: Self-administered versus interviewer administered, $r = 0.85$, weighted kappa 0.52
Validity	General construct: Correlates with interviewer assessment of performance
	Convergent and discriminant: High intercorrelations within dimensions and across instruments, e.g., HAQ and AIMS physical scales; lower intercorrelations across dimensions and across instruments, e.g., HAQ physical and AIMS psychologic scales; lower intercorrelations across dimensions and within an instrument, e.g., HAQ physical and pain
	Descriptive: Lower disability scores for osteoarthritis versus rheumatoid arthritis patients
	Predictive: Predicted greater or lesser disability but not rate of disease development
	Factor analytic: Support for 2 factors (physical and pain)
Sensitivity to change	Some indication of change over 6-month period
Comments and special limitations	Used mainly with arthritis patients; more information needed on reliabilities before using to assess individual change
References	49, 53, 54, 55

Name of instrument	Karnofsky Index of Performance Status (KPS)
Dimensions, superordinate categories	Performance status: (1) ability to work, (2) ability to perform normal activity, (3) need for assistance

Target population	Cancer patients (extending its use to noncancer patients lowered its reliability rating)
Number of items	11 items (levels of function)
Method of administration	Other
Length of administration	Can be completed quickly
Scoring	Numerical scale from 0 (dead) to 100 (normal, no complaint of complaints (c/o), no evidence of disease); uses 10-point increments
Reliability	Interrater: Correlation of physician with mental health professional on $n = 75$ patients—Pearson correlation, $r = 0.89$; Kappa = 0.53; another measure of interrater reliability via Cronbach coefficient alpha = 0.97 *Note:* Hutchinson et al.[56] achieved poor interrater reliability (34%–29% agreement) when used with noncancer patients in an emergency room setting; correlation of nurse versus social worker ratings, $r = 0.69$ Test–retest (1 week): Home versus clinic, $r = 0.66$
Validity	Convergent: Significant correlations with Cancer Inventory of Problem Situations, Katz ADL Index, National Hospice Study Severity Index and Physical Quality of Life Index Predictive: KPS with survival in days
Sensitivity to change	Yes; it is used to measure response to treatment
Comments and special limitations	Lack of standardized method of assessment and guidelines for training individuals in use of scale; these authors developed an interview guide of 6 items to improve consistency of assessment; predictive accuracy attained is insufficient to guide clinical practice and decision making; some reliability results understandably providing conservative estimates given variation in interviewer experience/training (e.g., nurse versus social worker) and setting (e.g., home versus clinic)
References	8, 56–60

Name of instrument	McMaster Health Index Questionnaire (MHIQ)
Dimensions, superordinate categories	Physical (mobility, self-care, communication, global physical); social (well-being, work/social role performance, family support, and participation); emotional (self-esteem, feelings about personal relationships, critical life events, global emotional functioning)
Target population	Wide variety of populations (e.g., physiotherapy outpatients, psychiatry outpatients, rheumatoid arthritis patients, chronic respiratory disease patients at home, elderly patients)
Number of items	59
Method of administration	Most administration at home by interviewer; can be self-administered
Length of administration	20 minutes
Scoring	Items with best clinical validity chosen for scales and weighted on this basis; Standardized 0–1 (good functioning) score; no total score; separate scores for 3 scales
Reliability	Test–retest (1 week): Physical (r ranged from 0.53 to 0.95 over 3 samples); emotional (r 0.70 and 0.77 for 2 samples); social (r 0.48 and 0.66 for 2 samples)
Validity	General construct: Better physical functioning for younger versus older Clinical/descriptive: Sensitivity, specificity, and predictive value regarding physician assessments of functional status
Sensitivity to change	Pilot study data (change in functional status occurring between hospitalization and convalescence but no data given)

Comments and special limitations	Different timeframes for 3 scales; reliabilities questionable for assessment of individual change; advantage is use with many different types of patients
References	61, 62–63

Name of instrument	Nottingham Health Profile
Dimensions, superordinate categories	Physical, social, emotional; Part I: Problems (6), e.g., pain, mobility; Part II: Effect of Part I on daily life (7), e.g., work, personal relationships
Target population	Most chronically ill populations
Number of items	45
Method of administration	Interviewer and self-administered
Length of administration	5–15 minutes
Scoring	Yes or no responses; Part I, items weighted for severity; weights total 100, with score range 0–100; Part II, not clear, but score accounts for both existence of problems and effect on 7 areas; profiles or graphic comparisons of scores; no total score; one score for each part; high scores = more problems, worse health
Reliability	Test–retest (time interval not reported): Based on patients with peripheral vascular disease and osteoarthritis; Part I, r ranged from 0.75 to 0.88; Part II, r ranged from 0.44 to 0.89
Validity	General construct: Correlated well with self-rated health (very good to very poor) and absence from work Descriptive: Distinguished between consulters and nonconsulters of medical care, younger versus older age groups, and groups of elderly people whose health states differed
Sensitivity to change	Reported 1984 but no data
Comments and special limitations	Use with individuals versus population questionable until more information on reliability (internal consistency) available; some sections not as sensitive to minor ailments so difficult to show change; those getting a zero for such sections cannot be shown to improve when, in fact, they feel better; however, did detect problems in group who were nonconsulters of care Authors say more likely to detect those ill or at risk who do not consider themselves sick because it does not directly ask about health
References	64–67

Name of instrument	Oars Multidimensional Functional Assessment Questionnaire (OMFAQ)
Dimensions, superordinate categories	Personal functioning (Part A): social, mental health, physical health, self-care capacity Service utilization (Part B): transportation, social/recreational, prepared meals, nursing, administrative, protective
Target populations	Older populations
Number of items	101
Method of administration	Trained interviewer
Length of administration	75 minutes
Scoring	Each item scored from excellent functioning (1) to totally impaired (6); each dimension can be summarized with a single score ranging from 1 to 6; additional scores include cumulative impairment scores, number of significant impairments, and patient state
Reliability	Part A only Interrater: Each of 5 researchers and 6 clinicians rated 30 interviews; all intraclass correlation coefficients were

	significant ($p = 0.001$): social = 0.823; economic = 0.783; mental health = 0.803; physical health = 0.662; self-care capacity = 0.865; the raters showed complete agreement on 74% of the ratings; 24% of the ratings differed by 1 point
Validity	Part A only
	Construct: Independent criteria available for 4 of the 5 areas of functioning (e.g., Karnofsky used for physical functioning); Used Kendell's tau and Spearman's rank order correlations, with all 4 areas demonstrating statistically significant agreement between OMFAQ and criterion: economic, tau = 0.62 and r = 0.68; mental health, tau = 0.60 and r = 0.67; physical health, tau = 0.75 and r = 0.82; self-care capacity, tau = 0.83 and r = 0.89
	Descriptive: Items retained from OARS that best discriminated between excellent and totally impaired functioning
Sensitivity to change	Yes; degree not specified; scores from repeated administration on different occasions can be used to develop a transition matrix that traces movement from one functional state to another
Comments and special limitations	The OMFAQ operationalizes the first two components of the OARS model; additional research is needed to examine the extent to which services impact movement between functional states (use of the transition matrix)
	The OMFAQ is a refinement of two earlier versions of the OARS approach: OARS Clinical Instrument; OARS Community Survey Questionnaire
	Only Part A (Personal Functioning) is reviewed
	The OMFAQ measures both adequate and inadequate functioning and provides a quick summary profile in 5 areas
	Additional OARS model instruments:
	1. The Functional Assessment Inventory[68] is an abbreviated version of the OMFAQ that takes only 30 minutes to administer; it has 11 sections
	2. The Philadelphia Geriatric Center Multilevel Assessment Inventory (MAI)[69] is also based on the OARS model; the MAI was developed to (1) include a better coverage of environmental factors, (2) provide scales of items based on sounder psychometric foundations, (3) provide a variety of instrument lengths appropriate for different assessment purposes and settings
References	68–71

Name of instrument	Quality of Life Index (QL Index)
Dimensions, superordinate categories	Physical, emotional, and social aspects of life
Target population	Sick people, especially with cancer and other chronic illness
Number of items	5
Method of administration	Other (physician)
Length of administration	Very brief, 1 minute
Scoring	(0–10) equal weighting items
Reliability	Internal consistency: Cronbach coefficient alpha = 0.775
	Interrater Spearman Rank rho = 0.81
Validity	General construct: High correlations among combinations of professional and nonprofessional
	Biologic: QL scores diminish on a gradient as one progresses from healthy subjects to those with definite disease and then to the seriously ill patients

Sensitivity to change	Not reported
Comments and special limitations	Same as Karnofsky: No standardized procedures for observing/scoring; loses convergent validity with healthy subjects
Reference	72

Name of instrument	Rand Health Insurance Experiment (HIE): Personal Functioning Index (PFI)
Dimensions, superordinate categories	Physical: self-care, mobility, physical activities and capacities
Target population	General population but used with chronic disease populations
Number of items	21
Method of administration	Self-administered
Length of administration	Brief
Scoring	6 levels for each item, with scale value based on mean General Health Rating Index score for persons at each of 6 levels of PFI; score 0–100; higher scores = fewer limitations; support to aggregate subscales of PFI; not to be aggregated with other Rand instruments
Reliability	Test–retest (1 year): Stability coefficient $r = 0.59$ Reproducibility: $r = 0.97$
Validity	Convergent and discriminant: Correlates in expected directions with other measures of physical, mental, and social health Predictive: Predicts general medical and mental health expenditures
Sensitivity to change	No data
Comments and special limitations	Authors separate role limitations from personal functioning because role limitations do not always match limitations in functioning
References	43, 73, 74–75

Name of instrument	Rand Health Insurance Experiment (HIE): Role Limitations
Dimensions, superordinate categories	Physical; freedom from acute or chronic limitations in performing usual role activities
Target population	General population but used with chronic disease populations
Number of items	3
Method of administration	Self-administered
Length of administration	Brief
Scoring	Dichotomous scoring: 1 = completely free of limitation; 0 = one or more limitations; not to be aggregated with other Rand instruments
Reliability	Test–retest (1 year): Stability coefficient $r = 0.50$ Reproducibility: $r = 0.92$
Validity	Convergent and discriminant: Correlates in expected direction with other measures of physical, mental, and social health Predictive: Predicts general medical and mental health expenditures
Sensitivity to change	No data
Comments and special limitations	See comment for Rand Health Insurance Experiment (HIE): Personal Functioning Index (PFI)
References	43, 73, 74–75

Name of instrument	Rand Health Insurance Experiment (HIE): Mental Health Index (MHI)

Dimensions, superordinate categories	Mental health: general positive aspect; emotional ties; psychologic distress
Target population	General population but used with chronic disease populations
Number of items	38
Method of administration	Self-administered
Length of administration	Brief
Scoring	Score 0–100; overall score, psychologic distress, psychologic well-being, 5 subscale scores; higher scores = higher level of variable (e.g., more distress, better mental health); strong psychometric support for overall index score; not to be aggregated with other Rand instruments
Reliability	Internal consistency: Alpha = 0.96 Test–retest: Stability coefficients $r = 0.60$–0.76 (1 year); $r = 0.54$–0.69 (2 year); $r = 0.54$–0.58 (3 year)
Validity	Convergent and discriminant: Correlated substantially with other measures of mental and emotional health and not as well with measures of physical and social health Descriptive: Differentiated patients treated for depression from those treated for arthritis, diabetes, cancer, renal disease, and dermatologic disorders Predictive: Predicts general medical expenditures and expenditures for outpatient mental health Factor analytic: Mental health subscales differ from scales measuring physical and social aspects of health
Sensitivity to change	Not reported
References	43, 73, 75–77

Name of instrument	Rand Health Insurance Experiment (HIE): Social Contacts
Dimensions, superordinate categories	Social well-being: Frequency of visits with friends and relatives
Target population	General population but used with chronic disease populations
Number of items	3
Method of administration	Self-administered
Length of administration	Brief
Scoring	Criterion method: Self-rated health, emotional ties, general positive affect used to determine scoring rules; three items were standardized and transformed to 0–100 scale; higher score = greater social well-being; not to be aggregated with other Rand instruments
Reliability	Internal consistency: Alpha = 0.72 Test–retest (1 year): Stability coefficient $r = 0.44$–0.57
Validity	Convergent and discriminant: Low but significant and positive correlations between Social Contacts scale and other measures of social well-being; these correlations were stronger than those between the Social Contacts Scale and other measures of health Predictive: Predicts improved mental health
Sensitivity to change	Not reported
Comments and special limitations	This scale is the weakest of the 5 Rand scales in terms of its reliabilities and its association with psychologic well-being (emotional ties); this scale is intended to be more distinct from the Mental Health Index than it turned out to be; Ware views social resources and contacts as a predictor versus a distinct component of health; sometimes a 9-item Social Resources Scale is included with the Social Contacts Scale
References	43, 73, 77

Name of instrument	Rand Health Insurance Experiment (HIE): General Health Rating Index (GHRI)
Dimensions, superordinate categories	Physical, mental (health and illness behaviors)
Target population	General population (shorter children's version available) but used with chronic disease populations
Number of items	22 (of 26 items in Rand Health Perceptions Questionnaire)
Method of administration	Self-administered
Length of administration	Approximately 7 minutes
Scoring	0–100 score; higher score = better perceived health status; subscale scores possible (e.g., current health, prior health); not to be aggregated with other Rand instruments
Reliability	Internal consistency: Alpha = 0.89 Test–retest (1 year): Stability coefficient $r = 0.68$
Validity	Convergent: GHRI related to many measures of mental and physical health Descriptive: Older persons and women rate health less favorably; distinguished between people with severe impairments in either the physical or emotional dimensions Clinical: GHRI correlated with clinical examination measures of chronic disease Factor analytic: Factor structure maintained in four general population studies Predictive: GHRI scores predict use of general and mental health care services
Sensitivity to change	Preliminary findings[43] indicate GHRI can detect changes over time in mental and physical functioning
Comments and special limitations	Psychometrically sound instrument that is brief and combines measures of both physical and mental health; Ware argues that a health perception measure reflects both an individual's values about his or her health and that individual's health state
References	43, 73, 78

Name of instrument	Rapid Disability Rating Scale (RDRS)
Dimensions, superordinate categories	Functioning of self-care independence
Target population	Older, chronically ill
Number of items	16
Method of administration	Nurses or other medically oriented staff with first-hand knowledge of patient's conditions
Length of administration	2 minutes
Scoring	3-point rating scale for each item
Reliability	Test–retest (average of 3½ days): Kendals tau = 0.913 Interrater: Product moment correlation = 0.831
Validity	General construct: Number of previous hospitalizations and number of deaths in a 6-month period Clinical: Prognostic judgments made by physicians
Sensitivity to change	No data
Comments and special limitations	The RDRS is similar to the Cumulative Illness Rating Scale; Rapid Disability Rating Scale-2 (RDRS-2) is a revised version with ratings based on performance and rated on a 4-point scale; three items were added; designed for use in research; clinical use has not been explored
Special limitations	Designed for use in research; clinical use has not been explored
References	79–80

Name of instrument	Thirty-Item Screening Scale
Dimensions, superordinate categories	Physical, mental, social well-being
Target Population	Low-level disability in a noninstitutionalized adult Canadian population
Number of items	30
Method of administration	Clinic samples interviewed; healthy sample self-administered
Length of administration	No information
Scoring	Scale weights yet to be developed; scores for each dimension: number of items with no disability converted to a stanine score; no total score; separate scores for each dimension
Reliability	Internal consistency: Item total r ranged from 0.06 to 0.59 for physical; 0.30 to 0.61 for social; 0.27 to 0.57 for psychologic; no r for total scale
Validity	Clinical: Most r between individual items and physician ratings reasonable
	Descriptive: Items appeared to differentiate between healthy sample and 2 clinic samples but no tests of significance reported
Sensitivity to change	No data
Comments and special limitations	Items are a mix of performance and capacity; difficult to evaluate instrument's claim to measure low-level disability because so little psychometric data reported; expected but unable to demonstrate positive health factor; reliabilities definitely not sufficient to assess individual change
Reference	81

REFERENCES

1. Lawton, M.P. The functional assessment of elderly people. *J Am Geriatr Soc,* 1971, *19*(6):465.
2. Tornberg, M.J. *The association of social dependency and self-esteem in advanced cancer patients.* Thesis, University of Washington, 1980.
3. Mumma, C.M. *The effects of disability following a cerebrovascular accident on older individuals and on their mental relationships.* Thesis, University of Washington, 1984.
4. Benoliel, J.Q., McCorkle, R.M., & Young, K. Development of a social dependency scale. *Res Nurs Health,* 1980, *3*:3.
5. Kuriansky, J., & Gurland, B. The performance test of activities of daily living. *Int J Aging Hum Dev* 1976, *7*(4):343.
6. World Health Organization. *The first ten years of the world health organization.* Geneva: The World Health Organization, 1958.
7. Katz, S., Ford, A.B., Moskowitz, R.W., et al. Studies of illness in the aged. *JAMA,* 1963, *185*(12):914.
8. Katz, S., Downs, T.D., Cash, H.R., & Grotz, R.C. Progress in development in the Index of ADL. *Gerontologist,* 1970, *10*(1, Part 1):20.
9. Katz, S., Hedrick, S.C., & Henderson, N.S. The measurement of long-term care needs and impact. *Health Med Care Serv Rev,* 1979, *2*(1):1.
10. Katz, S. Assessing self-maintenance: Activities of daily living, mobility, and instrumental activities of daily living. *J Am Geriatr Soc,* 1983, *31*(17):721.
11. Hedrick, S.C., Katz, S., & Stroud, M.W. Patient assessment in long-term care: Is there a common language? *Aged Care Serv Rev,* 1980/81, *2*(4):1.
12. Kane, R.A., & Kane, R.L. *Assessing the elderly: A practical guide to measurement.* Lexington, MA: Lexington Books, 1981.

13. Gentzsch, P. Mobility assessment tool. *Oncol Nurs Forum*, 1981, *8*(4):51.
14. Meissner, J.E. Evaluate your patient's level of independence. *Nursing*, 1980, *10*(9):72.
15. Mangen, D.J., & Peterson, W.A. *Research instruments in social gerontology. Vol. 3. Health, program evaluation, and demography*. Minneapolis: University of Minnesota Press, 1984.
16. Bombardier, C., & Tugwell, P. A methodological framework to develop and select indices for clinical trials: Statistical and judgmental approaches. *J Rheumatol*, 1982, *9*(5):753.
17. Bergner, L., Bergner, M., Hallstrom, A.P., et al. Health status of survivors of out-of-hospital cardiac arrest six months later. *Am J Public Health*, 1984, *74*(5):508.
18. Deyo, R.A., Inui, T.S., Leininger, J., & Overman, H. Physical and psychosocial function in rheumatoid arthritis. Clinical use of a self-administered health status instrument. *Arch Intern Med*, 1982, *142*(5):879.
19. Sugerbaker, P.H., Barofsky, I., Rosenberg, S.A., & Gianola, P.A-C. Quality of life assessment of patients in extremity sarcoma clinical trials. *Surgery*, 1982, *91*(1):17.
20. Heaton, R.K., Grant, I., McSweeny, A.J., et al. Psychologic effects of continuous and nocturnal oxygen therapy in hypoxemia chronic obstructive pulmonary disease. *Arch Intern Med*, 1983, *143*(10):1941.
21. McSweeny, A.J., Grant, I., Heaton, R.K., et al. Life quality of patients with chronic obstructive pulmonary disease. *Arch Intern Med*, 1982, *142*(3):473.
22. Ott, C.R., Sivarajan, E.S., Newton, K.M., et al. A controlled randomized study of early cardiac rehabilitation: The Sickness Impact Profile as an assessment tool. *Heart Lung*, 1983, *12*(2):162.
23. Barlow, P.B., Nelson, E.C., Howland, J., et al. Localizing community residents with chronic airway obstruction. A comparison of four strategies. *Am Rev Respir Dis*, 1984, *129*(3):361.
24. Deyo, R.A., & Inui, T.S. Toward clinical applications of health status measures: Sensitivity of scales to clinically important changes. *Health Serv Res*, 1984, *19*(3):275.
25. McLean, A. Jr., Dikman, S., Temkin, N., et al. Psychosocial functioning at one month after head injury. *Neurosurgery*, 1984, *14*(4):393.
26. Zeldow, P.B., & Pavlou, M. Physical disability, life stress, and psychosocial adjustment in multiple sclerosis. *J Nerv Ment Dis*, 1984, *172*(2):80.
27. Fink, A. *Social dependency and self-care agency: A descriptive-correlational study of ALS patients*. Thesis, University of Washington, 1985.
28. Snow, R., & Crapo, L. Emotional bondedness, subjective well-being, and health in elderly medical patients. *J Gerontol*, 1982, *37*(5):609.
29. Young, K. Quality of life and melanoma in the elderly (Abstract). *Am Public Health Assoc Proc, Energy, Health, and the Environment*, November 1981.
30. Deyo, R.A. Pitfalls in measuring the health status of Mexican Americans: Comparative validity of the English and Spanish SIP. *Am J Public Health*, 1984, *74*(6):569.
31. Gilson, B.S., Gilson, J.S., Bergner, M., et al. The Sickness Impact Profile. Development of an outcome measure of health care. *Am J Public Health*, 1975, *65*(12):1304.
32. Bergner, M., Bobbitt, R.A., Carter, W.B., & Gilson, B.S. The Sickness Impact Profile: Development and final revision of a health status measure. *Med Care*, 1981, *19*(8):787.
33. Conn, J., Bobbitt, R.A., & Bergner, M. *Administration procedures and interviewer training for the Sickness Impact Profile*. Seattle, WA: University of Washington Department of Health Services (USDHEW Grant No. HS-01769), July 1978.
34. Pollard, W.E., Bobbitt, R.A., Bergner, M., et al. The Sickness Impact Profile: Reliability of a health status measure. *Med Care*, 1976, *14*(2):146.
35. Bergner, M., Bobbitt, R.A., Kressel, S., et al. The Sickness Impact Profile: Conceptual formulation and methodology for the development of a health status measure. *Int J Health Serv*, 1976, *6*(3):393.
36. Carter, W.B., Bobbitt, R.A., Bergner, M., & Gilson, B.S. Validation of an interval scaling: The Sickness Impact Profile. *Health Serv Res*, 1976, *11*(4):516.
37. Liang, M.H., Cullen, K., & Larson, M. In search of a more perfect mousetrap (health status or quality of life instrument). *J Rheumatol*, 1982, *9*(5):775.
38. Bloom, J.R. Response to Ware's "Conceptualizing disease impact and treatment outcomes." Bringing the patient back in. Prepared for the Conference on Methodology for Behavioral & Psychosocial Cancer Research, American Cancer Soc., St. Petersburg, Florida, April 22, 1983.

39. Carter, W.B., & Deyo, R.A. The impact of questionnaire research on clinical populations: A dilemma in review of human subjects research resolved by a study of a study. *Clin Res,* 1981, *29*(4):287.
40. McCorkle, R., & Benoliel, J.Q. *Cancer patient responses to psychosocial variables.* Final Report of project supported by Grant No. NU00730, DHHS, University of Washington, 1981.
41. McCorkle, R., Benoliel, J.Q., & Donaldson, G. *A manual of data collection instruments.* Seattle, WA: University of Washington Department of Community Health Care Systems (DHHS Grant No. NU00730), 1981.
42. Mulhern, P. Personal communication to R. McCorkle, 1980–1985.
43. Ware, J.E. Jr. Overview of general health measures used in the Rand Health Insurance Experiment. Prepared for the Workshop on Advances in Health Status Assessment, First National Meeting of the Association of Health Services Research, Chicago, Illinois, June 1984.
44. Bush, J.W. General health policy model/Quality of Well-Being (QWB) Scale. Paper presented at Workshop on Advances in Health Status Assessment, Chicago, Illinois, June 1984.
45. Meenan, R.F., Gertman, P.M., & Mason, J. H. Measuring health status in arthritis. The Arthritis Impact Measurement Scale. *Arthritis Rheum,* 1980, *23*(2):146.
46. Meenan, R.F. The AIMS approach to health status measurement: Conceptual background and measurement properties. *J Rheumatol,* 1982, *9*(5):785.
47. Meenan, R.F., Mason, J.H., & Kazis, L.E. Psychosocial status in chronic illness. (Letter to the editor). *N Engl J Med,* 1984, *311*(24):1580.
48. Mason, J.H., Weener, J.L., Gutman, P.M., & Meenan, R.F. Health status in chronic disease: A comparative study of rheumatoid arthritis. *J Rheumatol,* 1983, *10*(5):763.
49. Brown, J.H., Kazis, L.E., Spitz, P.W., et al. The dimensions of health outcomes: A cross-validated examination of health status measurement. *Am J Public Health,* 1984, *74*(2):159.
50. Wylie, C.M., & White, B.K. A measure of disability. *Arch Environ Health,* 1964, *8*(6):834.
51. Linn, B.S., Linn, M.W., & Gurel, L. Cumulative illness rating scale. *J Am Geriatr Soc,* 1968, *16*(5):622.
52. Parkerson, G.R. Jr., Gehlbach, S.H., Wagner, E.H., et al. The Duke-UNC Health Profile: An adult health status instrument for primary care. *Med Care,* 1981, *19*(8):806.
53. Fries, J.F. Toward an understanding of patient outcome measurement. *Arthritis Rheum,* 1983, *26*(6):697.
54. Fries, J.F., Spitz, P., Kraines, R.G., & Holman, H.R. Measurement of patient outcome in arthritis. *Arthritis Rheum,* 1980, *23*(2):137.
55. Fries, J.F., Spitz, P.W., & Young, D.Y. The dimensions of health outcomes: The Health Assessment Questionnaire, Disability and Pain Scales. *J Rheumatol,* 1982, *9*(5):789.
56. Hutchinson, T.A., Boyd, N.F., & Feinstein, A.R., in collaboration with Gonda, A., Hollomby, D., & Rowat, B. Scientific problems in clinical scales, as demonstrated in the Karnofsky Index of Performance Status. *J Chronic Dis,* 1979, *32*(9/10):661.
57. Yates, J.W., Chalina, B., & McKegney, F.P. Evaluation of patients with advanced cancer using the Karnofsky Performance Status. *Cancer,* 1980, *45*(8):2220.
58. Chang, S.K., & Hawes, K.A. The adequacy of the Karnofsky Rating and Global Adjustment to Illness Scale as outcome measures in cancer rehabilitation and continuing care. In P.F. Engstrom, P.N. Anderson, & L.E. Mortenson (Ed.), *Advances in cancer control: Research and development. Progress in clinical and biological research,* Vol. 120. New York: Alan R. Liss, Inc., 1983, p. 429.
59. Mor, V., Laliberte, L., Morris, J.N., & Wiemann, M. The Karnofsky Performance Status Scale: An examination of its reliability and validity in a research setting. *Cancer,* 1984, *53*(9):2002.
60. Schag, C.C., Heinrich, R.L., & Ganz, P.A. Karnofsky Performance Status revisited: Reliability, validity, and guidelines. *J Clin Oncol,* 1984, *2*(3):187.
61. Chambers, L.W. Health program review in Canada: Measurements of health status. *Can J Public Health,* 1982, *73*(1):26.
62. Chambers, L.W., MacDonald, L.A., Tugwell, P., et al. The McMaster Health Index Questionnaire as a measure of quality of life for patients with rheumatoid disease. *J Rheumatol,* 1982, *9*(5):780.
63. Chambers, L.W. The McMaster Health Index Questionnaire. Prepared for the Workshop on Advances in Health Status Assessment, First National Meeting of the Association of Health Services Research, Chicago, June 1984.

64. Hunt, S.M., McKenna, S.P., McEwen, J., et al. A quantitative approach to perceived health status: A validation study. *J Epidemiol Community Health,* 1980, *34*(4):281.
65. Hunt, S.M., McKenna, S.P., McEwen, J., et al. The Nottingham Health Profile: Subjective health status and medical consultations. *Soc Sci Med,* 1981, *15*A(3,I):221.
66. Hunt, S.M. Nottingham Health Profile. Prepared for the Workshop on Advances in Health Status Assessment, First National Meeting of the Association of Health Services Research, Chicago, June 1984.
67. Hunt, S.M., McEwen, J., & McKenna, S.P. Perceived health: Age and sex comparisons in a community. *J Epidemiol Community Health,* 1984, *38*(2):156.
68. Pfeiffer, E., Johnson, T.M., & Chiofolo, R.C. Functional assessment of elderly subjects in four service settings. *J Am Geriatr Soc,* 1981, *29*(10):433.
69. Lawton, M.P., Moss, M., Fulcomer, M., & Kleban, M.H. A research and service-oriented multi-level assessment instrument. *J Gerontol,* 1982, *37*(1):91.
70. Duke University Center for the Study of Human Development. *Multidimensional functional assessment: The OARS methodology.* Durham, NC: Duke University, 1975.
71. Fillenbaum, G.G., & Smyer, M.A. The development, validity, and reliability of the OARS Multidimensional Functional Assessment Questionnaire. *J Gerontol,* 1981, *36*(4):428.
72. Spitzer, W.O., Dobson, A.J., Hall, J., et al. Measuring the quality of life of cancer patients. A concise QL-Index for use by physicians. *J Chronic Dis,* 1981, *34*(12):585.
73. Ware, J.E. Jr. Conceptualizing disease impact and treatment outcomes. Prepared for the Conference on Methodology for Behavioral and Psychosocial Cancer Research, American Cancer Society, St. Petersburg, Florida, April 22, 1983.
74. Ware, J.E. Jr., Brook, R.H., Williams, R.N., et al. *Conceptualizing and measurements of health for adults in the health insurance study: Vol. I. Model of health and methodology.* Santa Monica, CA: Rand Corporation, R-1987/1-HEW, 1980.
75. Nelson, E., Conger, B., Douglass, R., et al. Functional health status levels of primary care patients. *JAMA,* 1983, *249*(24):3331.
76. Ware, J.E. Jr., Johnston, S.A., Davies-Avery, A., & Brook, R.H. *Conceptualization and measurement of health for adults in the health insurance study: Vol. III: Mental health.* Santa Monica, CA: Rand Corporation, R-1987/3-HEW, 1979.
77. Williams, A.W., Ware, J.E. Jr., & Donald, C.A. A model of mental health, life events, and social supports applicable to general populations. *J Health Soc Behav,* 1981, *22*(4):324.
78. Davies, A.R., & Ware, J.E. Jr. *Measuring health perceptions in the health insurance experiment R-2711-HHS.* Santa Monica, CA: Rand Corporation, 1981.
79. Linn, M.W. A rapid disability rating scale. *J Am Geriatr Soc,* 1967, *15*(2):211.
80. Linn, M.W., & Linn, M.W. The Rapid Disability Rating Scale-2. *J Am Geriatr Soc,* 1982, *30:*378.
81. McDowell, I., & Roberts, J. The Thirty-Item Screening Scale: A survey measure of low-level disability. *Can J Public Health,* 1983, *74*(3):202.

CHAPTER 3

Measuring Mental Status and Level of Consciousness

Mary C. Fraser, R.N., M.A.

Many disease processes may induce alterations in mental status. These alterations may have profound effects on an individual's ability to communicate effectively. To assess a patient's orientation, attention, feeling states, thought patterns, and specific cognitive skills, the mental status examination has been developed. It is intended to provide specific and accurate information about a patient's current behavior and mental capabilities. An accurate assessment is necessary to evaluate a patient's capacity to function in a particular environment or to perform certain activities. Several instruments are useful for measuring an individual's mental functioning. However, these instruments vary in their performance and ability to measure mental status. In this chapter, the various instruments are described and their strengths and limitations discussed. In addition, examples of research studies using selected instruments and recommendations for further nursing research are presented.

Nursing evaluation of mentation seeks primarily to determine "the state of integrated human functioning" as opposed to locating a lesion or diagnosing a neurologic disease or psychiatric illness.[1-3] Because of this approach, standard neuropsychologic instruments designed for comprehensive, full-scale neurologic or psychologic testing of mental status, cognitive functioning, or adaptive and emotional behaviors that reflect the adequacy or inadequacy of cortical function are not included in this chapter. The mental status examinations included are those that are of most interest to the clinical nurse researcher, that is, those mental status measures that evaluate an individual's behavior or functioning that affect self-care abilities. If the mental status examination elicits evidence of dysfunction, the nurse should refer the patient for further exploration of mental functioning.

The concepts for defining mental status are highly abstract, and there is little agreement among health care practitioners on precise definitions for the terms. The definition of normal and abnormal states of mind is difficult because the terms used to describe these states have been given so many meanings. Compounding the difficulty is the fact that the pathophysiology of the confusional states delirium and dementia is not fully understood, and the definitions depend on their clinical relationships.[4]

Mental status examinations vary in their thoroughness. They are performed in a hierarchical manner, beginning with the most basic function—level of consciousness—and proceeding to the more complex areas of verbal reasoning and calculating ability.[1,5-8] The quantitative scales incorporate the simple questions in general clinical use for assessing the sensorium and memory and for eliciting descriptions of behavior.[1-15] Unlike the ordinary clinical examination to assess mental status, the order in which the questions are asked and the method of scoring are standardized in quantitative scales. The total score gives a measure of overall performance. Regardless of whether the instrument will be used for clinical assessment or to measure a variable for a research project, similar criteria should be used. This chapter focuses on the objective quantification or measurement of various aspects of mental status in adult populations to meet specific research goals.

COMPONENTS OF MENTAL STATUS

Health care practitioners rely on many different frameworks for assessing components of mental status. As shown in Table 3–1, Mitchell et al.[1] conceptualize the two main functional categories of mental status as consciousness and mentation.

Consciousness
Consciousness may be described as "the ability to appreciate sensory information, to react critically to it with thoughts and movements, and to permit the accumulation of memory traces" (p. 95).[14] It is the most rudimentary of all mental functions. Consciousness, as used in the biobehavioral sense, has two components: arousal and awareness of self.[1] The presence of sufficient arousal and awareness of self to attend to the examiner and to follow verbal directions is an active process that is prerequisite to subsequent examination. Arousal, also referred to as vigilance, is a function of the combined functions of the cerebral hemispheres and brainstem reticular activating system. Damage to these structures results in various degrees of alteration in the person's ability to be aroused or attentive to the environment. Awareness of both self and the environment is the other component of consciousness.[1] Many aspects of awareness, such as mood, judgment, and thinking, are evaluated as part of mentation. However, orientation to self and the environment is typically included with evaluating consciousness. Consciousness is difficult to measure accurately because the patient's behavior merely provides an estimate of his arousability and awareness of self at a given time. Consciousness is a dynamic state that is subject to change.[1,5,8]

Arousal is assessed by noting the patient's response to general environmental stimuli and

**TABLE 3–1. MENTAL STATUS
FUNCTIONAL CATEGORIES**

Category	Function
Consciousness	Arousal
	Self-awareness
Mentation/cognitive function	Thinking
	Remembering
	Perceiving
	Language
	Problem-solving

Adapted from Mitchell et al. Neurologic assessment for nursing practice, 1984, p. 7. Courtesy of Prentice Hall.

to verbal stimuli (Table 3–2). If there is no response to verbal stimuli, a painful stimulus is used. Responses include such behaviors as opening eyes, verbal utterances, and bodily movement, such as turning the head or obeying commands. Self-awareness or orientation can be evaluated by asking the patient questions about his name, the date, and the place.

Clinicians use many schemes for describing and defining gradations in the level of consciousness or level of arousal. The terms "alert," "awake," "lethargic," "obtunded," "stuporous," "semicomatose," and "comatose" are often used to denote decreasing levels of arousal, [1,4–8,14] although they may have various interpretations. Definitions of these terms are given in Table 3–3. Each term is qualitative in nature, encompassing a wide range of possible points on the continuum of consciousness, and thus there is much overlap.

TABLE 3–2. FUNCTIONAL CATEGORIES, ANATOMIC CORRELATES, AND TESTS USED TO EVALUATE MENTAL STATUS

Functional Category	Anatomic Correlate	Evaluative Tests
Consciousness		
Arousal	Reticular activating system (RAS) Brainstem reticular formation Diffuse projections to thalamus/cortex Diencephalon	Observe integrated function of Eye opening Verbal response Motor response
Self-awareness	Cerebral hemispheres	Verbal stimulus What is your name? Where are you? What is the date? Command: Raise your arms! Noxious stimulus Proximal nailbed pressure
Mentation		
Remembering	Limbic system, cortex Ascending activation via RAS and thalamic projection system	Digit span Recent and remote memory
Feeling (affective)	Limbic system	Observation of mood Emotional status
Language	Left hemisphere	Determine handedness Content and quantity of spontaneous speech Naming objects Repetition of phrases Reading ability (first determine educational level)
Spatial perception	Right hemisphere	Ability to copy figures Ability to draw clock face Right/left orientation Double simultaneous stimulation Observe dressing
Thinking	Cortex	Fund of information Calculations Social awareness and judgment Abstract thinking through interpretation of proverbs

Adapted from Mitchell et al. Neurologic assessment for nursing practice, *1984, p.94. Courtesy of Prentice Hall.*

TABLE 3–3. LEVELS OF CONSCIOUSNESS

Description	Definition
Alert	Normal, fully oriented
Awake	May sleep more than usual but is fully oriented when aroused or may be confused at times
Lethargic	Drowsy but obeys simple commands when stimulated
Obtunded	Exhibits mental blunting or torpidity (sluggishness, inactivity, slowness)
Stuporous	Very hard to arouse, generally unresponsive; looks around when stimulated, may obey commands at times; may curse or say "don't" when stimulated
Semicomatose	Purposeful movements when stimulated; does not obey commands or answer questions; does not talk at all
Coma	
Decorticate	Draws hands up onto chest when stimulated, but not purposefully
Decerebrate	Extends arms and legs, arches neck, and internally rotates hands and arms when stimulated
Unresponsive	No response to any stimulus

Adapted from Mitchell et al. Neurologic assessment for nursing practice, 1984, p. 30. Courtesy of Prentice Hall.

Plum and Posner[16] delineate five levels of responsiveness: alert wakefulness, clouding of consciousness or delirium, obtundation, stupor, and coma. They define delirium as a floridly abnormal mental state characterized by disorientation, fear, irritability, misperception of sensory, stimuli, and, often, visual hallucinations. They also specify that for all practical purposes the terms "clouding of consciousness" and "delirium" define equivalent alterations

TABLE 3–4. TERMINOLOGY FOR ACUTE AND CHRONIC ALTERATIONS IN CONSCIOUSNESS

Description	Definition
Acute alterations in consciousness (arousal)	
Clouding of consciousness	Reduced wakefulness and decreased attention
Confusional state	Disorientation, poor memory, defect in attention, impaired capacity to think with usual speed and clarity
Delirium	Disorientation, fearfulness, irritability, misperception of sensory stimuli, visual hallucination
Obtundation	Mental blunting, decreased alertness, decreased interest in environment
Stupor	Deep sleep, arousable only by vigorous and repeated stimuli
Coma	Unarousable by any stimulus, psychologic unresponsiveness
Subacute chronic alternations in consciousness (arousal)	
Vegetative state	Wakefulness with total apparent lack of cognitive function
Akinetic mutism (coma vigil)	Silent, alert but immobile, normal sleep–wake cycles
Alteration in awareness	
Disorientation in awareness	Errors in recognition of self, others, place, and/or time
Alteration in appearance of awareness	
Locked-in syndrome	Intact cognitive functions but unable to use voluntary motor system to execute responses

Adapted from Mitchell et al. Neurologic assessment for nursing practice, 1984, p. 102. Courtesy of Prentice Hall.

TABLE 3–5. DISORDERS COMMONLY CAUSING ALTERED AROUSAL

Structural	Metabolic
Trauma to head	Oxygenative deficiency
Major	Pulmonary disease, anemia, cardiopulmonary
Loss of consciousness for 24 hours or more	insufficiency, arrhythmia
Minor	Metabolic deficiency
Loss of consciousness for less than 20 minutes	Liver, renal failure, diabetes, fluid–electrolyte
Infection	imbalance, vitamin deficiency, gastroin-
Meningitis	testinal disease
Encephalitis	Exogenous toxins
Slow virus	Sedative/hypnotic overdose, alcohol over-
Creutzfelt-Jacob syndrome	dose, cyanide, salicylate poisoning, carbon
Pneumonia	monoxide poisoning
Septicemia, particularly streptococcal infections	
Neoplasm	
Primary, end-stage	
Metastatic	
Brainstem or pontine location	
Vascular	
Hemorrhage	
Subarachnoid, pontine, intraventricular, intra-cerebral, intracerebellar	
Hematoma	
Epidural, subdural, intracerebellar, intracerebral	
Occlusion	
Basilar artery	
Hydrocephalus	
Congenital end-stage	
Acquired	
Communicating/obstructive	
Noncommunicating/nonobstructive	

Adapted from Mitchell et al. Neurologic assessment for nursing practice, 1984, p. 101. Courtesy of Prentice Hall.

of arousal that commonly are preludes or sequels to stupor or coma, thus the term "delirium" can refer to either condition. Some authors define delirium as a state of confusion, with agitation and hallucinations, and generally consider this state separate from the continuum of confusion → stupor → coma.[17] Terminology often used to describe acute and chronic alterations in consciousness is shown in Table 3–4.

Deterioration in the level of consciousness is one of the most important and universally appreciated signs of deteriorating neurologic status in a variety of acute disorders.[1,5,8] The rapidity of the change in level of consciousness is an indicator of the acuity of the neurologic problem. Several disorders affecting the brain and central nervous system can progress rather rapidly to irreversible brain damage and death. Careful observation of small changes in the level of consciousness can often detect such worsening before irreversible brain damage has occurred, in time to institute definite medical and surgical treatment. Disorders that commonly cause such alterations are listed in Table 3–5.

Mentation

Mentation, also referred to as cognitive functioning, is the second main category of mental status.[1] Mentation includes many components. Those chosen for discussion in this chapter must display some degree of consciousness. As shown in Tables 3–1 and 3–2, the functions involved in mentation include attention, remembering, feeling (affective), language, spatial perception, and thinking.

The prerequisite for evaluating mentation is the ability of the patient to attend to and concentrate on the examiner without being distracted by extraneous environmental stimuli. Orientation to person, place, and time (examined under consciousness) is not required for examination of mentation. Patients who are disoriented can often answer questions and follow directions, although the content of the answers may not be accurate or appropriate.[1]

Remembering is closely associated with attention. Memory is defined as the ability to store and retrieve information.[1] It is crucial to all other aspects of mentation. Both short- and long-term memory should be evaluated. Short-term memory is evaluated by assessing the ability to recall new information. Long-term memories are those that have been part of the person's repertoire for longer than 24 hours and are apt to be disrupted least by disorders of attention or cognition.

Evaluation of feeling or affect is an important part of interpreting deficits in mentation. Depression can interfere with an individual's attention span and ability to concentrate as much as can degenerative brain damage. Evaluation of this component includes assessment of mood, facial expressions, body language, and the appropriateness to the situation of verbally and nonverbally expressed emotion.[1]

Language is a complex mental function involving the use of symbols to form, express,

---

TABLE 3–6. TERMINOLOGY FOR ABNORMAL MENTATION

Description	Definition
Thinking	
Dementia	Nonspecific term denoting generalized decline in mental processes, with preservation of arousal (consciousness)
Retardation	Nonspecific term denoting not having achieved expected level of mental development
Remembering	
Amnesia	Loss of the ability to form memories despite an alert state of mind
Feeling (emotion)	
Euphoria	A feeling of well-being, elation
Apathy	Lack of emotion, interest, or concern
Emotional lability	Sudden fluctuations in emotion, usually inappropriate to circumstances
Language	
Aphasia	Inability to understand or communicate using words, even though the sensory systems, mechanisms of phonation and articulation, and sensorium are relatively intact
Anomia	Inability to name objects
Neologisms	New and meaningless words
Alexia	Acquired inability to comprehend written language
Spatial perception	
Apraxia	Inability to perform a volitional act, even though the motor system and sensorium are relatively intact
Agnosia	Inability to understand the significance of sensory stimuli, even though the sensory pathways and sensorium are relatively intact

Adapted from Mitchell et al. Neurologic assessment for nursing practice, 1984, p. 116. Courtesy of Prentice Hall.

TABLE 3–7. A COMPARISON OF THE CLINICAL FEATURES OF CONFUSION, DEMENTIA, AND DEPRESSION

Feature	Confusion	Dementia	Depression
Essential feature	A clouded state of consciousness	Not based on disordered consciousness; based on loss of intellectual functions of sufficient severity to interfere with social and occupational functioning	
Onset	Acute/subacute, depends on cause	Chronic, generally insidious, depends on cause	Coincides with life changes, often abrupt
Course	Short, diurnal fluctuations in symptoms, worse at night, in dark, and on awakening	Long, no diurnal effects, symptoms progressive yet relatively stable over time	Diurnal effects, typically worse in the morning, situational fluctuations, not progressive
Duration	Hours to less than a month	Months to years	At least 2 weeks, can be several months or years
Awareness	Fluctuates, generally impaired	Generally normal	Often good
Alertness	Fluctuates, reduced or increased	Generally normal	Normal
Orientation	Fluctuates in severity, generally impaired, errors of commission	May be impaired; errors of commission	Selective disorientation, errors of commission
Memory	Recent and immediate impaired, unable to register new information or recall recent events	Recent and remote impaired, loss of recent first sign, some loss of common knowledge	Selective or patchy memory loss, often of the stressful area
Thinking	Disorganized, distorted, fragmented, slow or accelerated	Difficulty with abstraction	Intact
Perception	Distorted, based on state of arousal, mood, illusions, delusions, and hallucinations	Misperceptions often absent	Intact, delusions and hallucinations absent
Sleep–wake cycle	Disturbed, cycle reversed	Fragmented	Disturbed, often early morning rising
Electroencephalogram	Predominance of slow or fast cycles related to state of arousal	Normal or slow	Normal
Mini-Mental State Examination (MMSE)	Mean score 12	Mean score 7	Mean score 19
Associated features	Variable affective changes, with fear, apprehension, and bewilderment predominating Symptoms of autonomic hyperarousal	Affect tends to be superficial, inappropriate, and labile and includes apathy, depression, and euphoria with some degree of personality change, attempts to conceal deficits in intellect	Affect depressed, dysphoric mood, exaggerated and detailed complaints

From Foreman, M.D. The development of confusion in the hospitalized elderly. *Unpublished doctoral dissertation. University of Illinois at Chicago, College of Nursing, 1986.*

and communicate thoughts and feelings.[1,2] It is unique to humans and is the primary basis of human interaction. The functions of language include understanding spoken and written words and communicating by speaking and writing. The ability to use and understand language and intact memory must be present in order to test other more complex functions, such as problem solving, judgment, and calculations.

Spatial perception is a higher cognitive function, involving both recognition of space and shape and spatial memory.[1] Spatial perception is tested by having a person copy simple drawings. Spatial memory is evaluated by having the individual reproduce drawings of simple figures from memory.

Thinking comprises the sum total of cognitive activities in the brain.[1] It involves remembering, planning, foresight, judgment, abstraction, and the ability to transfer information about one situation to another.

The terminology used to describe abnormal mentation is shown in Table 3–6, and a comparison of the clinical features of confusion, dementia, and depression is given in Table 3–7.

Disorders that can produce alterations in mentation are even more wide-ranging than those that produce alterations in consciousness. Any primary neurologic disorder that affects the brain or any systemic disease that alters metabolic function of the brain can alter mentation.[1] Disorders can be classified in three ways (Table 3–8). First are acute and transient disorders, those that create sudden and often severe changes in mentation but disappear when the underlying cause is alleviated. Second are chronic disorders, which are generally related to permanent disruption of brain structure, for example, from cerebral infarct, head trauma, degenerative central nervous system disease, or acquired immune deficiency syndrome (AIDS). Third are developmental disorders, such as certain inborn errors of metabolism.[1]

TABLE 3–8. PHYSIOLOGIC DISORDERS CAUSING CHANGES IN MENTATION

Acute and transient
  Metabolic
    Systemic disease: Diabetes, pulmonary disease, hepatic disease, uremic failure, cardiopulmonary insufficiency, hypothyroidism
  Drug intoxication (therapeutic, substance abuse)
  Cerebrovascular: Transient ischemic attack
  Fluid—electrolyte/acid—base imbalance
  Nutritional deficiency: Vitamin B_{12}, thiamine, niacine, protein-calorie (kwashiorkor)
  Head trauma (brief loss of consciousness)
  Alterations in temperature regulation (hyperthermia, hypothermia)
  Physiologic stress (pain, surgery)
Chronic
  Head trauma
  Cerebrovascular: Stroke
  Neoplasm: Primary or metastatic
  Degenerative diseases: Alzheimer's disease, Pick's disease
  Acquired immune deficiency syndrome (AIDS)
Developmental
  Inborn errors of metabolism (e.g., phenylketonuria)
  Perinatal hypoxia

Adapted from Mitchell et al. Neurologic assessment for nursing practice, 1984, p. 115. Courtesy of Prentice Hall.

Effects of altered mentation can vary from minor annoyance over slight wordfinding difficulty to profound disruption in every aspect of living. Medical therapy for underlying non-neurologic acute systemic disorders often reverses the mental status changes seen in such situations, whereas the effects of the primary nervous system disorders may not be reversible.[1]

CONSIDERATIONS IN MEASUREMENT

Behavioral Terminology
To be considered valid and reliable, most data must fall into an understandable, objective, qualitative or quantitative means of classification. The components of mental status and level of consciousness, however, lend themselves less easily to the collection of standardized, objective data that can be quantified or qualitatively grouped in the same way as some other health variables, such as measuring blood pressure.[18] This is the reason for the shift in recent years to using more precise descriptions of a patient's behavior or functioning instead of, for example, classifying the patient as having a particular level of consciousness. Recording specific behavioral responses as incorporated on standardized mental status examinations provides better monitoring of a patient's progress and response to therapy and allows researchers and clinicians to compare more objectively the results of medical and nursing care.

Relationship Between Physical and Mental Status
Physical and mental functioning are known to be complex interdependent entities.[19,20] In addition to the patient's primary health condition, several other factors can influence mental status (Table 3–9).[21] Responsiveness can be altered by changes in sleep and activity patterns during hospitalization. For example, the patient who is feeling moderately fatigued may not have sufficient energy to complete the mental status examination. Physical impairments are often responsible for diminished performance on mental tests. Hearing losses have a notorious association with confusion in all age groups, especially the elderly. Visual problems compound the lack of sensory stimulation. Side effects of medications may create signs of mental status problems. If medical care is episodic and fragmentary, iatrogenic mental dysfunctioning can easily be overlooked. Another important factor is the patient's level of physical discomfort or pain. Any of these factors can influence the responses, resulting in answers that are not truly representative of a person's mental status functioning at that time.

Relationship Between Cognitive and Affective Status
Mental problems often can be confounded with one another. Cognitive and affective impairments especially are difficult to distinguish.[12,15,19] Although they occur separately, they also can coexist in the same person, and at times it is important to determine which problem is primary. These confounding problems reinforce the fact that a change in mental functioning may be a more important measurement than the capacity of mental functioning itself.

Relationship Between Personality Traits and Mental Functioning
Mental functioning is viewed as a characteristic that remains stable, improves, or deteriorates. In contrast, certain attributes are thought to be fixed human personality traits that relate to lifelong patterns of decision making, personal style, and reaction to stress.[19] This chapter excludes the measurement of personality traits except insofar as they become con-

---

TABLE 3–9. PSYCHOLOGIC AND ENVIRONMENTAL DISTURBANCES ASSOCIATED WITH MENTAL STATUS CHANGES

Psychologic disturbances
  Severe emotional stress—postoperative states, relocation, hospitalization
  Depression
  Anxiety
  Pain—acute and chronic
  Fatigue
  Grief
  Sensory/perceptual deficits—noise, alteration in functioning of senses
  Mania
  Paranoia
  Situational disturbances
Environmental disturbances
  Unfamiliar environment creating a lack of meaning in the environment
  Sensory deprivation/environmental monotony creating a lack of meaning in the environment
  Sensory overload
  Immobilization—therapeutic, physical, pharmacological
  Sleep deprivation
  Lack of temperospatial reference points

From Foreman. Nurs Res, 1986, 35(1):35.

founded with mental status measures. The confusion between measures of personality traits and measures of mental well-being often arises when rating scales for mental functioning include such items at "irritability," "bothersomeness," or "sociability" as well as the more classic affective components of mental status as "anxiety," "depressed mood," or "delusional statements." When such items are summed together to form a score, confounding may result because stable personality traits contribute to the totals.[19]

INSTRUMENTS USED TO MEASURE LEVEL OF CONSCIOUSNESS

The mental status examinations described in this section are used predominantly in critical care settings.

▪ GLASGOW COMA SCALE (GCS)

The Glasgow Coma Scale (GCS) (Table 3–10) is a widely used and accepted scale for assessing the depth and duration of impaired consciousness and coma. It was developed in 1974 at the University of Glasgow, Scotland, to standardize clinical observations of the level of consciousness in patients with head injuries.[22] It has been used since in a variety of settings in the United States and Europe and has proven to be a quick, accurate, and simple tool for evaluating neurologic status.[1,8,23–26] In addition, it can be combined with other clinical data to predict outcome both after head injury and nontraumatic coma.[27]

    The assumption underlying the use of this scale is that as a patient's level of responsiveness diminishes, there will be concomitantly fewer spontaneous responses and less purposeful responses to stimulation. The degree of impaired consciousness is assessed by three behaviors: eye opening, motor response, and verbal performance. A patient's performance

TABLE 3—10. GLASGOW COMA SCALE

	Examiner's Test	Patient's Response	Assigned Score
Eye opening (E)	Spontaneous	Opens eyes on own	4
	Speech	Opens eyes when asked to in a loud voice	3
	Pain	Opens eyes when pinched	2
	Pain	Does not open eyes	1
Best motor response (M)	Command	Follows simple commands	6
	Pain	Pulls examiner's hand away when pinched	5
	Pain	Pulls a part of body away when pinched	4
	Pain	Flexes body inappropriately to pain (decorticate posturing)	3
	Pain	Body becomes rigid in an extended position when pinched (decerebrate posturing)	2
	Pain	Has no motor response to pinch	1
Verbal response (talking) (V)	Speech	Carries on a conversation correctly and tells examiner where he is, who he is, and the month and year	5
	Speech	Seems confused or disoriented	4
	Speech	Talks so examiner can understand victim but makes no sense	3
	Speech	Makes sounds that examiner cannot understand	2
	Speech	Makes no noise	1

Coma score (E + M + V) = 3 to 15
Adapted from Rimel, J. In Rosenthal et al. Rehabilitation of the head injured adult, 1983, p. 9. Courtesy of F. A. Davis.

within each of these three areas is assigned a numerical value; however, the value does not take into account the level of stimulus required for its elicitation. The numbers are totaled to produce a numerical rating that is purported to correspond to the degree of arousal or responsiveness. The scale often is plotted graphically in the clinical setting, allowing for a quick assessment of serial (often hourly) evaluations.[22,24-26]

The GCS is extremely useful for evaluating patients at lower levels of responsiveness but lacks the sensitivity for measuring changes in cognitive function in mild deterioration in consciousness. The maximum score of 15 reflects a fully alert, well-oriented person, whereas a score of 3, the lowest possible score, indicates complete unresponsiveness. A score of 7 or less indicates coma.

Only a few studies have subjected the psychometric qualities of the GCS to rigorous and systematic empirical tests. The developers of the GCS conducted reliabilty studies on approximately 40 patients with head injuries. Studies of observer variability comparing responses of more than 50 nurses and physicians have shown that the GCS possesses adequate interrater reliability.[27] Additional data concerning other psychometric qualities of this scale have been published recently and are discussed in the next section.

▪ COMPREHENSIVE LEVEL OF CONSCIOUSNESS SCALE (CLOCS)

The Comprehensive Level of Consciousness Scale (CLOCS) was developed as an alternative to the GCS as a coma assessment instrument.[18] It is an eight-item behavioral scale designed to assess a wider range of behaviors related to the impairment of consciousness. The scales are:

1. Posture
2. Eye position at rest
3. Spontaneous eye opening
4. General motor functioning
5. Abnormal ocular movements
6. Pupillary light reflexes
7. General responsiveness
8. Best communicative effort

The developers of the CLOCS considered two goals in designing this instrument. The first goal was to facilitate interinstitutional comparison of empirical results by developing a highly standardized instrument. Thus, unlike the GCS, detailed instructions for the administration of the scale are readily available and are published in the original paper describing the CLOCS.[18] In addition, the stimuli applied by the examiner are well defined and are graded as to intensity. A glossary of technical terms accompanies the instrument to facilitate administration by nurses and other nonphysician staff members.

The second goal was to develop a scale of greater sensitivity to subtle changes in the patient's condition than is the GCS. Stanczak et al. reported the results of a study comparing the psychometric qualities of the GCS and the CLOCS.[18] In their series, 101 patients with impaired consciousness were evaluated serially with each instrument. Three forms of reliability were assessed: (1) the reliability coefficient (Chronbach coefficient alpha) for the GCS was 0.69 ($p < 0.0001$); the reliability coefficient for the CLOCS was 0.86 ($p < 0.0001$); (2) the interrater reliability analysis yielded a Pearson r of 0.95 ($p < 0.001$) for the GCS and 0.96 ($p < 0.001$) for the CLOCS; (3) test–retest reliability was assessed by calculating Spearman rank-order correlation coefficients (r_s), which resulted in an r_s of 0.85 ($p < 0.001$) for the GCS and 0.89 ($p < 0.001$) for the CLOCS. These data demonstrate that both instruments possess comparable interrater and test–retest reliability. However, the CLOCS (minus scale 2) is more internally consistent.

Two of the three measures of validity that were assessed are discussed here.[18] The assessment for construct validity yielded a Pearson r of 0.68 ($p < 0.001$) for the GCS, 0.71 ($p < 0.001$) for the CLOCS, and 0.75 for the CLOCS without scale 2 (eye position at rest). The assessment for predictive validity yielded a Pearson r of 0.56 for the GCS and 0.60 for the CLOCS (minus scale 2), indicating that the initial CLOCS scores accounted for approximately 4 percent more of the variance in outcome than did the initial GCS scores. These data show that the CLOCS and the GCS possess comparable construct and predictive validity. In addition, the CLOCS is a more reliable and sensitive instrument than the GCS for the assessment of acute, severe impairments in neurologic functioning.[18]

Based on their experience in using the CLOCS, the developers report that this new scale meets all the requirements of a practical, yet psychometrically sound, research instrument.[18] After a short period of familiarization with the scale, it can be administered in the same amount of time as the GCS, usually 3 to 5 minutes. Additionally, like the GCS, it is noninvasive and amenable to serial evaluations.

INSTRUMENTS USED TO MEASURE MENTAL STATUS

The instruments discussed in this section are used to measure the components of cognitive functioning, as shown in Table 3–1. Many of the instruments have been developed for or used extensively in measurement of cognitive functioning of the elderly. (For an excellent text on this topic, see Reference 19.) The list includes unidimensional and multidimensional tests, instruments that are completed in interview with the subject and those that are completed through ratings of performance, and instruments suitable for measuring differences both at the lower end and at the upper end of the cognitive-functioning spectrum.

The first two instruments discussed in this section were developed to measure mental status in postoperative patients.

▪ MENTAL STATUS ASSESSMENT TOOL

The Mental Status Assessment Tool, developed by Dodd after an extensive review of the literature,[28,29] was used in the intensive care setting to assess the mental status of five patients recovering from cardiac surgery. The tool[28] assesses the following behaviors: (1) general orientation items (e.g., name of hospital, month of year), (2) communication (verbal/nonverbal) about current experience of pain (criterion not used if patient is not experiencing pain), (3) recognition of visual stimuli, (4) recognition of tactile stimuli, (5) intactness of memory (recent, intermediate, and long-term), and (6) performing simple tasks on request (e.g., cough, turn, touch nose with index finger).

Instructions are provided for administering and scoring the tool[28,29] Specific criteria for each mental status category (orientation, confusion, disorientation, delirium), developed after consultation with other nurses and physicians, are listed on the tool. A check (√) is placed in the column for the criterion that best fits the patient's response. Checks are totaled at the bottom of each category column, and the column with the most checks reflects the patient's category of mental status.

Limited reliability and validity data are available. Two pilot studies involving approximately 25 nurses using the tool to assess the mental status of a total of 11 neurologic or postcardiac surgery patients yielded interrater reliability scores of 100 percent and 93 percent in assigning the mental status categories.[29] Some variations were observed in the distribution of checks for each category, but these differences were probably related to fluctuations of the patient's mental status rather than from misunderstanding of the criteria of the mental status tool.[29]

The tool is reported to be practical and convenient to use in the clinical setting; it can be reduced in size to a pocket-sized card, or the form can be used at the bedside as a separate vital signs sheet. In addition, many aspects of the tool can be easily adapted for patients who are unable to communicate verbally. Since the tool was published, nurses in a variety of clinical settings have used it and have adapted it to meet the needs of their populations of patients with a variety of medical and surgical diagnoses.[30]

▪ MENTAL STATUS EXAMINATION (MSE)

Adams et al.[31] developed the Mental Status Examination (MSE) to assess the mental status of patients undergoing coronary artery bypass surgery. This simple tool, which is printed in the original reference,[31] takes about 5 minutes to administer. It taps several dimensions of mental status: orientation, cognitive function, memory, feelings, and sensations. The interviewer asks the patient to answer 15 questions, which are recorded as correct or incorrect in the adjacent column. An additional 5 questions are observations of the patient's behavior. If the patient's response is abnormal, the examiner marks an X in the box corresponding to the component of mental status. Each X has a value of 1 point, except for the interviewer observation item "Patient unable to answer most or all questions because grossly confused, incoherent or agitated," which has a value of 13 points. Delirium scores can range from 0 to 13, with the higher scores indicating more severe delirium.

The MSE also measures components of euphoric response and catastrophic reaction. These items are scored separately from the questions measuring components of delirium. The authors report that the tool has internal validity,[31] but no reliability data have been published. The authors indicate that when the MSE is used preoperatively, it not only provides a baseline of the patient's mental status but frequently provides an opportunity for the patient to verbalize thoughts and concerns about the upcoming surgery. Postoperatively, the MSE serves to identify mental status of dysfunction.

INSTRUMENTS USED TO MEASURE MENTAL FUNCTIONING IN LONG-TERM CARE

The next four instruments discussed are those that Nelson et al. found to be the four most frequently cited bedside cognitive screening instruments.[32] These instruments were identified through their search of the Medline and Bibliographic Retrieval Service Psychological Abstracts Data Bases from 1975 and 1967, respectively, to 1985. Another instrument, the Matts Dementia Rating Scale, is not discussed in this review of brief cognitive mental status examinations, since it requires significantly more time for administration (30 to 45 minutes).[32]

▪ MINI-MENTAL STATE EXAMINATION (MMSE)

The Mini-Mental State Examination (MMSE) (Fig. 3–1), developed by Folstein et al.,[33] is a general purpose, simplified, and practical mental status examination. This instrument was developed originally to provide a quantitative assessment of cognitive performance in hospitalized psychiatric patients. The MMSE includes 11 questions, requires only 5 to 10 minutes to administer, and is, therefore, practical to use serially and routinely. The authors describe it as being mini because it concentrates on the cognitive aspects of mental functioning and excludes questions about mood, abnormal mental experiences, and the form of thinking. Yet within the cognitive realm it is thorough.

The test items cover orientation, memory, attention, and the ability to name, to follow verbal and written commands, to write a sentence spontaneously, and to copy a figure. Brief but detailed instructions for administering the test are given in the original paper.[33] The score is the sum of correct responses; the total score possible is 30 points. The authors suggest that patients scoring below 24 are cognitively impaired. An advantage of the MMSE is the large number of standardizations completed. Because this instrument is part of the National Institute of Mental Health (NIMH) Diagnostic Interview Schedule, it has been administered to approximately 15,000 people in five cities in the United States as part of the epidemiologic catchment area community survey program.[34] Since the MMSE is a graded measure of cognition, various cutoff scores can be used to satisfy the needs of sensitivity and specificity of the particular research design.

The MMSE has been subjected to several reliability and validity studies. Reliability scores ranged from 0.83 to 0.99 among groups of psychiatric, neurologic, and mixed-diagnoses patients.[32–36] These results were obtained when interrater and test–retest reliability were studied in combination. Considerable work has been done to establish that the MMSE distinguishes among people with the diagnoses of delirium or dementia, depression, schizo-

MINI-MENTAL STATE
Inpatient Consultation Form

Maximum Score	Score	
		ORIENTATION
5	( )	What is the (year) (season) (date) (day) (month)?
5	( )	Where are we: (state) (country) (town) (hospital) (floor)?
		REGISTRATION
3	( )	Name 3 objects: 1 second to say each. Then ask the patient all 3 after you have said them. Give 1 point for each correct answer. Then repeat them until the patient learns all 3. Count trials and record.
		TRIALS
		ATTENTION AND CALCULATION
5	( )	Serial 7s. 1 point for each correct. Stop after 5 answers. Alternatively spell "world" backwards.
		RECALL
3	( )	Ask for 3 objects repeated above. Give 1 point for each correct.
		LANGUAGE
9	( )	Name a pencil, and watch (2 points)
		Repeat the following "No ifs, ands, or buts." (1 point)
		Follow a 3-stage command: "Take a paper in your right hand, fold it in half, and put it on the floor." (3 points)
		Read and obey the following: "Close your eyes." (1 point)
		Write a sentence (1 point)
		Copy design (1 point)

TOTAL SCORE

Assess level of consciousness along a continuum.

| Alert | Drowsy | Stupor | Coma |

Figure 3–1. Mini-Mental State Examination form. *(From Folstein, Fetting, Lobo, et al.* Cancer, *1984, 53(10) (suppl.):2254.)*

phrenia, and elderly control subjects without any psychiatric diagnosis. Nelson et al. found eleven validation studies comprising 859 subjects.[32-35] The MMSE was reported to have high sensitivity (0.87) and high specificity (0.82) in a study of 97 patients admitted to a general medical unit. All patients who scored false positive had ≤8 years of formal education.

Concurrent validation of the MMSE as a measure of the delirious state has been accomplished by comparing it with the level of electroencephalogram slowing, with serum ammonia levels in patients with hepatic encephalopathy, and with the level of anticholinergic substances in the blood of postcardiac surgery patients. These studies indicated that the score on the MMSE falls as these physiologic abnormalities become more abnormal.[34]

The use of this test in clinical practice and research is increasing, as gauged by requests for copies and instructions for use and by the number of times it has appeared in publications in the last 20 years.[35] It is being widely used in research sponsored by the NIMH.

▪ COGNITIVE CAPACITY SCREENING EXAMINATION (CCSE)

The Cognitive Capacity Screening Examination (CCSE) was developed and reported by Jacobs et al. in 1977.[37] It was developed to diagnose diffuse organic mental syndromes in nonpsychiatric patients. It contains 30 items and is easy to administer, requiring only 5 to 15 minutes. Each correct item is scored 1 point. The content areas include orientation, digit span, concentration, serial 7s, repetition, verbal concept information, and short-term verbal recall. The authors suggest that patients who score below 20 are cognitively impaired.[37]

The CCSE has been reported to be a reliable and valid bedside cognitive screening instrument. The authors report 100 percent interrater reliability among three examiners with six patients.[37] No additional data about interrater or test–retest reliability have been published.

Several validation studies comprising more than 400 people have been reported.[32,37–41] These include patients with psychiatric, neurologic, and medical-surgical diagnoses, and two nonpatient populations, one of hospital staff and the other of community-dwelling elderly. Scores $\geq$ 20 were attained by more than 90 percent of individuals in the nonpatient groups. By comparison, almost all patients with clinically diagnosed organic mental syndromes and more than 75 percent of patients with strokes or hip fractures scored <20.[32]

Additional data about the psychometric properties of the CCSE were described recently by Foreman.[39] He conducted a study of 66 elderly hospitalized medical-surgical patients to compare the reliability and validity of the three most frequently used mental status questionnaires in this type of population: the CCSE, the MMSE, and the Short Portable Mental Status Questionnaire (SPMSQ). The various parameters of reliability and validity were relatively consistent among the questionnaires. The internal consistencies yielded reliability coefficients ranging from 0.90 to 0.97. Estimates of criterion-related validity were assessed by correlating the scores obtained on the three questionnaires with the clinical diagnosis of global cognitive impairment. The correlation coefficients, which were all significant at the $p < .001$ level, were: SPMSQ 0.71, MMSE 0.78, and CCSE 0.87.[39] All three questionnaires were shown to have excellent sensitivity and specificity. However, the CCSE was the only questionnaire that accurately classified all the patients and thus is the most clinically accurate measure of mental status.[39]

In Foreman's study, only those reliability and validity coefficients obtained with the CCSE consistently exceeded minimally acceptable standards, and, therefore, it is the most valid and reliable measure of mental status in this population.[39] However, he cautioned that factors other than psychometric properties must be considered when selecting an instrument to measure cognitive functioning. For example, a 30 item questionnaire, such as the CCSE, may impose too great a respondent burden for people with moderate to severe cognitive impairment. For such people, a shorter questionnaire, such as the MMSE, may prove to be a better instrument for measuring mental status.[39]

▪ MENTAL STATUS QUESTIONNAIRE (MSQ)

The Mental Status Questionnaire (MSQ)[19,42–44] is a brief, easily administered test that has been used extensively in geriatric research and practice. It has 10 questions that test orientation to time and place and knowledge of birth data, age, and past and current presidents. Sample questions include:

- What is this place?
- How old are you?
- What is the name of the President?

Each correct response is awarded 1 point. The score is associated with the severity of brain syndrome: 0 to 2 errors = none or minimal, 3 to 8 errors = moderate, and 9 to 10 errors = severe.[19,42]

No studies reporting interrater reliability data have been published. However, the simplicity of the items would appear to ensure satisfactory results.[32] Kahn et al. reported that the test–retest reliability was better than 0.8.[42] Test–retest reliability was evaluated also in a study in which the MSQ was administered four times at 3-week intervals to 55 elderly patients who were described as clinically stable. In 75 percent of the serial evaluations, the greatest change in score was only 1 point.[32]

Nelson et al. found three validation studies on more than 1300 subjects.[32,42,44] Two of the study populations were patients in nursing homes and psychiatric hospitals and community-dwelling elderly. The studies showed that less than 5 percent of patients without clinically diagnosed cognitive impairment made more than two errors. In contrast, using the same two-error cutoff, only 55 percent of patients with clinically diagnosed organic mental dysfunction were correctly classified.[42,44]

• SHORT PORTABLE MENTAL STATUS QUESTIONNAIRE (SPMSQ)

The Short Portable Mental Status Questionnaire (SPMSQ)[19,44–46] is included in the OARS (Older Americans Research Services) battery, a multidimensional tool for community-based assessment. The SPMSQ, which was developed with community-based elders and patients hospitalized with psychiatric illnesses, is suitable for administration apart from the more extensive OARS battery. The test contains 10 items and is easily administered.[45] The score is the total of incorrect responses. Examples of the questions, which are almost identical to those on the MSQ, are as follows:

- What is the date today (month/day/year)?
- What is your telephone number? (If no telephone, what is your street address?)
- What was your mother's maiden name?
- Subtract 3 from 20 and keep subtracting 3 from each new number you get until you get to, or as close to, zero.

The scoring is interpreted as follows: 0 to 2 errors = intact functioning, 3 to 4 errors = mild intellectual impairment, 5 to 7 errors = moderate impairment, and 8 to 10 errors = severe impairment. Based on extensive work in developing norms for the scale, the scores are adjusted for race and educational status.

In addition to borrowing several questions about orientation and memory items from the MSO, the SPMSQ includes items that test remote memory, partial survival skills for self-care in the community, and an indicator of mathematical ability. Despite the test's relative difficulty, Kane and Kane report that the scale generates a spread of scores from 0 to 10, even in nursing home populations, and is seemingly inoffensive when administered to a community-based sample.[19]

Test–retest reliability coefficients ranged from 0.82 to 0.83 when two groups of elderly people were retested at 4-week intervals.[45] Interrater reliability coefficients ranged from 0.62 to 0.87 ($p < .001$).[39,47] In Foreman's study of 66 elderly hospitalized patients, the internal consistency for the SPMSQ was 0.90.[39]

Several validation studies comprising more than 1600 subjects have been reported.[19,32,39,44,45,47] In three studies that compared SPMSQ results with psychiatrists' clinical diagnoses of organic mental disorder, the true positive rates ranged from 88 to 92 percent. False negative rates have ranged from 18 percent in a geropsychiatric clinic population to 28 percent in another patient population not defined in detail.[32]

• NEUROBEHAVIORAL COGNITIVE STATUS EXAMINATION (NCSE)

The Neurobehavioral Cognitive Status Examination (NCSE) is a newly developed, complete, neurologic mental status screening examination.[48,49] It was developed and copyrighted by the Northern California Neurobehavioral Group, Inc. Initially the instrument was called the "Neurobehavioral Mental Status Examination (NMSE)."[6] Its utility has been demonstrated in clinical use in psychiatry and neurology clinics and psychiatry and neurology inpatient services and in neuropsychologic screening of neurosurgical patients. The NCSE occupies a middle ground between very brief instruments that provide a global estimate of cognitive functioning and exhaustive neuropsychologic test batteries that offer a more thorough assessment.[48,49] It can be administered at the bedside in approximately 15 to 30 minutes. A major advantage of this test compared to other more brief instruments is that it provides a differentiated profile of the patient's cognitive status. It identifies intact areas of functioning, yet provides more detailed assessment in areas of dysfunction.

The NCSE consists of a test booklet (cover shown in Fig. 3–2) and an administration/scoring manual. (Copies of these materials can be requested from Ralph Kiernan, Ph.D., Northern California Neurobehavioral Group, Inc., Palo Alto, CA 94304.) The instrument assesses the level of consciousness, orientation, and attention, as well as five major ability areas: language, constructions, memory, calculations, and reasoning.[48,49] With the exception of the memory and orientation categories, the other tests begin with a screen item. The screen item is a demanding test of the skill involved, and 10 to 30 percent of the normal population fail the screen.[48] If the screen is answered correctly, the particular skill is considered intact, and no further testing of that skill is required. If the screen is failed, the metric, a series of test items of increasing complexity, is administered. Within each cognitive ability area, the number of correct responses is totaled and recorded on the front of the test booklet, resulting in independent scores for specific cognitive ability areas rather than a single overall score. Scores below a predetermined criterion are interpreted as reflecting impairment within that particular area of cognitive functioning.[48,49]

Normative data were collected on approximately 60 healthy adults, which showed that there was little variability and few errors among the categories.[49] Additional standardization data were obtained on 59 elderly volunteers. The mean test scores were within the normal range on the profile that was established for the nongeriatric standardization groups. However, the results in the areas of constructions, memory, and similarities were significantly lower than those of the standardization groups. These results characterize a slightly broader range of normal functioning on these three tests in the healthy geriatric population.[49]

In a study comparing the sensitivity of the NCSE with the MMSE and the CCSE, the NCSE was shown to be a more sensitive instrument for detecting cognitive impairment.[49] Thirty neurosurgical patients with verified brain lesions were tested with all three instruments. The results showed that the NCSE identified cognitive impairments in 28 patients (93 percent), the MMSE in 16 patients (53 percent), and the CCSE in 13 patients (43

Neurobehavioral Cognitive Status Examination Test Booklet

Name:_____   Date:_____
Examination Location:_____   Time:_____
Date of Birth:_____   Examiner:_____
Level of Education:_____

Mental Status Profile

	LOC	ORI	ATT	Language COMP	Language REP	Language NAM	CONST	MEM	CALC	Reasoning SIM	Reasoning JUD
*AVG. Range	-Alert-	--12--	-(S)8-	-(S)6-	--(S)-- --12--	--(S)-- --8--	--6-- -(S)5-	--12--	-(S)4-	--8-- -(S)6-	--6-- -(S)5-
Mild	--IMP--	--10-- --8--	--6-- --4--	--5-- --4--	--11-- --9--	--7-- --5--	--4-- --3--	--10-- --8--	--3-- --2--	--5-- --4--	--4-- --3--
Moderate		--6--	--2--	--3--	--7--	--3--	--2--	--6--	--1--	--3--	--2--
Severe		--4--	--0--	--2--	--5--	--2--	--0--	--4--	--0--	--2--	--1--
Write in Lower Scores											

Abbreviations:

S	-Screen	ATT	-Attention	CALC	-Calculations
LOC	-Level of Consciousness	COMP	-Comprehension	CONST	-Constructions
IMP	-Impaired	MEM	-Memory	SIM	-Similarities
ORI	-Orientation	REP	-Repetition	JUD	-Judgement
		NAM	-Naming		

Note: The validity of this examination depends on administration in strict accordance with the Neurobehavioral Cognitive Status Examination Manual.

*This average range is based on a standardization sample of normal subjects age 20–65. It cannot be taken as the appropriate standard for patients whose age is greater than 65.

Figure 3–2. Cover of the Neurobehavioral Cognitive Status Examination booklet. *(From the Northern California Neurobehavioral Group, Inc. © Copyright, 1983.)*

percent). In addition, the NCSE identified 14 patients as cognitively impaired who were not identified by either the CCSE or the MMSE. Discordant pair analyses showed that the differences in sensitivity were highly significant.[49] In contrast to the MMSE and the CCSE, the NCSE is thought to be more sensitive to cognitive deficits because it (1) scores each cognitive ability area separately, (2) increases the likelihood of detecting mild deficits by employing a graded series of test items within each cognitive domain, and (3) independently assesses a larger number of areas of cognitive function than does either of the other two examinations.[49]

▪ BRIEF NEUROPSYCHOLOGICAL MENTAL STATUS EXAM (BNMSE)

The Brief Neuropsychological Mental Status Exam (BNMSE) is a short but relatively comprehensive and practical instrument for measuring mental status.[50] This tool, which is still in its developmental stages, was constructed by health professionals in nursing, speech pathology, and neuropsychology at the Medical College of Virginia (MCV), Richmond, Virginia. It is intended for use with adult patients with organic brain dysfunction. This instrument, which takes approximately 15 minutes to administer, contains measures of orientation, concentration, sustained attention, insight, right–left orientation, receptive/expressive language functions, verbal memory, and arithmetic reasoning. Subtests of valid tests, including the Wechsler Adult Intelligence Scale, Wechsler Memory Scale, Babcock Story Recall, Ray Auditory Verbal Learning Test, and Halstead-Wepman Aphasia Screening Test were incorporated because of the availability of standardized norms for age or educational levels or both. In addition, the instrument contains a category for general nonsubstantiated behavioral observations, such as appropriateness of affect, awareness of impairment, speech fluency, and response latency. These behaviors are scored as present or absent. Criteria for scoring each type of behavior are included in an accompanying administration and scoring manual.

In each of the seven sections where the patient is requested to respond verbally or perform simple body movements, time limitations are specified on the examination form. If the patient answers correctly after the allotted time has elapsed, the answer is scored as incorrect. The authors note that, in general, elderly patients need more time than younger people to process the information; this observation should be considered when interpreting results of timed sections.[50]

This instrument was used in a pilot study of 18 adults with medically documented brain dysfunction who were hospitalized in various acute care units at MCV. The results strongly suggested that the instrument is sensitive to brain dysfunction related to cognitive deficits.[50] At least 50 percent of the patients demonstrated poor performance in three major categories: immediate and delayed story recall, attention, concentration, and mental tracking, and immediate auditory memory.[50]

In a pilot study using a revised version of the BNMSE, three of six patients without brain dysfunction demonstrated impairment in memory, sustained attention, and concentration. Their ages were between 48 and 65 years, and their educational levels were between 5 and 12 years.[50] This finding is of interest in that many patients who are assumed to be free of cognitive abnormalities may have limitations identified when mental status tests are used.

▪ BRIEF NEUROSCIENCE MENTAL STATUS EXAM

The Brief Neuroscience Mental Status Exam is similar to the BNMSE. However, this newer examination contains tests developed entirely at MCV.[5] This tool contains the eight measurement categories that are included in the BNMSE; an additional category to measure visuospatial perception is included. The Brief Neuroscience Mental Status Exam form and accompanying administration and scoring manual are copyrighted and can be obtained by contacting Jeffrey S. Kreutzer, Ph.D., Rehabilitation Psychology and Neuropsychology, MCV, Richmond, VA, 23298-0001.

The developers of the Brief Neuroscience Mental Status Exam have found it to be particularly useful in acute care clinical settings, especially with patients with suspected brain dysfunction. Studies are underway to collect normative data.[51]

▪ THE SET TEST

The Set Test,[52,53] developed in Scotland, is an easily used and practical method for identifying the presence and level of senile dementia. The test takes approximately 5 minutes to administer; often it is completed within 2 minutes. The patient is asked to name as many items as he can recall in each of four categories: animals, colors, fruits, and towns or cities.

One point is awarded for each correct item within a category. The maximum score is 10 per category, and the maximum total score for the test is 40. Norms have been developed in healthy old people who had a mean score of 31.2.[52] In a study in which the Set Test was administered to almost 200 elderly subjects, a total score under 15 corresponded closely to the status of patients with a clinical diagnosis of dementia, scores in the range of 15 to 24 showed a lesser degree of association with dementia, and scores of 25 or greater showed no dementia.[53] Hays,[54] a geriatric nurse practitioner, has found that people who score above 30 are usually in satisfactory mental health, whereas those who score less than 30 are experiencing cognitive dysfunction. She recommends from her own experience and those of colleagues in both community and hospital nursing services that using this test is a realistic screening device and a distinct asset in clinical practice.[55] Other reported advantages of this test are that physical illness, depression, and social class do not appear to influence test results. However, the test is not suitable for use with deaf or aphasic patients.

• VIRO ORIENTATION SCALE

The VIRO Orientation Scale was designed as a component of the *V*igor, *I*ntactness, *R*elationships, and *O*rientation method for rating geriatric patients on the basis of their responses and reactions during an interview situation.[19,56,57] This chapter discusses only the Orientation component of VIRO. The test contains eight items, of which six are straightforward orientation items and two assess recent memory. The total possible score is 24. Points are awarded for partially correct responses. Sample questions and scoring are as follows:

Knows age	Precisely	3
	Within 2 years	2
	Within 10 years	1
Knows year	Precisely	3
	Within 2 years	2
	Within 10 years	1
	All else	0
Remembers examiner's name	Yes	3
	Partially	2
	No	0
Estimation of interview length	Within 5 minutes	2
	Within 10 minutes	2
	Within 30 minutes	1
	All else	0

Reliability tests using this scale with two community-based samples of more than 500 subjects have shown coefficient alpha of 0.75 and 0.67. These reliabilities improved to 0.814 and 0.718 when the two items—the examiner's name and the length of the interview—were deleted from the scale, which suggests that those questions may touch upon a different area.[19]

• PHILADELPHIA GERIATRIC CENTER (PGC) MENTAL STATUS QUESTIONNAIRE

The Philadelphia Geriatric Center (PGC) Mental Status Questionnaire was developed by Fishback as a measure for determining the degree of senile dementia among residents of a geriatric center.[58] This instrument is capable of producing a spread of scores among those who would receive a 0 on the MSQ or SPMSQ. It contains 35 questions, including all the items on the MSQ and SPMSQ. In addition, it has items thought to be more pertinent to the nursing home patient, such as the season of the year and the last meal eaten. It also includes some items that probe the ability to perform activities of daily living (ADL). The inclusion of the ADL items may compromise the instrument.[19] The instructions do not clarify whether the respondent loses points on these items if the limitations are based on physical problems. Scoring, which awards 1 point for each correct answer, is as follows: 0 = total loss, 1 to 10 = severe loss, 11 to 20 = moderate loss, 21 to 33 = mild loss, 34 to 35 = not impaired, and 35 = perfect score. The instrument, along with Fishback's Visual Counting Test, was administered to 90 elderly patients. The test scores were well correlated with clinical findings.[58]

▪ PHILADELPHIA GERIATRIC CENTER (PGC) EXTENDED MENTAL STATUS QUESTIONNAIRE

The Philadelphia Geriatric Center (PGC) Extended Mental Status Questionnaire (EMSQ) was developed by staff at the Philadelphia Geriatric Center, a Jewish home for the aged.[59] This instrument is a further modification of the PGC Mental Status Questionnaire. It contains 10 items that measure orientation to time, place, person, and remote memory. It also includes 14 additional items that assess both lower and higher levels of cognitive functioning: recall of family names, orientation to immediate environmental context, recall of meaningful religious/cultural events or information, and numerical calculations. An advantage of this instrument is that it does not include ADL items and thus remains free of the possible confounding of Fishback's instrument.[19] Of particular interest are questions that are designed especially for the resident population of the Philadelphia Geriatric Center. The rationale is that patterns of memory retention and loss may be socially and culturally determined.

Wheliham et al. reported a study in which the EMSQ and the PGC Delayed Memory Test were administered to 70 elderly patients with organic brain syndrome who were admitted to the PGC.[59] (Copies of these tests are available from William M. Whelihan, Ph.D., Philadelphia Geriatric Center, 5301 Old York Road, Philadelphia, PA 19141). The Delayed Memory Test is similar to the Wechsler Memory Scale Logical Memory subtest, in which a patient is read a short paragraph and then asked to recall the information. The primary difference between the two measures is that the PGC Delayed Memory Test consists of material that is culturally relevant to residents of the PGC. The results of detailed analyses indicate that the EMSQ and the PGC Delayed Memory Test were the best combined predictors of clinical judgment of senile dementia among a multidisciplinary set of variables. The EMSQ differentiated patients with moderate/severe dementia from patients classified as nondemented or mildly demented.[59] Patients who were mildly demented were incorrectly classified, but with the addition of the PGC Delayed Memory Test, 75 percent of the patients with mild dementia were classified correctly.

▪ MEMORY AND INFORMATION TEST (MIT)

The Memory and Information Test (MIT) is a British test that was adapted for use in the Newcastle-upon-Tyne population surveys.[60] These surveys assessed the psychiatric morbidity among representative samples of people aged 65 years or over who were living in their homes outside institutions. The MIT consists of 11 questions, with a maximum score of 20. Sample questions and scoring are:

When is your birthday?	2
(month, date)	
What is today's date?	2
(year, month)	
(day of month, day of week)	2
Present monarch?	2
(name and number)	
Name of Prime Minister?	1
Date of World War II?	2
(year started, year ended)	

Although this test seems more difficult than either the MSQ or the SPMSQ, in the British survey it was used (with a cutoff between 12 and 13) to discriminate those people with the clinical diagnosis of dementia. In addition, it correlated with 4-year mortality rates.[19]

• FACE-HAND TEST

The Face-Hand Test, designed by Fink et al., is based on the patient's ability to recognize simultaneous tactile stimulation to the cheek and palms of the hand.[61] The rationale of the test is that double simultaneous stimulation is necessary, since patients with mental changes may experience perceptual errors that are not demonstrated on routine stimulation. The patient is touched on the hands and cheek simultaneously in 10 trials. Because the patient can become familiar with the testing pattern, only the last 4 of 10 paired stimuli count for the score. An advantage of the Face-Hand Test is that it is minimally influenced by language, culture, and verbal skills. It has been widely used in gerontologic research, although it is questionable if the test provides additional information to the mental status battery.[62] Fink et al. have demonstrated the Face-Hand Test to be a reliable test for brain damage and useful for discriminating between psychotic patients and those with brain damage.[17,61]

• VISUAL COUNTING TEST

The Visual Counting Test, reported by Fishback, is based on the assumption that counting extended fingers is one of the first skills learned by a young child and one of the last to disappear in disoriented adults.[19,58] The examiner holds up fingers in four different combinations and asks the subject to indicate the number of fingers. Each correct response is scored 25 points. This test has the advantage of being simple, insensitive to culture and language, and easy to administer to all but deaf patients. Fishback reports that this test correlated well with his own PGC Mental Status Questionnaire, but no additional reports of the Visual Counting Test can be found in the literature.[19,58]

• THE MISPLACED OBJECTS TEST

The Misplaced Objects Test is a brief, simple test of memory dysfunction in the aged.[63] The subjects are required to place magnetized representations of common objects frequently misplaced in the home (e.g., eyeglasses, umbrella, keys) on a board that is imprinted with a cross-section of a seven-room house. No more than two objects may be placed in one room.

Five to thirty minutes later, after intervening distraction, the subject is asked to recall the location of each object. One point is awarded for each object correctly recalled. The task has obvious face validity, and discriminate validity was demonstrated in a study in which 60 aged persons with memory impairment recalled significantly fewer objects than were recalled by 44 unimpaired aged persons or young adults. Test–retest reliability on successive days demonstrated a correlation of 0.84. The developers of the test reported also that subjects appeared to enjoy the gamelike structure of the test and were not threatened by the test procedures. The measure is appropriate for subjects of many ages, since performance requirements are minimal and readily apparent.[6] Kane and Kane reported that this test is worthy of further exploration to develop norms and refinements of scoring.[19]

▪ WECHSLER MEMORY SCALE

The Wechsler Memory Scale measures primarily memory functions, both recent and remote, apart from other areas of cognitive performance.[19,64,65] The objective of the test battery was to create a measure that correlated well with intelligence tests, without duplicating them. The seven subtests include personal and current information, orientation, mental control (backward counting, alphabet, and counting by 30), logical memory (two passages read and subject scored on average number of items retained when repeating), digit span (forward and backward), visual reproduction (draw geometric figures from memory), and associate learning (learning 10 word pairs in three trials).

The scoring results in memory quotient scores corrected for age. There are some suggestions that scoring is most useful on three factors: memory, attention, and concentration. Scoring instructions published by Wechsler[64] and Klonoff and Kennedy[66] show norms for people in their 80s and 90s. The test is easy to administer, but Kramer and Jarvik report that the measure has not been entirely satisfactory.[62] Questions on validity center on whether the test measures motivation, cooperation, and willingness to memorize material of little value rather than recall of learned material. More recently, Baker et al. have reported the value of using this test as part of a neurobehavioral test battery for monitoring people who have had occupational exposures to neurotoxins.[67]

▪ GERIATRIC INTERPERSONAL RATING SCALE (GIES)

The Geriatric Interpersonal Rating Scale (GIES) was developed by Plutchik et al. to test the cognitive and perceptual functioning of psychogeriatric patients.[68] Like the MMSE, it was designed to sample thoroughly the cognitive domain, has face validity, and is administered quickly. The items, which are in a semistructured interview format, include simple orientation questions, tests of appropriate social behavior in the testing situation, copying a figure, tests of immediate and remote memory, tests of quantitative and verbal aspects of cognitive functioning, and digits-forward sequences. Correct answers are scored as pluses and summed for a possible score of 46. In a study of 78 geriatric patients, split-half reliability testing of the GIES equaled 0.93.[68] Item analyses showed that most of the items significantly discriminated between a high-scoring group and a low-scoring group.

▪ COGNITIVE ASSESSMENT SCREENING TEST (CAST)

The Coginitive Assessment Screening Test (CAST) was developed recently by a multi-disciplinary team at the Hebrew Rehabilitation Center for Aged in Boston, Massachusetts (written communication, M. Albert, July 30, 1985). It is designed to provide an overview of the major aspects of cognition, rather than an indepth assessment. The test may help clarify what aspects of behavior are due to cognitive disability, as opposed to psychological disturbance.

The test items have been carefully selected and modified for the institutionalized elderly. There are seven categories of multiple task items. The first four tasks, attention, memory, abstraction (visual), and orientation, are those tasks most useful for identifying serious cognitive impairment, and are worth a possible 58 points. The remaining tasks are: abstraction (verbal), naming, copying, and word generation, which provide information concerning quality and severity of impairment, for a subtotal of 28 points. The total possible score is 86.

Test-retest reliability was reported to be .86 (personal communication, M. Smith, March 1987). The developers are in the process of validating this instrument against other standard mental status tests. Recent data comparing the CAST with the MMSE yielded a correlation coefficient of 0.78. For a copy of the CAST and instructions for use, contact Marilyn Albert, Ph.D., Department of Psychiatry, Massachusetts General Hospital, Boston, MA, 02114.

▪ FROMAJE

The acronym FROMAJE stands for *F*unction, *R*easoning, *O*rientation, *M*emory, *A*rithmetic, *J*udgment, and *E*motional status.[18,19,23,69] This instrument, which was developed to assist physicians in assessing the mental status of the elderly, is a structured interview approach that includes an optional scoring format. Function refers to self-care ability related to mental status; the information for this rating is obtained from relatives or significant others. Reasoning is measured through proverb interpretation. Questions about person, place, and time measure orientation. Memory is assessed by questions to tap the immediate memory, recent memory, and distant memory. To assess arithmetic, the patient is asked to count forward and backward and to subtract serial 7s. For judgment, a realistic problem is presented, and the patient is asked to solve it. Emotional status is assessed by evaluating general behavior during the interview and some probing about behaviors, such as crying, hallucinations, and mood swings.

During the 15 to 20-minute interview, each component is tested and scored individually. A score of 1 is awarded for no problem, 2 for a moderate problem, and 3 for a severe problem. A score of 9 to 10 signifies minimal mental dysfunction, 11 to 12 moderate mental dysfunction, and 13 or more, severe mental dysfunction. The FROMAJE approach is not appropriate for aphasic patients, who would show false positives for dementia. The authors report 100 percent interrater reliability among three examiners with six subjects. These six subjects included three with and three without a diagnosed organic mental syndrome.

In its present format, this instrument is more appropriate for use as a clinical assessment tool[19] than as a measurement tool in a research study. The clinician is permitted much judgment is selecting the questions and interpreting the responses. The author points out that the final rating is a product of the examiner's subject assessment.[19,20]

▪ GALVESTON ORIENTATION AND AMNESIA TEST (GOAT)

The Galveston Orientation and Amnesia Test (GOAT) is a brief quantitative rating scale that measures directly disorientation and amnesia during the recovery phase after closed head injury.[70] It is a practical, reliable scale that can be used at the bedside or in the emergency room.

The GOAT consists of 10 questions that evaluate (1) the major spheres of orientation (time, place, and person), (2) an estimation of the interval following injury for which the patient is unable to recall any events, that is, the duration of posttraumatic amnesia, and (3) an estimation of the interval antedating the injury for which no events are recalled. The core of the GOAT is four questions assessing temporal orientation, including day of the week, day of the month, year, and time of day.

The maximum GOAT score is 100.[70] The test form contains a column for recording error points; the total number of error points are subtracted from 100 to determine the GOAT score. Clinicians can plot a graph of serial scores that conveniently depicts the recovery of a closed head injury patient who is no longer comatose.

Standardization studies of the GOAT have been performed on 50 patients ages 16 to 50 years, who sustained mild closed head injuries.[70] The results showed that the median GOAT score was 95. The defective range was defined as a score below 66, and the borderline abnormal range was considered to be scores between 66 and 75. Correlates of performance on the GOAT were determined by computing the Kendall rank-order correlation coefficient (r). The results showed no significant relationship between GOAT score and age ($r = 0.10$), education ($r = 0.13$), or injury–test interval ($r = 0.07$).[70]

Reliability studies were reported on 13 patients hospitalized after closed head injury of varying severity and have shown that the GOAT has satisfactory interrater reliability, with a Kendall r correlation coefficient of 0.99 ($p < 0.001$).

In a validity study of 52 young adults with closed head injuries, the duration of impaired GOAT scores was strongly related to the acute neurosurgical ratings of eye opening, motor responding, and verbal responding on the GCS. The analyses confirmed highly significant relationships between these three behavioral areas and GOAT scores, yielding Chi-square values ranging from 18.98 to 21.09, $p < 0.00001$.[70] In addition, the relationship between the interval of impaired GOAT performance and long-term recovery category was highly significant (Chi-square $= 18.0$, $p < 0.0001$).

INSTRUMENT SELECTION

When considering if mental status behavioral rating scales have adequate research utility, several criteria must be met. (The reader is referred to textbooks about nursing research, e.g., Chapter 6 in Reference 19 for detailed discussions about using a tool for clinical assessment versus for research and evaluation purposes.) A primary question is, "Does the instrument measure the phenomenon or variable of interest to the nurse researcher?" This is particularly important when measuring a concept that has many components, such as mental status. Both instruments that measure a single cognitive dimension, such as memory or orientation, and, more commonly, instruments that measure several attributes of the cognitive domain are available. The multidimensional instruments, of course, provide a more complete assessment of cognitive functioning.

For the reader who is interested in instruments for measuring mental status that are not included in this chapter, two excellent references are suggested, *Neuropsychological Assessment*[71] and several chapters in *Assessing the Elderly: A Practical Guide to Measurement*.[19] Additional methodologic considerations for designing a research project to measure acute confusional states are found in a review by Foreman.[21]

Regardless of the setting or the mental status instrument(s) being used, it is particularly important for the researcher to be mindful of the privileged nature of the relationship with the patient and of the impact specific questions may have on the patient. Mueller's recommendations to clinicians who are performing mental status examinations apply to the research setting as well.[6] Initially, the person administering the tool should explain to the patient the purpose of the mental status examination (which would also be covered in obtaining informed consent), indicating that it is part of every complete patient evaluation. It may help to reduce the patient's anxiety and avoid offending the patient by adding, "You may find some of the questions very easy and some quite difficult to answer."[6]

APPLICATIONS FOR THE CLINICAL SETTING

In an acute care setting, when measuring the level of consciousness in patients with a life-threatening condition, the instrument should (1) require brief administration time, (2) be unobtrusive and noninvasive, and (3) be amenable to serial examinations. Many of these same characteristics are desirable when measuring cognitive/mental functioning in long-term care.

The complete nursing assessment of patients with any type of medical, surgical, or psychiatric diagnosis includes the evaluation of the patient's capacity to think, as shown by the patient's grasp of a situation, memory, attention, and ability to understand and express himself or herself. The results of this evaluation enable the nurse and other members of the health care team to appreciate the patient's capacity to (1) relate his or her history accurately, (2) understand and adhere to the clinicians' suggestions for treatment, for managing the actual and potential disease-related problems, and for health promotion activities, (3) give informed consent for diagnostic and therapeutic procedures, and (4) give informed consent for participation in clinical trials and other biomedical research projects.[34] There are many types of populations in which there is a great need for further characterizing the patient's mental status. Two such types are oncology and AIDS.

Oncology

Alterations in mental status in oncology patients can be related to multiple etiologies, such as the disease process, the treatment, or other factors, for example, metabolic encephalopathy. Many clinicians have emphasized the importance of performing a cognitive assessment of cancer patients.[34,72–75] Levine et al. recommend that mental status examinations, including bedside tests of cognitive functioning, be part of the clinical routine for all cancer patients.[73] Cognitive assessment is particularly important for cancer inpatients because cognitive dysfunction is prevalent in this population, is associated with a poor prognosis, and creates problems of patient management.[34]

The most common primary tumors that metastasize to the brain are carcinomas of the lung and breast and malignant melanoma.[72,73,76,77] Posner reported that 60 percent of patients with cerebral and meningeal metastases experience impaired intellectual functioning.[76] Many of these patients have clouding of consciousness indicative of delirium.[73]

Folstein et al., who have had a long-standing interest in measuring mental status, administered the MMSE to a total of 160 oncology inpatients in two different surveys.[34] The results showed that 14 to 29 percent of the patients scored in the cognitively impaired range on the MMSE. These investigators are studying methods to operationalize the cognitive impairment of delirium and other syndromes. In addition to using the MMSE, their methods include unipolar and bipolar analog scales for rating consciousness, which have shown acceptable levels of interrater reliability, and a hand-held tachistoscope that measures perception time. Patients with delirium are unable to perceive the simple stimulus quickly.[34]

Deterioration in level of consciousness and alterations in mental status can result from neurologic effects of chemotherapy and radiotherapy.[72–84] In recent years, with more aggressive therapy regimens being used, it has become increasingly evident that acute and chronic neurotoxicity has become a significant problem. Grading systems for scoring changes in level of consciousness and mental status are being used and further refined.[79–81,83]

Several studies have documented the effects of cancer chemotherapy on cognitive functioning.[73–76,82–84] In a study of 50 oncology patients, 23 of whom were receiving chemotherapeutic agents, Silberfarb et al. administered the CCSE as part of a battery of measures. Their results showed that impaired cognition was quite common in this population.[74] Brown et al. used the MMSE in a study to assess the neurotoxicity in patients exhibiting mental status changes after receiving the agent spiromustine.[84] Recently, several investigators have reported that a significant number of patients receiving experimental therapy with interleukin 2/lymphokine-activated killer cells experience mental status changes.[85–87] Thus, this group of patients is another example of a population in which research studies are needed greatly to detect, quantify, and characterize mental status dysfunctions.

A study by Moore et al. was conducted to characterize the late effects of therapy on cognitive functioning in children treated for acute leukemia.[88] This study is an illustration of a collaborative effort of investigators from nursing, psychology, and medicine. To conduct a study of this scope, substantial involvement from people with formal neuropsychologic training is necessary. Particularly in the absence of an interdisciplinary/collaborative effort, it seem prudent to consult with neuropsychologists, psychiatrists, or people with similar training when a study protocol is being formulated.

Aids
Neurologic complications occur more frequently in patients with AIDS than in the general oncology patient population.[89] There are multiple etiologies, including human immunodeficiency virus (HIV) infection of neural tissue, opportunistic infections of the nervous system, malignant involvement of the central nervous system, or side effects of treatment with known neurotoxic agents.[89,90] The most common neurologic dysfunction is subacute encephalitis, which occurs in about one third of patients with AIDS.[91] This condition is characterized by subtle cognitive changes that may progress to a debilitating dementia in several weeks to months. Many clinicians have advocated frequent evaluations of mental status to detect cognitive impairment.[89–94] Several of the mental status instruments reviewed in this chapter would be particularly useful in this population to quantify cognitive changes, whether early and subtle or associated with a dementia syndrome.

SUMMARY

A review of selected instruments for measuring levels of consciousness and mental status has been presented. Recommendations for specific tests depend on the particular research application. Altered mental status is experienced by many types of patients. Nurses spend more time caring for patients than any other health professional and are in an ideal position to conduct research studies to further characterize the patient's mental status. Ultimately, these contributions may help document the disease course, provide for more effective treatment, improve the quality of life for affected patients, and provide for the development of new instruments.

ACKNOWLEDGMENTS

The author is indebted to Mark Foreman, R.N., M.S.N., for helpful discussions and comments on earlier drafts of this chapter; she thanks Dr. Margaret Tucker, Dr. Margaret Dear, and Susan Simmons-Alling for their reviews and suggestions; and she is grateful to Kathleen

Barry of NCI and Ellen Chiazze and Christine Lick of Westat, Inc. for their excellent technical assistance.

REFERENCES

1. Mitchell, P.H., Cammermeyer, M., Ozuna, J., & Woods, N.F. *Neurologic assessment for nursing practice.* Reston, VA: Prentice-Hall, 1984.
2. Ozuna, J. Alterations in mentation: Nursing assessment and intervention. *J Neurosurg Nurs,* 1985, *17*(1):66.
3. Mitchell, P.H., & Irvin, N.J. Neurological examination: Nursing assessment for nursing purposes. *J. Neurosurg Nurs,* 1977, *9*(1):23.
4. Adams, R., & Victor, M. Delirium and other acute confusional states. In K.J. Isselbacher, R.D. Adams, E. Braunwald, et al. (Eds.), *Harrison's principles of internal medicine* (9th ed.). New York: McGraw-Hill, 1980, p. 122.
5. Strub, R.L., & Black, F.W. *The mental status examination in neurology* (2nd ed.). Philadelphia: F.A. Davis, 1985.
6. Mueller, J. The mental status examination. In H.H. Goldman (Ed.), *Review of general psychiatry.* Los Altos, CA: Lange, 1984, p. 206.
7. Price, M., & DeVroom, H. A quick and easy guide to neurological assessment. *J Neurosurg Nurs,* 1985, *17*(5):313.
8. Hickey, J. *The clinical practice of neurological and neurosurgical nursing* (2nd ed.). Philadelphia: Lippincott, 1986, p. 116.
9. Ninos, M., & Makohon, R. Functional assessment of the patient. *Geriatr Nurs,* 1985, *6*(3):139.
10. Reynolds, J., & Logsdon, J. Assessing your patient's mental status. *Nursing,* 1979, *79*(8):26.
11. Richardson, K. Assessing communications: Confusion-recognition and remedy. *Geriatr Nurs,* 1983, *4*(4):237.
12. Wilson, H., & Kneisl, C. *Psychiatric nursing.* Menlo Park, CA: Addison-Wesley, 1979, p. 81.
13. Goldenberg, B., & Chiverton, P. Assessing behavior: The Nurse's Mental Status Exam. *Geriatr Nurs* 1984, *5*(2):94.
14. Alcorn, M.H. Altered levels of responsiveness: Decreased response. In M. Snyder (Ed.), *A guide to neurological and neurosurgical nursing.* New York: Wiley, 1983, p. 95.
15. Hagerty, B. *Psychiatric-mental health assessment.* St. Louis: Mosby, 1984.
16. Plum, F., & Posner, J.B. *The diagnosis of stupor and coma* (3rd ed.). Philadelphia: F.A. Davis, 1980, p. 1.
17. Bates, B. *A guide to physical examination.* Philadelphia: Lippincott, 1979, p. 359.
18. Stanczak, D.E., White, J.G., Gouview, W.D., et al. Assessment of level consciousness following severe neurological insult: A comparison of the psychometric qualities of the Glascow Coma Scale and the Comprehensive Level of Consciousness Scale. *J Neurosurg,* 1984, *60*(5):955.
19. Kane, R.A., & Kane, R.L. *Assessing the elderly: A practical guide to measurement.* Lexington, MA: Lexington Books D.C. Heath, 1981.
20. Habot, B., & Libow, L.S. The interrelationship of mental and physical status and its assessment in the older adult: Mind-body interaction. In J.E. Birren, & R.B. Sloane (Eds.), *Handbook of mental health and aging.* Englewood Cliffs, NJ: Prentice-Hall, 1980, p. 701.
21. Foreman, M. Acute confusional states in hospitalized elderly: A research dilemma. *Nurs Res,* 1986, *35*(1):34.
22. Teasdale, G., & Jennett, B. Assessment of coma and impaired consciousness. A practical scale. *Lancet,* 1974, *2*(7872):81.
23. Henderson, M.L. Altered presentations. *Am J Nurs,* 1985, *85*(10):1104.
24. Rimel, R.W., & Jane, J.A. Characteristics of the head-injured patient. In M. Rosenthal, E.R. Griffith, M.R. Bond, and J.D. Miller (Eds.), *Rehabilitation of the head injured adult.* Philadelphia: F.A. Davis, 1983, p. 9.
25. Jones, C. Glasgow Coma Scale. *Am J Nurs,* 1979, *79*(9):1551.
26. Scherer, P. Assessment: The logic of coma. *Am J. Nurs,* 1986, *86*(5):542.

27. Teasdale, G., Knill-Jones, R., & Van Der Sande, J. Observer variability in assessing impaired consciousness and coma. *J. Neurol Neurosurg Psychiatry,* 1978, *41*(7):603.

28. Dodd, M. The confused patient: Assessing mental status. *Am J Nurs,* 1978, *78*(9):1501.

29. Dodd, M. A study to compare pulmonary values to mental status in postcardiotomy patients in an intensive care unit. Master's Thesis, University of Washington, 1973.

30. Dodd, M. Personal communication, August 1985.

31. Adams, M., Hanson, R., Norkool, D., et al. The confused patient: Psychological responses in critical care units. *Am J Nurs,* 1978, *78*(9):1504.

32. Nelson, A., Fogel, B.S., & Faust, D. Bedside cognitive screening instruments: A critical assessment. *J Nerv Ment Dis,* 1986, *174*(2):73.

33. Folstein, M., Folstein, S., & McHugh, P. Mini-Mental State. A practical method for grading the cognitive state of patients for the clinician. *J Psychiat Res,* 1975, *12*(3):189.

34. Folstein, M.F., Fetting, J.H., Lobo, A., et al. Cognitive assessment of cancer patients. *Cancer,* 1984, *53*(10) (suppl.):2250.

35. Anthony, J., LeResche, L., Niaz, U., et al. Limits of the Mini-Mental State as a screening test for dementia and delirium among hospital patients. *Psychol Med,* 1982, *12*(2):397.

36. Dick, J.P.R., Guiloff, R.J., Stewart, A., et al. Mini-Mental State examination in neurological patients. *J Neurol Neurosurg Psychol,* 1984, *47*(5):496.

37. Jacobs, J.W., Bernhard, M.R., Delgado, A., & Strain, J.J. Screening for organic mental syndromes in the medically ill. *Ann Intern Med,* 1977, *86*(5):40.

38. Kaufman, D.M., Weinberger, M., Strain, J.J., & Jacobs, J.W. Detection of cognitive deficits by a brief mental status examination. *Gen Hosp Psychiatry,* 1979, *30*(1):247.

39. Foreman, M.D. A comparison of the reliability and validity of three mental status questionnaires in elderly hospitalized medical-surgical patients. *Nur Res,* in press.

40. Omer, H., Foldes, J., Toby, M., & Menczel, J. Screening for cognitive deficits in a sample of hospitalized geriatric patients: A re-evaluation of a brief mental status questionnaire. *J Am Geriatr Soc,* 1983, *31*(5):266.

41. McCartney, J.R., & Palmeteer, L.M. Assessment of cognitive deficit in geriatric patients: A study of behavior. *J Am Geriatr Soc,* 1985, *33*(1):457.

42. Kahn, R., Goldfarb, A.I., Pollack, M., & Peck, A. Brief objective measures for the determination of mental status in the aged. *Am J Psychiatry,* 1960, *117*(4):326.

43. Kahn, R.L., Goldfarb, A.I., Pollack, M., & Peck, A. Relationship of mental and physical status in institutionalized aged persons. *Am J Psychiatry,* 1960, *117*(4):120.

44. Fillenbaum, G.G. Comparison of two brief tests of organic brain impairment: The MSQ and the Short Portable MSQ. *J Am Geriatr Soc,* 1980, *28*(1):381.

45. Pfeiffer, E. A short portable mental status questionnaire for the assessment of organic brain deficit in elderly patients. *J Am Geriatr Soc,* 1975, *23*(10):433.

46. Duke University Center for the Study of Aging and Human Development. *Multidimensional Functional Assessment: The OARS Methodology.* Durham, NC: Duke University, 1978.

47. Fillenbaum, G.G., & Smyer, M.A. The development, validity, and reliability of the OARS multidimensional functional assessment questionnaire. *J Gerontol,* 1981, *36*(5):428.

48. Kiernan, R.J., Mueller, J., Langston, J.W., & Van Dyke, C. The Neurobehavioral Cognitive Status Examination. Part I: A brief but quantitative approach to cognitive assessment. *Ann Neurol,* submitted for publication.

49. Schwamm, L.H., Van Dyke, C., Kiernan, R.J., et al. The Neurobehavioral Cognitive Status Examination. Part II: Comparison with the CCSE and MMSE in a neurosurgical population. *Ann Neurol,* submitted for publication.

50. Turner, H.B., Kreutzer, J.S., Lent, B., & Brockett, C.A. Developing a brief neuropsychological mental status exam: A pilot study. *J Neurosurg Nurs,* 1984, *16*(5):257.

51. Kreutzer, J.S. Personal communication, January 1987.

52. Isaacs, B., & Akhtar, A.J. The Set Test: A rapid test of mental function in old people. *Age Aging,* 1972, *1*(4):222.

53. Isaacs, B., & Kennie, A.T. The Set Test as an aid to the detection of dementia in old people. *Br J Psychiatry,* 1973, *12*(3):467.

54. Hays, A. The Set Test to screen mental status quickly. *Geriatr Nurs,* 1984, *5*(2):96.
55. Hays, A., & Borger, F. A test in time. *Am J Nurs,* 1985, *85*(10):1107.
56. Kastenbaum, R., & Sherwood, S. VIRO: A scale for assessing the interview behavior of elderly people. In D. Kent, R. Kastenbaum, & S. Sherwood (Eds.), *Research planning and action for the elderly: The power and potential of social science.* New York: Behavioral Publications, 1972, p. 166.
57. Schaie, K.W., & Schaie, J.P. Clinical assessment and aging. In J.E. Birren & K.W. Schaie (Eds.), *Handbook of the psychology of aging.* New York: Van Nostrand Reinhold Company, 1985, p. 692.
58. Fishback, D.B. Mental Status Questionnaire for organic brain syndrome, with a New Visual Counting Test. *J. Am Geriatr Soc,* 1977, *25*(4):167.
59. Whelihan, W.M., Lesher, E.L., Kleban, M.H., & Granck, S. Mental status and memory assessment as predictors of dementia. *J Gerontol,* 1984, *39*(5):572.
60. Kay, D. The epidemiology and identification of brain deficit in the elderly. In C. Eisendorfer, & R. Friedel (Eds.), *Cognitive and emotional disturbance in the elderly.* Chicago: Year Book, 1977, p. 11.
61. Fink, M., Green, M., & Bender, M.B. The Face-Hand Test as a diagnostic sign of organic mental syndrome. *Neurology,* 1952, *2*(1):46.
62. Kramer, N.A., & Jarvik, L.F. Assessment of intellectual changes in the elderly. In A. Raskin, & L.F. Jarvik (Eds.), *Psychiatric symptoms and cognitive loss in the elderly.* New York: Wiley, 1979, p. 221.
63. Crook, T., Ferris, S., & McCarthy, M. The Misplaced-Objects Task: A brief test for memory dysfunction in the aged. *J Am Geriatr Soc,* 1979, *27*(6):284.
64. Wechsler, D. A standardized memory scale for clinical use. *J Psychol,* 1945, *19*:87.
65. Erickson, R.C., & Scott, M.L. Clinical memory testing: A review. *Psychol Bull,* 1977, *84*(6):1130.
66. Klonoff, H., & Kennedy, M. Memory and perceptual functioning in octogenarians and non-agenarians in the community. *J Gerontol,* 1965, *20*(5):328.
67. Baker, E.L., Feldman, R.G., White, R.F., et al. Monitoring neurotoxins in industry: Development of a neurobehavioral test battery. *J Occup Med,* 1983, *25*(2):125.
68. Plutchik, R., Conte, H., & Lieberman, M. Development of a scale (GIES) for assessment of cognitive and perceptual functioning in geriatric patients. *J Am Geriatr Soc,* 1971, *19*(7):614.
69. Libow, L.S. A rapidly administered, easily remembered status evaluation: FROMAJE. In L.S. Libow, F.T. Sherman (Eds.), *The core of geriatric medicine: A guide for students and practitioners.* St. Louis: Mosby, 1981, p. 85.
70. Levin, H.S., O'Donnell, V.M., & Grossman, R.G. The Galveston Orientation and Amnesia Test: A practical scale to assess cognition after head injury. *J Nerv Ment Dis,* 1979, *167*(11):675.
71. Lezak, M.D. *Neuropsychological assessment* (2nd ed.). New York: Oxford University Press, 1983.
72. Klein, P. Neurologic emergencies in oncology. *Semin Oncol Nurs,* 1985, *1*(4):278.
73. Levine, P.M., Silberfarb, P.M., & Lipowski, Z.J. Mental disorders in cancer patients: A study of 100 psychiatric referrals. *Cancer,* 1978, *42*(3):1385.
74. Silberfarb, P.M., Philibert, D., & Levine, P.M. Psychosocial aspects of neoplastic disease: II. Affective and cognitive effects of chemotherapy in cancer patients. *Am J Psychiatry,* 1980, *137*(5):597.
75. Silberfarb, P.M. Chemotherapy and cognitive defects in cancer patients. *Ann Rev Med,* 1983, *34*(1):35.
76. Posner, J. Neurological complications of systemic cancer. *Med Clin North Am,* 1971, *55*(1):625.
77. Ryan, L.S. Nursing assessment of the ambulatory patient with brain metastases. *Cancer Nurs,* 1981, *4*(4):281.
78. Doogan, R.A. Hypercalcemia of malignancy. *Cancer Nurs,* 1981, *4*(4):299.
79. Kaplan, R.S., & Wiernik, P.H. Neurotoxicity of antitumor agents. In M.C. Perry, & J.W. Yarbro (Eds.), *Toxicity of chemotherapy.* Orlando, FL: Grune & Stratton, 1984, p. 365.
80. Miller, A.B., Hoogstraten, B., Staquet, M., & Winkler, A. Reporting results of cancer treatment. *Cancer,* 1981, *47*(1):207.
81. Castellanos, A.M., and Fields, W.S. Grading of neurotoxicity in cancer therapy (Letter to Editor). *J Clin Oncol,* 1986, *4*(8):1277.
82. Nand, S., Messmore, H.L. Jr., Patel, R., et al. Neurotoxicity associated with systemic high-dose cytosine arabinoside. *J Clin Oncol,* 1986, *4*(4):571.

83. Pratt, C.B., Green, A.A., Horowitz, M.E., et al. Central nervous system toxicity following treatment of pediatric patients with Ifosfamide/Mesna. *J Clin Oncol,* 1986, *4*(8):1253.
84. Brown, T.D., Ettinger, D.S., & Donehower, R.C. A phase I trial of Spirohydantoin Mustard (NSC 172112) in patients with advanced cancer. *J Clin Oncol* 1986, *4*(8):1270.
85. Jassak, P.F., & Sticklin, L.A. Interleukin 2: An overview. *Oncol Nurs Forum,* 1986, *13*(6):17.
86. Seipp, C.A., Simpson, C., & Rosenberg, S.A. Clinical trials with IL-2. *ONF,* 1986, *13*(6):25.
87. Corey, B.S., & Collins, J.L. Implementation of an RIL-2/LAK cell clinical trial: A nursing perspective. *Oncol Nurs Forum* 1986, *13*(6):31.
88. Moore, I.M., Kramer, J., & Ablin, A. Late effects of central nervous system prophylactic leukemia therapy on cognitive functioning. *ONF,* 1986, *13*(4):45.
89. Donehower, M.G. Malignant complications of AIDS. *ONF,* 1987, *14*(1):57.
90. Levy, R.M., Bredesen, D.E., & Rosenblum, M.L. Neurological manifestations of the acquired immunodeficiency syndrome (AIDS): Experience at UCSF and review of the literature. *J Neurosurg,* 1985, *62*(4):475.
91. Carne, C.A., & Adler, M.W. Neurological manifestations of human immunodeficiency virus infection. *Br Med J,* 1986, *293*:462.
92. Snider, W.D., Simpson, D.M., Nielson, S., et al. Neurological complications of acquired immune deficiency syndrome: Analysis of 50 patients. *Ann Neurol,* 1983, *14*:403.
93. Holland, J.C., & Tross, S. The psychosocial and neuropsychiatric sequele of the acquired immunodeficiency syndrome and related disorders. *Ann Intern Med,* 1985, *103*(5):760.
94. Sunder, J.A. AIDS: A neurological nursing challenge. *Top Clin Nurs,* 1984, *6*(2):67.

CHAPTER 4

Single Instruments for Measuring Quality of Life

Marilyn Frank-Stromborg, R.N., Ed.D.

With the advent of aggressive chemotherapy and radiation therapy, there have been numerous indications that health professionals have added a new dimension to their list of concerns when discussing the care of the patient with cancer. Increasingly, the value of cancer treatments is judged not only on survival but on the quality of that survival. This new concern is broadly titled "quality of life." Articles on cancer have repeatedly alluded to this concept, although it was not until 1977 that the term "quality of life" first received a separate heading in *Index Medicus*.[1] Oncology is not the only discipline that has focused on the impact of new treatments and procedures on quality of life. Interest in this area has surfaced in the cardiology, renal, geriatric, and surgical literature as well.

DEFINITIONS OF QUALITY OF LIFE

Quality of life has been defined in purely objective terms by measuring such items as income, housing, physical function, and purity of air.[2,3] Other authors have focused on the subjective dimensions by investigating individual aspirations, frustrations, attitudes, and perceptions.[4] Several researchers have attempted to measure both the objective and subjective dimensions that bear on the quality of life.[5-8] Hornquist writes that quality of life should include measurement of both individual needs and the available resources.[9] The multiple objective and subjective dimensions that have been used in studies to assess quality of life are listed in Table 4–1.

However, the division between subjective and objective measurements of quality of life may be artificial, since what has emerged in the research literature is that objective and subjective dimensions do not seem congruent with each other. For instance, Evans et al.'s study of quality of life of patients with end-stage renal disease found that "patients on dialysis were clearly not functioning like people who were well, despite the fact that they were enjoying life" (p. 557).[10] Because the definitions of quality of life and approaches to measurement vary considerably from study to study, meaningful comparisons between studies are difficult to make.

TABLE 4—1. DIMENSIONS USED IN STUDIES TO ASSESS QUALITY OF LIFE

Dimension	Representative Studies
Subject's opinion of quality of life or life satisfaction	Andrews and Withey,[1] Bortner and Hultsch,[2] Cantril,[3] Campbell,[4,5] Campbell and Converse,[6] Campbell et al.,[7] Crandall and Putnam,[8] Fry and Ghosh,[9] Johnson et al.,[10] Kazak and Linney,[11] Kilpatrick and Cantril,[12] Hatz and Powers,[13] Jackle,[14] Laborde and Powers,[15] Levy and Wynbrandt,[16] Neugarten et al.,[17] Padilla et al.,[18] Palmore and Kivett,[19] Palmore and Luikart,[20] Penckhofer and Holm,[21] Soper,[22] Sophie and Powers,[23] Watts,[24] Webb and Powers[25]
Socioeconomic status (including occupation, education, income and/or financial status)	Bonney et al.,[26] Campbell,[4,5] Campbell and Converse,[6] Campbell et al.,[7] Johnson et al.,[10] Kaplan De-Nour and Shanan,[27] Levy and Wynbrandt,[16] Padilla et al.[18]
Physical health (including activity level and/or physical symptoms)	Bonney et al.,[26] Campbell,[4,5] Campbell and Converse,[6] Campbell et al.,[7] Johnson et al.,[10] Kaplan De-Nour and Shanan,[27] Levy and Wynbrandt,[16] Padilla et al.[18]
Affect	Campbell,[4,5] Campbell and Converse,[6] Campbell et al.,[7] Conte and Salamon,[28] Crandall and Putnam,[8] Glenn and McLanahan,[29] Johnson et al.,[10] Keon and McDonald,[30] Levy and Wynbrandt,[16] Neugarten et al.[17]
Perceived stress	Campbell,[4,5] Campbell and converse,[6] Campbell et al.[7]
Friendships (including social support)	Campbell,[4,5] Campbell and Converse,[6] Campbell et al.,[7] Johnson et al.,[10] Levy and Wynbrandt[16]
Family (including children)	Campbell,[4,5] Campbell and Converse,[6] Campbell et al.,[7] Johnson et al.,[10] Kaplan De-Nour and Shanan,[27] Levy and Wynbrandt[16]
Marriage (including sex)	Bonney et al.,[26] Campbell,[4,5] Campbell and Converse,[6] Campbell et al.,[7] Johnson et al.,[10] Kaplan De-Nour and Shanan,[27] Levy and Wynbrandt,[16] Padilla et al.[18]
Achievement of life goals	Levy and Wynbrandt,[16] Neugarten et al.[17]
Satisfaction with housing and neighborhood	Campbell,[4,5] Campbell and Converse,[6] Campbell et al.[7]
Satisfaction with city and nation	Campbell,[4,5] Campbell and Converse,[6] Campbell et al.,[7] Cantril,[3] Kilpatrick and Cantril[12]
Satisfaction with self (including self-esteem)	Campbell,[4,5] Campbell and Converse,[6] Campbell et al.,[7] Conte and Salamon,[28] Kaplan De-Nour and Shanan,[27] Neugarten et al.[17]
Depression, psychologic defense mechanisms, and coping	Bonney et al.,[26] Kaplan De-Nour and Shanan,[27] Levy and Wynbrandt[16]

From Ferrans, Powers. Adv Nurs Res, 1985, 8(1):15. See Appendix A for references.

The major challenge to the use of the term quality of life . . . is that the term is too broad and inclusive to be meaningful. Central to this position was the definitional problem, that is, that the term is operationally defined in very different ways by different investigators. Thus, the failure to achieve a shared definition results in the use of measures that are assessing different things (p.2327).[11]

Examples illustrating this criticism are found in the work of Palmer et al.[12] and Cookfair et al.[13] Palmer's measurement of quality of life consists of asking women with primary breast cancer who had adjuvant chemotherapy, "How much did the full course of treatment interfere with your life?"[12] Cookfair's quality of life assessment was based on the measurement of three variables (employment, functional status, and nursing needs) of 1902 cancer patients of

TABLE 4–2.   METHODOLOGIC APPROACHES TO QUALITY OF LIFE RESEARCH

	General Strategy of Approach	When Data Collected	Benefits	Limitations
Most optimal	Prospective	Several times in course of treatment, usually from diagnosis through posttreatment period	Offers true process evaluation of same group of patients; offers baseline to follow-up comparisons; higher reliability estimate of quality of life	Expensive, data takes long time to obtain; patient attrition
	Single data collection/patient same time posttreatment	Researcher assesses at same time posttreatment for each patient, e.g., 1 year posttreatment	Offers uniformity of posttreatment evaluation of patients	Limited view of quality of life, possible low reliability
	Cross-sectional/separate groups	At different phases of illness or treatment with patients with same illness, e.g., three groups of patients with breast cancer, at diagnosis, recurrence, near death	Offers some view of flow of quality of life in relation to illness with less expense than prospective design; possibly increases reliability about quality of life	Patients may not really be well matched other than on disease variable; therefore, true phase comparisons risky
Least optimal	Single data collection/patients at variable times posttreatment	Researcher assesses patients at variable times after their treatment, e.g., patients range 1–10 years postmastectomy	Offers ability to assess maximal number of patients, least expensive method of collecting quality of life data	Severe limit on comparability of patient responses due to history effects, variability of time since diagnosis, treatment

From Wellisch. Cancer, *1984, 53:2292.*

varying diagnosis and demographic characteristics.[13] Obviously, there can be no comparison of quality of life in these two studies.

Wellisch[14] has written an excellent review of the issues involved in measuring quality of life. One of the important points he makes is that the optimal measurement approach to quality of life is the prospective design in which the same group of patients is interviewed sequentially. Evans et al. make the same recommendation, since they believe that the subjective quality of life (i.e., the individual's attitudes) is a state rather than a trait and is thus subject to variation over time.[10] If measurement takes place at only one point in the patient's experience, the true picture of quality of life may not emerge. Wellisch's recommended

TABLE 4–3. RESEARCH STRATEGIES AND TECHNOLOGIES FOR QUALITY OF LIFE RESEARCH

	Tools	Administrator	Advantages	Disadvantages
Least optimal	Unstructured interview/clinical	Treating physician	Low cost, easy, and plentiful patient access	Physician bias severe; patient often skews response set to please doctor; no objective measures, low reliability
	Semistructured interview	Usually treating physician	Low cost, easy, and plentiful patient access	Less bias than in unstructured condition, but physician and patient bias still problem, low validity, questionable reliability
	Analog rating scales	Can be physicians, i.e., GIAS or Index or patient, i.e., linear analog self-assessment scale	Very brief, can be closely tailored to specific tumor types, sites, regimens	Overly constrictive view of patient life, validity problems
	Psychologic tests	Self-administered	In-depth look at emotional status of patient	Often are very poorly standardized for cancer patients, confounded with pre-illness issues; only covers emotional issues
Most optimal	Combination structured interviewing, analog, scales, behavioral functioning/activities	Some patient self-administered, some administered by project staff (not treating physician)	Very comprehensive; can be both general and tailored to specific illness/ treatment, better content, and construct validity	Expensive to design; can be lengthy to administer, convergent validity (between measures) can suffer

From Wellisch. Cancer, 1984, 53: 2293.

methodologic approaches and research strategies for quality of life research are shown in Tables 4–2 and 4–3.[14]

HEALTH AS A DIMENSION OF QUALITY OF LIFE

Regardless of the approach, research has indicated clearly the importance of health in determining life satisfaction.[5–17] As a result of these findings, health indices have been developed that attempt to define quality of life as it applies to the state of wellness of the individual. Most health indices have tended to concentrate on the physical functions of patients and to be cross-sectional (one time period) analyses of the health status of the person. The literature indicates that this narrow functional definition of health status may be changing. For instance, Ware advocates the use of a multidimensional conceptual model to measure health status, mental status, social status, general status (i.e., self-ratings of health, physical symptoms, psychosomatic symptoms) and diagnostic indicators (i.e., blood pressure).[18]

Thus, what emerges from a review of the literature about health indices for determining quality of life is the general consensus that attributes of mind, body, and spirit all need to be included in any comprehensive approach. This approach is recommended because there are numerous domains of social and physiologic function that may be substantially affected by changes in health status. For instance, Berg et al. constructed a values scale that included cognitive, emotional, social, and physical functions. Berg's results indicate that any attempt to define health operationally, as it relates to quality of life, must include more than just physical functions.[5,19]

OTHER DIMENSIONS OF QUALITY OF LIFE

Although health is definitely an important component of quality of life, other dimensions have been more difficult to define. An attempt to define the dimensions that constitute quality of life has been made by Flanagan, who studied 3000 Americans of varying ages and health status in terms of their perceptions of what constitutes quality of life.[16] Using the critical incident technique, he identified those factors a healthy population considers to be important for quality of life.[16] One example follows:

> Think of the last time you did something very important to you or had an experience that was especially satisfying to you. What did you do or what happened that was so satisfying to you? (p. 57)[16]

Flanagan asked two critical incident questions of groups of people and obtained 6500 critical incidents. Categorization by independent judges resulted in 15 factors that included all of the 6500 critical incidents. A sample of 3000 people (30 to 70 years of age) was then asked a question about each of these 15 factors: "At this time in your life, how important is _____?" Flanagan found that six dimensions were regarded as being extremely important to overall quality of life: health, having and raising children, material comforts, work, close relationship with a spouse, and understanding oneself.

SELECTING A QUALITY OF LIFE INSTRUMENT

The assessment of quality of life is still an evolving area of clinical research. The researcher desiring to measure this area must consider multiple issues and choices in instrument selection.

Multiple versus Single Instruments

The first issue is whether the concept can be measured by a single instrument or requires multiple instruments. Fletcher and Bulpitt point out that there are serious restrictions on the use of multiple instruments to measure quality of life,[20] including feasibility, design, and costs. Using a large battery of tests requires a variety of staff, and patients may be reluctant to spend the time involved in filling out the instruments. They point out that since many short-term trials that are designed to assess the efficacy of drugs are using quality of life measurements, some measures (i.e., social support and spiritual well-being) are unlikely to be sensitive to the effects of the drug treatment.[20] This chapter discusses single instruments, and Chapter 5 details the use of multiple instruments to measure quality of life.

Qualitative versus Quantitative Data

The researcher is confronted with the issue of whether to pick an instrument that results in qualitative (descriptive) data or one that provides quantitative data (data yielding scores appropriate for statistical testing). Many of the qualitative instruments discussed identify the specific areas that have been affected by the disease and thus change the person's overall quality of life. In contrast, the quantitative instruments yield an overall quality of life assessment score. In an effort to validate their instruments, many researchers have compared the single quality of life scores obtained on their instruments with scores on comparable research tools. One criticism of a single global index is that it conveys no clues about why functioning may be impaired and may neglect important quality of life dimensions.

Objective versus Subjective Instrument

The third choice the researcher has is whether to use an objective instrument (the patient's quality of life is evaluated by the health professional) or a subjective instrument (the patient evaluates his or her own quality of life). One of the criticisms of past research in the area of quality of life has been that most studies tended to reflect the health professional's perception of the patient's quality of life rather than the patient's own evaluation.[21,22] As seen in Table 4–3, objective instruments emerge as the least optimal method of obtaining a quality of life assessment. This criticism has resulted in the development of many objective instruments.[23–26]

Objective versus Subjective Dimensions of Quality of Life

The last choice is whether to use an instrument that focuses on measuring objective dimensions (housing, work, education, environment, socioeconomic status) or one that measures subjective dimensions (psychosocial). Evans et al.'s study of patients with end-stage renal disease illustrates the use of objective and subjective indicators. Their objective indicators were functional impairment and ability to work. The subjective indicators of quality of life were well-being, psychologic effect, and life satisfaction.[10] Another example of a study measuring both dimensions is the U.S. government 1977 report, *Social Indicators*.[27] The objective indicators surveyed were economic productivity, crime rates, family income, health indices, and accident rates. The subjective factors were satisfaction with housing, health care, and recreational opportunities.[27] The majority of instruments detailed in this chapter focus on measuring the subjective aspects of a person's life to determine quality of life.

Overall, the choice of the instrument will depend on the goal of the research, as well as pragmatic considerations (e.g., resources available to do content analysis of qualitative data, computer availability, stamina of the sample being assessed that may influence the length of the instrument desired). Sugarbaker et al.'s approach to measuring quality of life is considered by some authors to be the state-of-the-art.[28] It was a cooperative, multidisciplinary effort using multiple quality of life assessment methodologies (e.g., they measured both objective and subjective dimensions and used interview and self-reports). Practically (Table 4–3), this all-inclusive approach may not always be possible. Thus, single quality of life instruments may be the only realistic option for the researcher.

OBJECTIVE SCALES YIELDING QUANTITATIVE DATA

• KARNOFSKY PERFORMANCE STATUS SCALE

Early attempts to measure quality of life in patients focused on one dimension of the patient's life—the ability to perform activities of daily living (ADL). Karnofsky and Burchenal developed a scale that rates physical activity from 1 percent to 100 percent in increments of 10 percent.[29] Although designed as an objective measure of quality of life, one researcher used the Karnofsky Scale as a subjective tool; with it, patients evaluated their own physical status.[30] Examples from Karnofsky and Burchenal's scale are:

+50 Requires considerable assistance and frequent medical care
+40 Disabled, requires special care and assistance
+30 Severely disabled, hospitalization is indicated although death not imminent
+20 Hospitalization necessary, very sick, active supportive treatment necessary[29]

Grieco and Long reevaluated the Karnofsky Performance Status Scale and report that:

Tests of inter-rater reliability, concurrent validity, and discriminant validity indicate that, with standardized observational procedures based on a mental status exam, the Karnofsky Scale is acceptably reliable and valid as a global measure, but it does not adequately capture the conceptual domain of quality of life (p. 129).[21]

• ZUBROD SCALE

The Zubrod Scale (a scale of 0 to 4 in increments of 1) evaluates the ability of the patient to remain ambulatory and to perform ADL.[31] Both the Karnofsky and Zubrod Scales have been used extensively by cooperative cancer research groups because they show a correlation with tumor response to treatment and survival.

• QL-INDEX

An objective scale that has been used primarily by physicians, but as a broader orientation than the Zubrod or Karnofsky Scales, was developed by Spitzer et al.[32] The QL-Index measures not only health but also family support, activity, daily living, and outlook. The range of scores is 0 to 10, and it takes about 1 minute for the health professional to complete. An example from one category on the QL-Index is:

During the last week, the patient:

has been appearing to feel well or reporting feeling "great" most of the time (+2)
has been lacking energy or not feeling entirely up to par more than just occasionally (+1)
has been feeling very ill or "lousy," seeming weak and washed out most of the time or was unconscious (+0)

Spitzer reports that the instrument has discriminant construct validity, content validity, high internal consistency (Cronbach coefficient alpha = 0.775), and statistically significant inter-rater Spearman rank correlation (r_{ho} = 0.81, $p < 0.001$). The QL-Index was piloted by more than 150 physicians who rated 879 patients. It was standardized on cancer patients with several levels of seriousness of diagnosis as well as on people with several other chronic diseases as controls. Grieco and Long state that the QL-Index has the advantage of brevity but, like the Karnofsky Scale, lacks standardized observational procedures.[21] In other words, there are no standardized instructions for scoring these two instruments.

SUBJECTIVE SCALES YIELDING QUANTITATIVE DATA

▪ QUALITY OF LIFE INDEX (QLI)

Padilla et al. developed a subjective self-evaluation questionnaire (14 linear analog scale items comprise the instrument), the Quality of Life Index (QLI).[23,24] They viewed quality of life as a broad concept, and the scale includes three general areas: psychologic well-being (general quality of life, fun, satisfaction, usefulness, sleep), physical well-being (strength, appetite, work, eating, sex), and symptom control (pain, nausea, vomiting). Their tool was a revision of one created earlier by Present et al.[25] The QLI was tested with four subject groups: oncology outpatients receiving chemotherapy (n = 43) or radiation therapy (n = 39), oncology inpatients receiving chemotherapy (n = 48), and nonpatient volunteers (n = 48). Three representative questions from the QLI are:

With respect to your general physical condition, please describe:
How much STRENGTH have you had?
None _____ A great deal
Is the amount of time you sleep sufficient to meet your needs?
Not at all sufficient _____ Completely sufficient
Have you felt satisfied with your life?
Not at all _____ Extremely

Test–retest reliability coefficients were high ($r > 0.60$, $p < 0.01$), internal consistency was 0.88 ($p < 0.01$), and the QLI scores and physician estimates of Karnofsky ratings, prognosis, and patient self-ratings of quality of life were poor. Ryan used the QLI in her study of 422 veterans with lung or colon cancer from 11 Veterans Administration medical centers.[33] She reported internal consistency of the items of the QLI using Cronbach coefficient alpha as significant, $r = 0.93$, $p < 0.01$. In test–retest, the percentage of retest responses within 1 cm on the original linear analog scale response was 72 percent in a group of veterans before treatment and 70 percent in a similar veteran group after cancer treatment.[33]

▪ FERRANS AND POWERS QUALITY OF LIFE INDEX (QLI)

Ferrans and Powers Quality of Life Index (QLI) was developed to measure the quality of life of healthy people as well as those who are experiencing an illness (the QLI was piloted with dialysis patients).[34,35] There are 35 items on this instrument that assess 18 areas, including life goals, general satisfaction, stress, physical health. The instrument consists of two sections. One section measures satisfaction with various domains of life, and the other measures the importance of the domain to the subject. This approach to quality of life measurement is unique among all the tools. Sample questions from the tool are:

	Very Dissatisfied 1	Moderately Dissatisfied 2	Slightly Dissatisfied 3	Slightly Satisfied 4	Moderately Satisfied 5	Very Satisfied 6

Part I
How satisfied are you with your health?
How satisfied are you with your family's health?

	Very Unimportant 1	Moderately Unimportant 2	Slightly Unimportant 3	Slightly Important 4	Moderately Important 5	Very Important 6

Part II
How important is your health to you?
How important is your family's health to you?

The psychometric properties of the QLI are strong. Test–retest reliability coefficient with a healthy population (69 graduate students, 2-week interval) was 0.87, and it was 0.81 with an ill group (20 dialysis patients, 1-month interval). Cronbach coefficient alpha (measuring internal consistency) for the total instrument was 0.93 with graduate students and 0.93 with 349 dialysis patients. The alphas for the subscores were 0.87 for the healthy and functioning, 0.82 for socioeconomic, 0.90 for psychologic/spiritual, and 0.77 for the family subscale. Criterion-related validity was established by comparing the QLI with a question on overall satisfaction with life. Subjects were asked to rate their overall satisfaction with life on a 6-point rating scale, which ranged from "very satisfied" to "very dissatisfied." The correlation between scores from the QLI and the life satisfaction question for graduate students was 0.75 and for the dialysis patients 0.77. Construct validity was explored using factor analysis. Four underlying dimensions were found for the QLI: health and functioning, socioeconomic, psychologic/spiritual, and family. Scoring information is given in Reference 34, and the computer program that performs the calculations was written by Ferrans and is available on request. Send correspondence to Marjorie Powers, R.N., Ph.D., Professor, Medical–Surgical Nursing, College of Nursing, University of Illinois, Chicago, IL 60680.

▪ QUALITY OF LIFE QUESTIONNAIRE (QLQ)

In Young and Longman's pilot study of quality of life in people with melanoma, they developed a short Quality of Life Questionnaire (QLQ) and correlated this scale with several other instruments (i.e., Social Dependency Scale, Symptom Distress Scale, Behavior-Morale Scale).[4] Their instrument uses a Likert-type scale, and subjects are instructed to rate their current quality of life from 1 (poor) to 6 (excellent). In another question, subjects are asked to rate, on a scale from 1 (not at all satisfied) to 10 (very satisfied), their feelings of satisfaction with their current quality of life. These two questions were found to be strongly associated (0.81) and statistically significant ($p < 0.0001$).[36] The QLQ correlated positively with behavior-morale and negatively with symptom distress and social dependency. As quality of life was ranked higher, symptom distress and social dependency were ranked lower.

• SICKNESS IMPACT PROFILE (SIP)

The Sickness Impact Profile (SIP) has been used by researchers to measure quality of life. The SIP was initially developed by Bergner et al. in 1972 and, after pilot testing on a sample of 278 subjects and revisions, resulted in a measure that contains 136 items that are grouped into 12 categories of life activities.[26] The categories are physical dimension (body movement, mobility, ambulation), psychosocial dimension (intellectual function, social interaction, emotional behavior, communication), sleep and rest, taking nutrition, usual daily work, household management, leisure and recreation. Two typical statements on the SIP are:

- I laugh or cry suddenly.
- I just pick or nibble at my food.

The instrument takes between 20 and 30 minutes (a conservative estimate) to administer, and "scores that range from zero to one hundred percent disruption can be calculated for each scale category, for each dimension of the scale, or categories can be disregarded and one total disruption score calculated" (p. 37).[37] Investigators report that the SIP scores discriminate among subsamples, and correlations between criterion measures and SIP scores provide evidence for the validity of the instrument. The SIP has been used with patients with coronary artery disease, pulmonary disease, and hyperthyroidism as an outcome measure in evaluating treatments.[38–40] Johnson et al. used the SIP with radiation oncology patients and believe that this instrument is an acceptable measure of quality of life.[37] Recently, the criticism has been made that since the SIP assesses a fairly broad functional state, it may not discriminate among more subtle changes produced by the disease state or treatment.[41] The lack of ability to detect change becomes important in studies attempting to show "before" and "after" quality of life changes.

• SELF-ANCHORING LIFE SATISFACTION SCALE

Another approach to measuring quality of life is to measure satisfaction with life. Cantril's Self-Anchoring Life Satisfaction Scale was designed to measure a general sense of well-being.[42] The subjective scale asks the subject to identify the best possible life he could imagine and define the worst possible life he could imagine. These two extremes are related to a ladder, with the best possible life on rung 10 and the worst possible life on rung 1. Subjects are then asked to indicate where on the ladder they would place themselves 5 years ago, at present, and 5 years hence. The same procedure is used for assessing health status. This approach to measuring quality of life has been used successfully with patients undergoing dialysis or coronary revascularization or with severe osteoarthritis.[43,44] Content validity, face validity, and reliability for the instrument have been established.

• LINEAR ANALOG SELF-ASSESSMENT (LASA)

Priestman and Baum developed a Linear Analog Self-Assessment (LASA) for patients to make their own assessments about their quality of life during and after treatment.[45] In their study, the patients were asked to evaluate ten areas of life: feeling of well-being, mood, level of activity, pain, nausea, effectiveness of treatment, appetite, ability to perform housework, social activities, and level of anxiety. For each one of these areas, a 10 cm line is drawn, and on each end of the line are descriptive words of extremes of that area. The patient is asked to mark the line at a point most appropriate to his or her feelings at that moment; the distance, in centimeters, along the line to the mark gives a score out of ten. This approach (the linear or visual analog scale) is also being used successfully to measure nausea and vomiting, as well as the subjective feeling of pain.[46] Reliability and validity information is missing from the article, but they report that LASA tests measuring well-being correlate well with the patient's clinical status.

▪ DANOFF ET AL. QUESTIONNAIRE

Danoff et al. developed an interview questionnaire that consists of four sections: descriptive demographic items, medical data, perceptual quality of life questions (patient's perception of various life concerns), and health status questions.[22] It differs from the other described quality of life instruments in that they define quality of life in both objective (education, income, housing, employment) and subjective (psychosocial) terms. The patient is asked to rate his feelings about 41 perceptual quality of life questions on a 7-point scale that ranges from "delighted (1)" to "terrible (7)." The authors interviewed by telephone 399 cancer patients who were alive without evidence of disease 3 or more years after initial radiation treatment. Examples of perceptual quality of life items are given below:

How do you feel about . . .

the people you see socially?
the income you (and your family) have?
your own health and physical condition?

Danoff et al. compared the demographic, perceptual, and health status data on their instrument with a national data baseline obtained from several national surveys. They believe that an advantage of their instrument is that it has been standardized, allowing for data replication and comparison with future studies and baselines.

▪ FUNCTIONAL LIVING INDEX—CANCER (FLIC)

Schipper et al.'s Functional Living Index—Cancer (FLIC) is another subjective tool yielding quantitative data. This tool is specifically for people with cancer.[47] It is designed for easy, repeated patient self-administration. The FLIC is a 22-item questionnaire that has been validated on 837 patients in two Canadian cities over a 3-year period. Each item on the FLIC is answerable in Likert format with a 1 to 7 range. Factor analysis was stable through separate clinical trials, indicating strong construct validity. The FLIC has five factors: physical well-being, psychologic state, family situational interaction, social ability, and somatic sensation. Concurrent validity was tested against the Karnofsky Index, Beck Depression Scale, Spielberger State and Trait Anxiety Scale, and Katz Activities of Daily Living Index, the McGill/Melzack Pain Index, and the General Health Questionnaire.

> The physical function and ability factor of the FLIC correlates well with those concurrent validation studies measuring physical attributes or their consequences, but does not correlate strongly with the psychosocial measures. Analogously, FLIC's emotional function factor correlates strongly with measures of depression and anxiety, but weakly with physical ability measures. These data provide clear evidence that the FLIC measures a composite of distinct factors contributing to overall functional living (p. 481).

Sample questions from this instrument follow:

Rate your ability to maintain your usual recreation or leisure activities.

1	2	3	4	5	6	7

How much of your usual household tasks are you able to complete?

1	2	3	4	5	6	7

• ROMSAAS ET AL. QUESTIONNAIRE

Romsaas et al.[48] developed an instrument that is a checklist of 15 categories (information, fatigue, pain, nutrition, speech and language, respiration, bowel and bladder, transportation, mobility, self and home care, vocational and educational, interests and activities, emotional, family, and interpersonal relationships). Typical questions on this patient participation tool follow:

How often are you having problems with breathing or with feeling short of breath?
Always
Sometimes
Never

Are you concerned about your ability to participate in any of the following? (Please check all that apply)
Home activities and hobbies
Sexual activity or interest
Community activities
Social relationships
Exercise or sports
Other

Although it is primarily a checklist, there are open-ended questions inviting concerns not included on the checklist. The purpose of this tool is to identify the rehabilitation and continuing care needs of ambulatory cancer patients and to enable them to develop interventions designed to improve quality of life.

SUBJECTIVE SCALES YIELDING QUALITATIVE DATA

• CAIN AND HENKE SURVEY

One of the first qualitative nursing studies to investigate the area of quality of life in cancer patients was one conducted by Cain and Henke in 1978.[49] They developed a survey that assessed primarily the nonmedical needs of 50 ambulatory cancer patients. The survey, which took approximately 20 minutes to complete, asked about pain, nausea and vomiting, work, leisure activity, dependency needs, future concerns, religious beliefs, and overall quality of life. This survey served to identify specific areas that had changed the quality of life of the patients with cancer.

The rest of the qualitative instruments discussed in this chapter are all similar in that they result in a description of the changes that have occurred in the person's life (rather than a single score) and thus indirectly assess overall quality of life. Most of the qualitative instruments are a result of a desire by clinicians to have a tool that systematically assesses the impact of cancer on the lives of patients and targets the specific areas that have changed, thus enabling them to develop appropriate, focused interventions.

• FREIDENBERG ET AL. QUESTIONNAIRE

One such tool yielding descriptive data was developed by Freidenberg et al. to measure the psychosocial problems of cancer patients and thus indirectly assess the quality of life.[50] Their tool is a structured problem-oriented interview that assesses 122 potential cancer-related problems grouped into 13 areas of life functioning: physical discomfort, medical treatment, hospital service, mobility, housework, vocational, financial, family, social, worry, affect, body image, and communication. Patients were asked to report the severity of each acknowledged problem on a 10-point scale (1 = mild, 10 = severe). The instrument takes 1/2 to 1 hour to administer. Two typical questions on this instrument are:

Are there any changes in activities with friends? If so, how severe is the change?

Are there any changes in family role? If so, how severe is the change?

• HEALTH SURVEY

Stromberg and Wright's instrument, Health Survey, differs from the other qualitative instruments in that it not only identifies the specific areas altered by the diagnosis of cancer but also obtains patients' perceptions of the severity of the change and their attitude toward the alteration in lifestyle.[51] Ratings on severity of the change were obtained from seven options on a Likert-type scale ranging from "extremely negative" to "extremely positive." The Health Survey employs both open-ended and closed-ended questions and consists of the following sections: (1) demographic data (measured by 18 items), (2) physical impact data (measured by 18 items, such as taste, weight, activity), (3) psychosocial impact data (measured by 12 items, such as sex, finances, self-image), (4) patient/health professional relationship data (measured by 5 items, such as who they communicate with, how often, and why). An example of one question area from the Health Survey is:

Has your physical activity changed?   Yes_____   No_____
What kinds of change?
What is your attitude toward your change in physical activity?
Strongly negative _____ Strongly positive
How have your daily activities been affected by changes in physical activity?

Content validity for the Health Survey is reported, and it was piloted on 340 ambulatory cancer patients.

SUMMARY

Early quality of life tools (i.e., Karnofsky) focused on one dimension, functional status. More recently developed instruments have a broader concept of quality of life and measure other dimensions as well as functional status (e.g., work, self-esteem). In the evolution of quality of life instruments, it has been recognized that it involves multiple dimensions, as shown by Flanagan's study.[16] Whether the dimensions now recognized as contributing to quality of life hold true over time and disease state is dependent on further research.

REFERENCES

1. Luce, J., & Dawson, J. Quality of life. *Semin Oncol,* 1975, *2*(4):323.
2. House, P., Livingston, R., & Swinburn, C. Monitoring mankind: The search for quality. *Behav Sci,* 1975, *20*(1):57.
3. Patrick, D., Bush, J., & Chan, M. Toward an operational definition of health. *J. Health Soc Behav,* 1973, *14*(1):6.
4. Young, K., & Longman, A. Quality of life and persons with melanoma: A pilot study. *Cancer Nurs,* 1983, *6*:219.
5. Berg, R., Hallauer, D., & Berk, S. Neglected aspects of the quality of life. *Health Serv Res,* 1976, *11*(4):391.
6. Gitter, S., & Mostofsky, D. The social indicator: An index of the quality of life. *Soc Biol,* 1973, *20*:289.
7. Charnes, A., Cooper, W., & Kozmetsky, G. Measuring monitoring and modeling quality of life. *Management Sci,* 1973, *19*:1172.
8. Patterson, W.B. The quality of survival in response to treatment. *JAMA,* 1975, *233*(3):280.
9. Hornquist, J.O. The concept of quality of life. *Scand J Soc Med,* 1982, *10*:57.
10. Evans, R., et al. The quality of life with end-stage renal disease. *N Engl J Med,* 1985, *312*(9):553.
11. Bard, M. Summary of the informal discussion of functional states: Quality of Life. *Cancer,* 1984, *53*(10):2327.
12. Palmer, B., Walsh, G., McKinna, J., & Greening, W. Adjuvant chemotherapy for breast cancer: Side effects and quality of life. *Br Med J,* 1980, *281* (6253):1594.
13. Cookfair, D., & Cummings, K. Quality of life among cancer patients. *Advances in Cancer Control: Research and Development.* New York: Alan R. Liss, 1983, p. 445.
14. Wellisch, D. Work, social, recreation, family, and physical status. *Cancer,* 1984, *53*(10):2290.
15. Palmore, E., & Kivett, V. Change in life satisfaction: A longitudinal study of persons aged 46–70. *J Gerontol,* 1977, *32*(3):311.
16. Flanagan, J. Measurement of quality of life: Current state of the art. *Arch Phys Med Rehabil,* 1982, *63*:56.
17. Rippers, V. Scaling the seriousness of illness: A methodological study. *J Psychosom Res,* 1976, *20*(6):567.
18. Ware, J. Conceptualizing disease impact and treatment outcomes. *Cancer,* 1984, *53*(10):2316.
19. Lerner, M. Conceptualization of health and social well-being. *Health Sci Res,* 1973, *8*(1):6.
20. Fletcher, A., & Bulpitt, C. The treatment of hypertension and quality of life. *Qual Life Cardiovasc Care,* 1985, *1*(3):140.
21. Grieco, A., & Long, C. Investigation of the Karnofsky Performance Status as a measure of quality of life. *Health Psychol,* 1984, *3*(2):129.
22. Danoff, B., Kramer, S., Irwin, P., & Gottlieb, A. Assessment of the quality of life in long-term survivors after definitive radiotherapy. *Am J Clin Oncol,* 1983, *6*:339.
23. Padilla, G., Presant, C., Grant, M., et al. Quality of life index for patients with cancer. *Res Nurs Health,* 1983, *6*(2):117.
24. Padilla, G., & Grant, M. Quality of life as a cancer nursing outcome variable. *Adv Nurs Sci,* 1985, *8*(1):45.

25. Presant, C., Klahr, C., & Hogan, L. Evaluating quality-of-life in oncology patients: Pilot observations. *Oncol Nurs Forum*, 1981, *8*(3):26.
26. Bergner, M., Bobbitt, R., Pollard, W., et al. The sickness impact profile: Validation of a health status measure. *Med Care*, 1976, *14*(1):57.
27. U.S. Department of Commerce, Bureau of the Census. *Social indicators, 1976.* Superintendent of Documents, Washington, DC: U.S. Government Printing Office, 1977.
28. Sugarbaker, P., Barofsky, I., Rosenberg, S., & Gianola, F. Quality of life assessment of patients in extremity sarcoma clinical trials. *Surgery*, 1981, *91*(1):17.
29. Karnofsky, D., & Burchenal, J. The clinical evaluation of chemotherapeutic agents in cancer. In C.M. MacLeod (Ed.), *Evaluation of chemotherapeutic agents.* New York: Columbia Press, 1949.
30. Waterhouse, J., & Metcalfe, M. A tool for measuring sexual adjustment in postoperative cancer patients. *Proceedings of the Oncology Nursing Society's Nineth Annual Congress,* Toronto, Canada, May 2–5, 1984.
31. Zubrod, C.G., et al. Appraisal of methods for the study of chemotherapy of cancer in man: Comparative therapeutic trial of nitrogen mustard and triethylene thiophosphoramide. *J Chron Dis,* 1960, *11*:703.
32. Spitzer, W., et al. Measuring the quality of life of cancer patients: A concise QL-Index for use by physicians. *J Chron Dis,* 1981, *34*(12):585.
33. Ryan, L. Quality of life and lung or colon cancer: A prospective study to determine the impact of an experimental treatment. Paper presented at the Tenth Annual Oncology Nursing Society Congress, May 1985, Houston, Texas.
34. Ferrans, C., & Powers, M. Quality of life index: Development and psychometric properties. *Adv Nurs Res,* 1985, *8*(1):15.
35. Ferrans, C. Psychometric assessment of a quality of life index for hemodialysis patients. Doctoral dissertation, University of Illinois, Chicago.
36. Longman, A. Personal communication on quality of life questionnaire tool development (Phase I), May 9, 1984.
37. Johnson, J., King, K., & Murray, R. Measuring the impact of sickness on usual functions of radiation therapy patients. *Oncol Nurs Forum,* 1983, *10*(4):36.
38. Oh, C., et al. A controlled randomized study of early cardiac rehabilitation: The sickness impact profile as an assessment tool. *Heart Lung,* 1983, *12*(2):162.
39. Nocturnal Oxygen Therapy Trial Group. Continuous or nocturnal oxygen therapy in hypoxemic chronic obstructive lung disease. *Ann Intern Med,* 1980, *93*:391.
40. Rockey, P., & Griep, R. Behavioral dysfunction in hyperthyroidism. *Arch Intern Med,* 1980, 140:1194.
41. Deyo, R. Measuring functional outcomes in therapeutic trials in chronic disease. *Controlled Clin Trials,* 1984, *5*:223.
42. Cantril, H. *The pattern of human concerns.* New Brunswick, NJ: Rutgers University Press, 1965.
43. Laborde, J., & Powers, M. Satisfaction with life for patients undergoing hemodialysis and patients suffering from osteoarthritis. *Res Nurs Health,* 1980, *3*(1):19.
44. Penckofer, S., & Holm, K. Early appraisal of coronary revascularization on quality of life. *Nurs Res,* 1984, *33*(2):60.
45. Priestman, T., & Baum, M. Evaluation of quality of life in patients receiving treatment for advanced breast cancer. *Lancet,* 1976, *1*(7965):899.
46. Cotanch, P. Measuring nausea and vomiting in clinical nursing research. *Oncol Nurs Forum,* 1984, *11*(3):92.
47. Schipper, H., Clinch, J., McMurray, A., & Levitt, M. Measuring the quality of life of cancer patients: The functional living index-cancer: Development and validation. *J Clin Oncol* 1984, *2*(5):472.
48. Romsaas, E., Juliani, L., Briggs, A., et al. A method for assessing the rehabilitation needs of oncology outpatients. *Oncol Nurs Forum,* 1983, *10*(3):17.
49. Cain, M., & Henke, C. Living with cancer: A random sample of 50 patients in a hematology-oncology clinic. *Oncol Nurs Forum,* 1978, *5*(3):4.

50. Freidenbergs, I., Gordon, W., Hubbard, M., & Diller, L. Assessment and treatment of psycho-social problems of the cancer patient: A case study. *Cancer Nurs,* 1980, *3*(2):111.
51. Stromborg, M., & Wright, P. Ambulatory cancer patients' perceptions of the physical and psycho-social changes in their lives since the diagnosis of cancer. *Cancer Nurs,* 1984, *7*(2):117.

APPENDIX A (References for Table 4–1)

1. Andrews, F., & Withey, S. *Social indicators of well-being.* New York: Plenum Press, 1976.
2. Bortner, R., & Hultsch, D. A multivariate analysis of correlates of life satisfaction in adulthood. *J Gerontol,* 1970, *25*:41.
3. Cantril, H. *The patterns of human concerns.* New Brunswick, NJ: Rutgers University Press, 1965.
4. Campbell, A. *The sense of well-being in America.* New York: McGraw-Hill, 1981.
5. Campbell, A. Subjective measures of well-being. *Am Psychol,* 1976, *31*:117.
6. Campbell, A., & Converse, P. *Human meaning of social change.* New York: Russell Sage Founda-tion, 1972.
7. Campbell, A., Converse, P., & Rogers, W. *The quality of American life.* New York: Russell Sage Foundation, 1976.
8. Crandall, J., & Putnam, E. Relations between measures of social interest and psychological well-being. *J Individ Psychol,* 1980, *36*:156.
9. Fry, P., & Ghosh, R. Attributional differences in the life satisfactions of the elderly: A cross-cultural comparison of Asian and United States subjects. *Int J Psychol,* 1980, *15*:201.
10. Johnson, J., McCaulley, C., & Copley, J. The quality of life of hemodialysis and transplant patients. *Kidney Int,* 1982, *22*:286.
11. Kazak, A., & Linney, J. Stress, coping, and life change in the single-parent family. *Am J Community Psychol,* 1983, *11*:207.
12. Kilpatrick, F., & Cantril, H. Self-anchoring scaling: A measure of individual's unique reality worlds. *J Individ Psychol,* 1960, *16*:158.
13. Hatz, P., & Powers, M. Factors related to satisfaction with life for patients on hemodialysis. *J Am Nephrol Nurs Technician,* 1980, *1*:290.
14. Jackie, M. Life satisfaction and kidney dialysis. *Nurs Forum,* 1974, *13*:360.
15. Laborde, J., & Powers, M. Satisfaction with life for patients undergoing hemodialysis and patients suffering from osteoarthritis. *Res Nurs Health,* 1980, *3*:19.
16. Levy, N., & Wynbrandt, G. The quality of life on maintenance hemodialysis. *Lancet,* 1975, *1*:1328.
17. Neugarten, G., Havinghurst, R., & Tobin, S. The measure of life satisfaction. *J Gerontol,* 1961, *16*:134.
18. Padilla, G., Present, C., Grant, M., et al. Quality of life index for patients with cancer. *Res Nurs Health,* 1983, *6*:117.
19. Palmore, B., & Kivett, V. Change in life satisfaction: A longitudinal study of persons aged 46–70. *J Gerontol,* 1977, *32*:311.
20. Palmore, E., & Luikart, C. Health and social factors related to life satisfaction. *J Health Soc Behav,* 1972, *13*:68.
21. Penckhofer, S., & Holm, K. Early appraisal of coronary revascularization on quality of life. *Nur Res,* 1984, *33*:60.
22. Soper, W. Relationships between subjectively and statistically determined contributors to life satisfaction for male university faculty. *Psychol Rep,* 1980, *46*:731.
23. Sophie, L., & Powers, M. Life satisfaction and social function: Post-transplant self-evaluation. *Dial Transplant,* 1979, *8*:1198.
24. Watts, W. The future can fend for itself. *Psychology Today,* 1981, *15*:36.
25. Webb, S., & Powers, M. Evaluation of life satisfaction and sexual function in female patients post renal transplant. *Dial Transplant,* 1982, *11*:799.
26. Bonneyu, S., Finkelstein, F., Lytton, B., et al. Treatment of end-stage renal failure in a defined geographic area. *Arch Intern Med,* 1978, *138*:1510.

27. Kaplan De-Nour, A., & Shanan, J. Quality of life of dialysis and transplanted patients. *Nephron*, 1980, *25*:117.
28. Conte, V., & Salamon, M. An objective approach to the measurement and use of life satisfaction with older persons. *Measure Fval Guidance*, 1982, *15*:194.
29. Glenn, N., & McLanahan, S. The effects of offspring on the psychological well-being of older adults. *J Marriage Family*, Vol. 43, May 1981, 409.
30. Keon, T., & McDonald, B. Job satisfaction and life satisfaction: An empirical evaluation of their interrelationship. *Hum Relations* 1982, *35*:167.

CHAPTER 5

Multiple Instruments for Measuring Quality of Life

Hannah Dean R.N.C., Ph.D.

Health care providers want to improve the quality of life of the people they serve. They make decisions on the basis of what they suppose to be the expected quality of life for patients. They interpret the admonition to "Do no harm" in terms of the expected quality of life outcome of treatment or no treatment, surgery or no surgery, and this treatment or an alternative treatment.

IMPORTANCE OF MEASURING QUALITY OF LIFE

The conceptualization and measurement of quality of life are vital to health policy, evaluation research, and clinical decision making. Kaplan and Bush[1] argue the importance of health-related quality of life for evaluation research and policy analysis. They indicate the need for a means to compare the outcomes of different interventions for different disease groups in different populations. Vaisrub alludes to the importance of quality of life as a measure of the usefulness of cardiac revascularization when he says, "The attained 'quality of life' [after cardiac revascularization] is apt to be void of social usefulness" (p. 236).[2]

Two recent evaluation studies startled the hospice community when their results failed to indicate significant differences in the quality of life between dying persons in hospice and nonhospice settings.[3,4] Such findings, if considered valid and replicable, could lead to limitations in funding for programs. It is incumbent on researchers to ensure that the measures used are valid and sufficiently sensitive to detect differences in quality of life in dying persons.

Schipper et al.[5] suggest that patients should be informed about the quality of life and the survival statistics as part of informed consent regarding the management of their cancers. Lynch[6] moderated a grand rounds in critical care in which Engelhardt discussed the "quality of life" versus the "quality of morbidity." Engelhardt makes a strong case for the importance of providing patients with a clear picture of the impact of treatment. Informed consent requires that patients have information upon which to decide whether increased lifespan is worth the morbidity associated with their conditions or their treatment or both. For example, Sugarbaker et al.[7] report evidence that suggests that amputation for sarcoma is less disruptive to quality of life than is a limb-sparing procedure involving surgery and irradiation.

Clinical decision making also requires attention to factors that influence compliance. An extensive study of the effects of antihypertensive therapy on the quality of life compared three antihypertensive agents. Croog et al.[8] report this excellent quality of life study using multiple instruments and a comparative design. The resulting data provide health care professionals with information that will assist them in choosing medications to improve compliance with the medical regimen for hypertension.

Significant health policy and clinical decisions may depend on the perceived effect on quality of life of various approaches to providing care. The data on which such decisions are made must be replicable, valid, and sufficiently sensitive to yield meaningful results.

APPROACHES TO MEASURING QUALITY OF LIFE

This chapter focuses on the use of multiple instruments to measure quality of life as a multidimensional, complex concept. The multiple instrument approach is advocated because of the need for reliable, comparable, valid, and sensitive measurements. Use of multiple instruments allows flexibility in the conceptualization of quality of life while permitting comparability of specific dimensions across studies. Employing increasingly sensitive measures for specific domains may be more feasible with the use of multiple instruments.

Frank-Stromborg[9] reports on selecting a single instrument to measure quality of life. She emphasizes four decisions a researcher must make in choosing an instrument: qualitative versus quantitative measures, subjective versus objective reporters, subjective versus objective dimensions, and single versus multiple instruments. Other choices emerge from the literature, such as global versus domain-specific measures, societal versus individual perspectives, and cognitive versus affective evaluations.

Global measures of quality of life include those that seek responses, such as the following:

> Please mark with an X the appropriate place within the bar to indicate your rating of this person's quality of life during the past week. (100 mm bar with "lowest quality" on the left and "highest quality" on the right) (p. 589).[10]

This approach assumes that the respondent can provide a valid overall assessment of quality of life. A global approach implies unidimensionality. Domain-specific approaches seek assessments of variables related to a multidimensional concept. Domain-specific data may be achieved by either single or multiple instruments.

Societal versus individual perspectives of the quality of life may vary considerably. The researcher should clarify which approach is being used. Conclusions should reflect limitations to generalizations based on the approach used. Campbell[11] alludes to this distinction when he argues that the individual's experience of quality of life may not relate directly to societal indicators, such as education, mortality, and employment.

George[12] distinguishes between cognitive and affective evaluations of life quality. Cognitive evaluations are those based on the facts of a person's circumstances. Affective evaluations reflect how respondents feel about their quality of life irrespective of the objective facts. Both approaches have value in measuring quality of life.

CONCEPTUALIZING QUALITY OF LIFE

In spite of frequent references to quality of life in relation to health care issues in the professional and public press, the definition of the concept remains elusive. A review of the literature reveals a variety of terms equated with quality of life, such as life satisfaction,[13–15] self-esteem,[16] well-being,[17–19] health,[7,20,21] happiness,[22] adjustment,[23] value of life,[24] meaning of life,[25,26] and functional status.[27,28]

Additionally, the dimensions of the concept of quality of life vary from study to study. Hutchinson et al.[29] identify physical, social, and emotional dimensions. Flanagan[30] describes 15 aspects in 5 categories, including physical and material well-being, relations with other people, social, community, and civic activities, personal development and fulfilment, and recreation. McSweeney et al.[31] define quality of life as emotional functioning, social role functioning, and participation in activities of daily living and recreational pastimes. Linn and Linn[32] operationalize quality of life as scores on scales of depression, self-esteem, life satisfaction, alienation, and locus of control. Levy and Wynbrandt[33] report on quality of life in terms of income, sexual activity, and lifestyle.

Acceptance of the premise that quality of life is a multidimensional concept demands a conceptual framework identifying the elements of which it is comprised. Two authors present specific frameworks that may prove useful in clinical nursing research.

The Ware Framework

Ware[34] proposes five elements to be used as guides in selecting instruments to measure quality of life: disease, personal functioning, psychologic distress/well-being, general health perceptions, and social/role functioning. Disease is central because it is the focus of our interest, the reason we are interested in a particular population for study. Ware recommends disease-specific measures because of the heterogeneity of the concept. Personal functioning is defined as the performance of or capacity to perform the activities of daily living (ADL), such as self-care, mobility, and physical activities.

Ware insists that the third element, psychologic distress and well-being, be measured using specific measures of psychologic status. General health perceptions refers to self-rated measures of general health and well-being. Finally, role functioning is distinguished from personal functioning and refers to the performance of or capacity to perform activities associated with an individual's usual role, such as father, mother, companion, helpmate.

The George and Bearon Framework

George and Bearon[35] selected four dimensions to define quality of life, including both subjective evaluations and objective conditions. Their subjective evaluations include life satisfaction and self-esteem; their objective conditions include general health/functional status and socioeconomic status. They present detailed accounts of 21 instruments for and methods of measuring the proposed dimensions, with descriptions, measurement properties, and recommendations for use of each.

INSTRUMENTS USED TO MEASURE ELEMENTS OF QUALITY OF LIFE

Frank-Stromborg[9] describes 13 methods of measuring quality of life with a single instrument. Some of the instruments described by her might also be suitable in a multiple instrument approach. For example, the Sickness Impact Profile (SIP), the Karnovsky Performance

Status Scale, and Cantril's Self-Anchoring Striving Scale can serve as measures of elements within a conceptual framework.

The instruments described in this chapter are organized according to major studies in which they were used as measures of quality of life. This arrangement illustrates conceptual frameworks and multiple instruments in quality of life research. Three additional instruments are included because they relate to quality of life research.

Burckhardt Study

Burckhardt[36] studied the impact of physical, psychologic, and social factors on the perception of quality of life among 94 people with arthritis in a community. She created a quality of life index using a single question rating the subject's overall quality of life, the Life Satisfaction Index (LSI-Z), and the Domain Satisfaction Scale.

· LIFE SATISFACTION INDEX (LSI-Z)

Wood et al.[37] developed the LSI-Z as a short form of the Life Satisfaction Rating (LSR), devised by Neugarten et al. in 1961. The LSI-Z consists of 13 items to which the subject is asked to respond with "agree," "disagree," or "?." Sample items are:

This is the dreariest time of my life.

I am just as happy as when I was younger.

"Agree" answers score 2 points and "?" answers score 1 point. All items must be answered. The validity and reliability coefficients between the original LSR and the LSI-Z were 0.57 and 0.79, respectively.

· DOMAIN SATISFACTION SCALE

Burckhardt describes the Domain Satisfaction Scale as developed from empirical data by Flanagan,[30] using a 7-point rating scale developed by Andrews and Withey.[38] She refers to Campbell et al.[39] when describing the reliability and validity of the tool.

· INDEX OF DOMAIN SATISFACTIONS

The Index of Domain Satisfactions was developed by Campbell et al.[39] Respondents rate their satisfaction with each domain on the a 7-point rating scale ranging from "completely satisfied" to "completely dissatisfied." The domains explored include marriage, family life, health, neighborhood, friendships, housework, job, life in the United States, city or county, nonwork, housing, usefulness of education, standard of living, amount of education, and savings. The nonwork item follows several questions about leisure time:

Overall, how satisfied are you with the ways you spend your spare time?
Which number comes closest to how satisfied or dissatisfied you feel?

(1 = completely satisfied; 7 = completely dissatisfied.)

Results are reported with overall distribution of responses on each scale and average score values. Campbell et al. report stability correlations ranging from 0.42 to 0.67 for the individual domains and 0.76 for the sum of 14 domain satisfactions.[39] Validity is not addressed explicitly. However, the domains selected relate to everyday life and are similar to those identified by Flanagan[30] and Andrews and Withey.[38]

The Evans et al. Study

Evans et al.[40] report a study of quality of life of 859 patients with end-stage renal disease. Objective measures of functional ability were obtained using the Karnovsky Index and the patient's response to the question:

Are you *now able* to work for pay full time, part time, or not at all?

Subjective indicators were drawn from the work of Campbell et al.,[39] including the Index of Psychological Affect, the Index of Overall Life Satisfaction, and the Index of Well-Being.

▪ INDEX OF PSYCHOLOGICAL AFFECT

The Index of Psychological Affect (called the Index of General Affect by Campbell et al.[39]) consists of eight semantic differential items, including boring/interesting, miserable/enjoyable, useless/worthwhile, lonely/friendly, empty/full, discouraging/hopeful, rewarding/disappointing, and brings out the best in me/doesn't give me much chance.[40] Respondents place an X in one of seven boxes between the bipolar items indicating their feelings about their present lives. Campbell et al. report a reliability coefficient of 0.89 on the Index of General Affect.[39] Correlations with the overall life satisfaction item ($r = 0.55$) and the happiness item ($r = 0.52$) provide indications of validity.

▪ INDEX OF OVERALL LIFE SATISFACTION

Evans et al. are unclear about their use of the Index of Overall Life Satisfaction.[40] Campbell et al. measure the Index of Domain Satisfactions, and they include an overall life satisfaction item:

We have talked about various parts of your life, now I want to ask you about your life as a whole. How satisfied are you with your life as a whole these days? Which number on the card comes closest to how satisfied or dissatisfied you are with your life as a whole?

(1 = completely satisfied; 7 = completely dissatisfied.)

In a repeat interview with 285 subjects 8 months after the initial data collection, the stability correlation for the Index of Overall Life Satisfaction was 0.43.[40] Campbell et al. do not address validity explicitly.

▪ INDEX OF WELL-BEING

The Index of Well-Being [40] is a composite of the Index of Overall Life Satisfaction and the Index of General Affect. The estimated reliability is reported to be 0.89. Validity is not addressed.

The Lewis Study

Lewis' study of late-stage cancer patients is the third major study from which instrument examples are drawn.[41] Lewis chose the Rosenberg Self-Esteem Scale, the Crumbaugh Purpose-in-Life Test, and the Lewis et al. Anxiety Scale as indicators of the psychosocial aspects of quality of life.

• ROSENBERG SELF-ESTEEM SCALE

The Rosenberg Self-Esteem Scale purports to measure a basic feeling of self-worth. It consists of 10 items to which the subject responds on a 4-point scale from "strongly agree" to "strongly disagree." Lewis reports reliability coefficients from 0.85 to 0.92 and validity correlations ranging from 0.56 to 0.83 with similar measures.

• CRUMBAUGH PURPOSE-IN-LIFE TEST (PIL)

The Crumbaugh Purpose-in-Life Test[42] is a 20-item instrument to which subjects respond on a 7-point scale. Sample items include the following:

> In life I have no goals or aims at all (1) . . .
>> very clear goals and aims (7).

> I am a very irresponsible person (1) . . .
>> a very responsible person (7).

The Purpose-in-Life Test is designed to measure the degree to which the subject experiences a sense of meaning and purpose in life. Split-half correlations are reported to be 0.85 in a sample of church parishioners. PIL scores correlated with therapist ratings (0.38, $n = 50$) and minister ratings (0.47, $n = 120$).

• LEWIS ET AL. ANXIETY SCALE

The Lewis et al. Anxiety Scale[43] was developed for use with cancer patients. Subjects respond to nine items on a 5-point scale (1 = none of the time; 5 = all of the time), including:

> I feel more nervous than usual.
> I get irritable over small matters.
> I am jittery.

Lewis[41] reports stability reliability at 0.90 and split-half reliability at 0.79. According to Lewis, validity was established by its inverse relation with an attitude scale measuring perceived functional effectiveness.

Three Additional Instruments

Three additional instruments that may have utility in multiple instrument studies as measures of psychologic well-being include the Philadelphia Geriatric Center (PGC) Morale Scale, the Bradburn Affect Balance Scale (ABS), and the Spielberger State-Trait Anxiety Inventory (STAI).

• PHILADELPHIA GERIATRIC CENTER (PGC) MORALE SCALE

The Revised Philadelphia Geriatric Center (PGC) Morale Scale is a 17-item instrument requiring mostly "yes" or "no" answers.[44] Designed to measure morale in aging populations, the PGC Morale Scale assumes morale to be multidimensional. The revised PGC Morale Scale was tested on 828 elderly people. Sample items include:

I get upset easily.
I sometimes feel that life isn't worth living.

The items factor into three dimensions: agitation (6 items), attitude toward own aging (5 items), and lonely dissatisfaction (6 items), each with a high degree of internal consistency (Cronbach coefficient alpha 0.85, 0.81, and 0.85, respectively). The original PGC Morale Scale[45] was validated by comparing scores with ratings by professionals of institutionalized patients' morale (criterion validity coefficient was 0.47) and with the Neugarten et al. Life Satisfaction Rating. The correlation between PGC Morale Scale and Life Satisfaction Rating was 0.57.

• BRADBURN AFFECT BALANCE SCALE (ABS)

George and Bearon[35] report on the ABS, a ten-item measure of feelings toward life. Respondents answer "yes" or "no" to questions about five positive and five negative feelings experienced in the previous few weeks. The positive and negative dimensions are separate. The instrument is constructed to compare the number of positive affect responses to the number of negative affect responses. Scores range from -4 to $+4$, with positive scores representing greater degrees of happiness. Reliability is demonstrated by a test–retest correlation of 0.76. Correlations with an 18-item version of the LSI-A* and Rosow Morale Scale ($r = 0.66$ and 0.61, respectively) indicate validity for the ABS. George and Bearon describe the ABS as the best available measure of affect.

• SPIELBERGER STATE-TRAIT ANXIETY INVENTORY (STAI)

The STAI[46] provides self-report measures of both state and trait anxiety as a means of measuring psychologic well-being. Subjects respond on a 4-point scale (not at all, somewhat, moderately so, and very much so) to 20 items according to the way they feel at the moment as a measure of state anxiety. Trait anxiety is measured by responses on a 4-point scale (almost never, sometimes, often, and almost always) to 20 items that indicate how subjects generally feel. Items on the state form include, for example:

I feel at ease.
I feel nervous.
I am worried.

---

*One of the versions of the Life Satisfaction Index designed by Neugarten, Havighurst, and Tobin in 1961.

Trait form items include the following:

> I feel satisfied with myself.
> I am happy.
> I am a steady person.

According to Dreger,[47] the STAI is among the best of the standardized anxiety measures. He reports alpha reliability coefficients of 0.83 to 0.92 for state anxiety scores and 0.86 to 0.92 for trait scores for the normative samples. Correlations with the IPAT Anxiety Scale* (0.75), the Manifest Anxiety Scale (0.80), and the Adjective Check List (0.52) provide estimates of validity.

SUMMARY

The use of multiple instruments has the potential for solving problems of comparability and sensitivity. The researcher must consider the problems that may result from such a strategy, however, such as administration, time requirements, and directions. Administration of instruments varies; instruments may require completion by the researcher, by a health care professional, by the subject, or by a significant other. When choosing multiple instruments to measure elements of quality of life, the researcher must attend to variations in administration. The time required of respondents affects willingness to participate in research. The cumulative time required to complete multiple instruments is a prime consideration. Flanagan[48] cautions about ensuring that directions to respondents are clear. The use of multiple instruments may increase the possibility of confusion about the directions for completion.

Choosing multiple instruments for measuring quality of life has the advantage of allowing flexibility in the conceptualization of the quality of life. As the concept is refined and clarified, researchers using multiple instruments will be able to compare specific dimensions. As more sensitive instruments are developed, substitutions may be made without having to change all instruments in a battery.

REFERENCES

1. Kaplan, R., & Bush, J. Health-related quality of life measurement for evaluation research and policy analysis. *Health Psychol*, 1981, *1*(1):61.
2. Vaisrub, S. Quality of life manque. *JAMA*, 1976, *236*(4):387.
3. Wales, J., Kane, R., Robbins, S., et al. UCLA hospice evaluation study. *Med Care*, 1983, *21*(7):734.
4. Greer, D., & Mor, V. *A preliminary report of the National Hospice Study*, Washington, DC: Health and Human Services, 1984.
5. Schipper, H., Clinch, J., McMurray, A., & Levitt, M. Measuring the quality of life of cancer patients: The Functional Living Index—Cancer: Development and validation. *J Clin Oncol*, 1984, *2*(5):472.
6. Lynch, E. To treat or not to treat—The dilemma. *Heart Lung*, 1978, *7*(3):499.
7. Sugarbaker, P.H., Barofsky, I., Rosenberg, S.A., & Gianola, F.J. Quality of life assessment of patients in extremity sarcoma clinical trials. *Surgery*, 1982, *91*(1):17.
8. Croog, S.H., Levine, S., Testa, M.A., et al. The effects of antihypertensive therapy on the quality of life. *N Engl J Med*, 1986, *314*(26):1657.

*One of the standardized measures of anxiety developed by the Institute for Personality and Ability Testing, Inc.

9. Frank-Stromborg, M. Selecting an instrument to measure quality of life. *Oncol Nurs Forum*, 1984, *11*(5):88.
10. Spitzer, W., Dobson, A., Hall, J., et al. Measuring the quality of life of cancer patients. *J Chronic Dis*, 1981, *34*(12):585.
11. Campbell, A. Subjective measures of well-being. *Am Psychologist*, 1976, *31*(2):117.
12. George, L. Subjective well-being: Conceptual and methodological issues. In C. Eisdorfer (Ed.), *Annual review of gerontology and geriatrics, Vol. 2* New York: Springer, 1981, p. 345.
13. Brown, J., Rawlinson, M., & Hilles, N. Life satisfaction and chronic disease: Exploration of a theoretical model. *Med Care*, 1981, *19*(11):1136.
14. Laborde, J., & Powers, M. Satisfaction with life for patients undergoing hemodialysis and patients suffering from osteoarthritis. *Res Nurs Health*, 1980, *3*(1):19.
15. Ferrans, C.E., & Powers, M.J. Quality of life index: Development and psychometric properties. *Adv Nurs Sci*, 1985, *8*(1):15.
16. Ziller, R. Self-other orientations and quality of life. *Social Indicators Res*, 1974, *1*:301.
17. Fletcher, A., & Bulpitt, C. The treatment of hypertension and quality of life. *Qual Life Cardiovasc Care*, 1985, *1*(3):140.
18. House, P., Livingston, R., & Swinburn, C. Monitoring mankind: The search for quality. *Behav Sci*, 1975, *20*:57.
19. Carstensen, L., & Cone, J. Social desirability and the measurement of psychological well being in elderly persons. *J Gerontol*, 1983, *38*(6):713.
20. Bergner, M., Bobbitt, R., Pollard, W., et al. The sickness impact profile: Validation of a health status measure. *Med Care*, 1976, *14*(1):57.
21. Lerner, M. Conceptualization of health and social well-being. *Health Services Res*, 1973, *8*:6.
22. Shinn, D., & Johnson, D. Avowed happiness as an overall assessment of quality of life. *Social Indicators Res*, 1978, *5*:475.
23. Crewe, N. Quality of life: The ultimate goal in rehabilitation. *Minn Med*, 1980, Aug:586.
24. Bayles, M. The value of life—By what standard? *Am J Nurs*, 1980, *80*(12):2226.
25. Berg, R., Hallauer, D., & Berk, S. Neglected aspects of quality of life. *Health Serv Res*, 1976, *11*(4):391.
26. Mount, B., & Scott, J. Wither hospice evaluation? *J Chronic Dis*, 1983, *36*(11):731.
27. Hochberg, F., Linggood, R., Wolfson, L., et al. Quality and duration of survival in glioblastoma multiforme. *JAMA*, 1979, *241*(10):1016.
28. Gilbert, H., Kagan, A., Nussbaum, H., et al. Evaluation of radiation therapy for bone metastases: Pain relief and quality of life. *Am J Roentgenol*, 1977, *129*(6):1095.
29. Hutchinson, A., Farndon, J., & Wilson, R. Quality of survival of patients following mastectomy. *Clin Oncol*, 1979, *5*:391.
30. Flanagan, J. A research approach to improving our quality of life. *Am Psychologist*, 1978, *33*(2):138.
31. McSweeney, A., Grant, I., Heaton, R., et al. Life quality of patients with chronic obstructive pulmonary disease. *Arch Intern Med*, 1982, *142*(3):473.
32. Linn, B., & Linn, M. Late stage cancer patients: Age differences in their psychophysical status and response to counseling. *J Gerontol*, 1981, *36*(6):689.
33. Levy, N., & Wynbrandt, G. The quality of life on maintenance hemodialysis. *Lancet*, 1975, *1*(7920):1328.
34. Ware, J. Conceptualizing disease impact and treatment outcomes. *Cancer*, 1984, *53*(10):2316.
35. George, L., & Bearon, L. *Quality of life in older persons: Meaning and measurement.* New York: Human Sciences Press. 1980.
36. Burckhardt, C. The impact of arthritis on quality of life. *Nurs Res*, 1985, *34*(1):11.
37. Wood, V., Wylie, M., & Sheafor, B. An analysis of a short self-report measure of life satisfaction: Correlation with rater judgements. *J Gerontol*, 1969, *24*:465.
38. Andrews, F., & Withey, S. *Social indicators of well-being.* New York: Plenum Press, 1976.
39. Campbell, A., Converse, P., and Rodgers, W. *The quality of American life.* New York: Russell Sage, 1976.
40. Evans, R., Manninen, D., Garrison, L., et al. The quality of life of patients with end stage renal disease. *N Engl J Med*, 1985, *312*(9):553.

41. Lewis, F. Experienced personal control and quality of life in late-stage cancer patients. *Nurs Res,* 1982, *31*(2):113.
42. Crumbaugh, J. Cross validation of purpose-in-life test based on Frankl's concepts. *J Individ Psychol,* 1968, *24*(1):74.
43. Lewis, F., Firsich, S., & Parsell, S. Clinical tool development for adult chemotherapy patients: Process and content. *Cancer Nurs,* 1979, *2*(2):99.
44. Lawton, M. The Philadelphia Geriatric Center morale scale: A revision. *J Gerontol,* 1975, *30*(1):85.
45. Lawton, M. The dimensions of morale. In D. Kent, R. Kastenbaum, & S. Sherwood (Eds.), *Research, planning and action for the elderly.* New York: Behavioral Publications, 1972, p. 144.
46. Spielberger, C. STAI—Self-evaluation questionnaire. Palo Alto, CA: Consulting Psychologists Press, 1977.
47. Dreger, R. Review of the State-Trait Anxiety Inventory. In O. Buros (Ed.), *The eighth mental measurements yearbook.* Highland Park, NJ: Gryphon Press, 1978, p. 1094.
48. Flanagan, J. Measurement of quality of life: Current state of the art. *Arch Phys Med Rehabil,* 1982, *63*(2):56.

CHAPTER 6

Social Support: Conceptualizations and Measurement Instruments

Ada M. Lindsey, R.N., Ph.D.

It has been observed that people diagnosed with the same condition, of approximately similar severity who are being treated with the same prescribed therapeutic regimen have considerable variation in recovery patterns and in adaptation or adjustment to living with the condition. These observations have led clinicians and investigators to consider the possible contribution of other variables in influencing the responses to illness.

One such variable that is receiving increasing attention is social support. For example, there are recent reviews of social support,[1-5] descriptions of the properties of social support,[1-2,6-8] studies including social support as a variable,[9-16] and reports of development of instruments to measure social support.[17-23]

The importance of social support as a variable is that it may influence health outcomes. The quality and availability of social support may have an important role in recovery processes after illness. Current theories suggest that social support may have a protective function, serve a stress-buffering or moderating role in health maintenance, and be related to positive health outcomes.[24-28] Loss or lack of social support has been linked with a variety of conditions and illnesses.[11,29-32]

Cassel[33] is one of the few investigators who has proposed a mechanism for the role of social environment in disease etiology, suggesting that the social environmental stressors alter the neuroendocrine balance and thus increase susceptibility to disease. People deprived of meaningful social contact do not receive adequate information or feedback. Cassel speculated that this is a key property of those with inadequate social environments. In contrast, people with adequate social support are helped in coping with crisis and adapting to change.

Socially competent individuals are likely to have well-developed social networks and, as a result, may be more resistant to the effects of stressors.[34] People considered to be well-integrated and functioning well will receive more assistance from others.[35] Cobb[36] suggests there is evidence that high levels of social support have an influence on recovery from illness, and this facilitation may be accomplished through increased compliance with the prescribed medical regimen.

Caplan[37] proposed that having social support implies that the person has an enduring pattern of relationships over time. A social support network provides "psychosocial supplies" for the individual, and these "supplies" provide for the maintenance of health of the individual. "A common impression of social support is that it provides armor to individuals who need it, can find it and use it . . ." (p. 158).[5]

The quality and availability of social support may have an important role in an individual's recovery from or adaptation to an illness or surgery. For example, social support perceived to be adequate may facilitate a person's coping with stressful life events or a major crisis, in maintaining health, or in adapting to changes.

CONCEPTUALIZATIONS OF SOCIAL SUPPORT

Further study is necessary to determine whether social support influences health, what types of support are more important under what specific circumstances, and the mechanisms by which social support exerts an influence. Because of the increased interest in social support as a moderator variable, definitions, conceptualizations, identification of distinguishing characteristics, and creation of instruments to measure social support have evolved in recent years.

Several of the major conceptualizations of social support are reviewed in detail elsewhere.[1-6,8] They are briefly summarized here to provide a context for selection of an instrument to measure social support.

The definition provided by Cobb[24] states that social support is provision of information that leads people to believe they are cared for, loved, esteemed, valued, and a member of a network of communication and mutual obligation. Caplan[38] recognized that support is from continuing, enduring relationships. Significant others help in mobilizing psychologic resources and mastering emotional burdens; they are a refuge or sanctuary for stability and comfort. They share tasks and provide material supplies, skills, and cognitive guidance to improve the individual's handling of situations.

The perception of having a confidant or at least one, close, confiding relationship is considered to be a strong indicator of social support.[39-41] Weiss[42] used the construct, social relationships, as the major focus and acknowledged the multiple functions of the construct. The six functions of social relationships described by Weiss are social integration, reliable alliance, guidance, opportunity for nurturance, reassurance of worth, and attachment/ intimacy. Social integration is provided through a network of relationships in which participants share concerns, information, and ideas; a sense of reliable alliance is provided primarily through relationships with kin in which the person is assured of continuing assistance. Obtaining guidance occurs during stressful situations when the individual seeks emotional support and cognitive guidance from a trustworthy and authoritative figure. Opportunity for nurturance refers to an adult taking responsibility for the well-being of another. Reassurance of worth occurs through recognition of a person's competence in a social role. Attachment or intimacy refers to gaining a sense of security and place.

The conceptualization of social support proposed by House[43] has four supportive behavior categories that reflect four types of support: informational, appraisal, instrumental, and emotional. The emotional type of support is the provision of empathy and demonstration of love, trust, and caring. Instrumental support is the access of the individual to behaviors that directly help in time of need. Informational support occurs through the provision of information that the person can use in coping with personal and environmental problems. Appraisal support is the transmission of information relevant to self-evaluation.

Kahn[44] conceptualized social support as consisting of interpersonal transactions that include the expression of positive affect of one person toward another, the affirmation of another's behaviors, perceptions, or expressed views, and the giving of symbolic or material aid to another person. The term "convoy" is used to denote the set of significant people through whom support is given or received. The characteristic of reciprocity is included in the conceptualization of social support by both Kahn[44] and Caplan.[38]

Bloom[3] presents a conceptual overview of social support systems and cancer and addresses well the problem of differences and imprecisions in definitions of the multidimensional construct of social support. In Bloom's review, five components of social support were identified: feedback to the individual about himself or herself, the expression of acceptance and affection, tangible material support, information, and affiliative aspects.

Examples of differences in approaches to conceptualizations of social support are given for two studies conducted in elderly persons. Rundall and Evashwick[9] make a distinction between social network and support network in their study of social network and help-seeking among 883 elderly persons. These investigators developed a typology of four categories: engaged, abandoned, trapped, and disengaged. The typology includes the level of interaction with the network and the satisfaction with the level of interaction. The use of health and social services by these subjects was found to vary according to the behavior category (e.g., engaged versus abandoned). The adequacy of social support was measured in 331 older adults ($\geq$65 years) living in a community.[12] Social support was conceptualized from the perspective of three parameters: roles and available attachments, perceived support, and frequency of social interaction. These three components of social support were found to predict the 30-month mortality.

An individual's social support system is comprised of multiple networks. These include the kinship network (spouse or partner, family members, and other relatives), social and role networks (friends, neighbors, and work associates), professional networks (health care providers and other professionals), and community networks (church and community groups and agencies).[4]

Social support also has been examined in the context of family functioning. Caplan[45] acknowledges that support system functions depend on stability, intactness, and integration of the family. Eight support system functions of the contemporary American family were identified; examples of these functions are family as collector and disseminator of information, as source of practical service and concrete aid, as source and validation of identity, and as haven for rest and recuperation.[38]

The social support system is a composite of interpersonal relationships that satisfy specific personal social needs.[4] Social support is a component of human relationships. These relationships are the formal and informal social support systems.

There are distinctions between the support network and perceived or actual social supportive behaviors. The network is the group of people with whom the person has social connections; these relationships may be formal or informal and can be described by size, density, and complexity. The network serves such functions as the provision of information and aid. The impact these network functions are perceived to have on the person is the social support.[21] The extent the person believes or feels the supportive behaviors provided by the network have met his or her needs is the perceived level of social support. Quantitative descriptions of the social network and network analysis are beyond the scope of this chapter and are available elsewhere.[46,47]

The perception of support and the actual support provided may be incongruent. Individual traits, attitudes, and moods may influence both the perceived and the actual support available and provided. In stressful circumstances, a person may include available social support in the appraisal process, and the subsequent seeking of support may be a response to obtain information or other support to deal with the stressful event.[21] The social support available may thus influence the individual's subsequent coping or adapting to the circumstance.

Social support has both qualitative and quantitative dimensions and includes both subjective and objective perceptions. Social support varies according to age and life situation.[31] Social support varies with availability of sources of support, accessibility to those sources, nature and intensity of the relationship, and changes in level of functioning. Thus, measuring social support at one point in time will not reflect this variability. Past experiences, perceived need, and other demands may influence provision and perception of social support available.

Social support is derived from people, places, and activities. Factors influencing the giving or receiving of social support include interpersonal, cultural, environmental, and physical; for example, geographical proximity of persons in the individual's support network may facilitate or constrain the provision of supportive behaviors. Ability to generate support for self would influence the perceived adequacy of social support available. Measurement instruments must be sufficiently sensitive to capture these subtle differences.

There is a need to determine levels of social support in healthy people to use as normative data for comparison with levels of social support in people who are ill. There is a need to study the reciprocity of social support, not just the receiving aspect. There are a number of unresolved issues; for example, what are the critical supportive behaviors, and how do they differ in relation to different stressful life events? What types of support and sources of support are most important in which set of circumstances? What are the most important structural properties of social support networks for the provision of social support perceived to be adequate? What is the nature of the support relationships that leads to improved coping or adjustments? Are the same elements of social support perceived to be important in all cultures? It is apparent that many very important questions about social support remain unanswered.

Norbeck[8] developed a model that includes elements of social support and nursing practice and proposed relationships between the two that need to be studied. Properties of the individual and of the situation and the influences of these on the need for social support and on the availability of support are described.

If, in fact, social support is a moderator variable influencing maintenance of health and health outcomes, determining the level of perceived social support, the availability of support, and changes in support over time become important clinical considerations. Enhancing or facilitating the quality or quantity of support may be a crucial intervention strategy. If this is the case, there is need for a measure of social support to document baseline support in health as well as at the time of diagnosis and throughout the illness and treatment trajectory.[48]

INSTRUMENTS TO MEASURE SOCIAL SUPPORT

Social support is a multidimensional construct. As yet, there is no universally accepted definition or conceptualization of social support. Thus efforts to create instruments to measure social support also reflect this range of diversity.

Murawski et al.[6] suggest that measurement of social support should include determination of the individual's interpersonal support system, characteristics of his or her social roles in the primary support group, beliefs about sources of support that would be available during an illness, patterns of social affiliation, and need for social affiliation. They perceive these aspects to be critical elements of social support.

A variety of approaches has been used in studies of social support. For example, questions were embedded in studies to assess social support resources, such as marital status, frequency of contacts with parents, children, friends, living arrangements, and other indicators of social ties. Approaches to the measurement of social support have included assessment of the respondent's perceptions of the supportive aspects of their social environments,[49,50] of receiving supportive behaviors,[20] of satisfaction with support available,[19] and of affect, affirmation, and aid potentially available.[17,18]

As recently as 1977, Dean and Lin[26] were unable to locate any measures of social support with known or acceptable reliability or validity data. The following section is a brief summary of instruments that purport to measure social support or some aspect of it. Published reliability and validity data are given, and examples of items are included.

• PERSONAL RESOURCE QUESTIONNAIRE (PRQ)

Brandt and Weinert,[19] nurse researchers, developed the Personal Resource Questionnaire (PRQ) as a measure of the multidimensional characteristics of social support. The instrument has two parts. Information about the person's resources and the person's satisfaction with the resources is obtained from part one. Information about the existence of a confidant is obtained from one item in part one. The second part is based on the social relationship dimensions described by Weiss.[42] There is a 25-item Likert scale and a 5-item self-help ideology scale included as part two of the PRQ. The authors report a high internal consistency reliability coefficient ($\alpha = 0.89$) for part two. They suggest that the moderate intercorrelations obtained for intimacy, social integration, worth, and assistance subscales reflect some overlap. The nurturance subscale is thought to be independent because there were low intercorrelations between that scale and the other four. Additional reliability or validity data are not reported.

Eight life situations were created for part one of the PRQ. The situations include circumstances in which the person may need assistance, and the respondent is asked who or what they could turn to for help (e.g., no one, spouse, child, relative, friend, spiritual advisor, professional person, agency, books, or prayer). Following identification of the sources of support, the individual is asked if he or she has actually experienced the situation recently and, if so, what was the extent of satisfaction felt with the assistance obtained.

Part two has 5 items for each of Weiss' five social relationship dimensions[42] (intimacy, social integration, nurturance, worth, and assistance). A 7-point Likert scale is used for the respondent to rate each of 25 items from "strongly agree" to "strongly disagree." A few sample items are given in the report of the development of this instrument.[19]

Sometimes I can't count on my relatives and friends to help me with important problems.

There is someone I feel close to who makes me feel secure (p. 278).[19]

The last section (5 items) of part two of the PRQ was included as an estimate of the respondents' ideologic stance toward self-help. These items were used to determine if the PRQ was measuring the constructs of social support.[19] Development of the PRQ is reported as part of a study in which the PRQ was used as a measure of social support; the stress of long-term illness (multiple sclerosis) on the well spouses and family functioning was investigated.

• NORBECK SOCIAL SUPPORT QUESTIONNAIRE (NSSQ)

The Norbeck Social Support Questionnaire (NSSQ)[17,18] is another instrument that has been developed by nurse researchers to measure the multidimensional construct of social support. It is a short, self-administered questionnaire. The instrument taps three major components:

functional aspects, network, and loss. Affect, affirmation, and aid are the functional aspects assessed, and number in the network, duration of relationships, and frequency of contact are the network properties measured. Total loss includes the number of source of support categories in which a loss occurred and the perceived amount of support lost.

Conceptual definitions of social support proposed by Kahn[44] were used as the theoretical basis for the NSSQ. Social support is defined as "interpersonal transactions that include one or more of the following: the expression of positive affect of one person toward another; the affirmation or endorsement of another person's behaviors, perceptions, or expressed views; the giving of symbolic or material aid to another" (p. 85).[44] The term "convoy" was suggested by Kahn as representing the vehicle for provision of social support. "An individual's convoy at any point in time thus consists of the set of persons on whom he or she relies for support and those who rely on him or her for support" (p. 84).[44] The NSSQ includes items to tap the three supportive transaction components (affect, affirmation, and aid) and to assess representative convoy or network properties (number in network, frequency of contact, and duration of relationships).

The first item on the NSSQ asks the respondent to "list each significant person in your life" considering "all the persons who provide personal support for you or who are important to you." For the next set of six questions, the respondent is asked to identify the extent of support provided by each of the individuals listed in the network. For example, one of the questions used for affect is:

How much does this person make you feel liked or loved?

An item used to tap affirmation is:

How much does this person agree with or support your actions or thoughts?

To assess long-term aid, the question used is:

If you were confined to bed for several weeks, how much could this person help you?

The rating scale is 1, not at all; 2, a little; . . . 5, a great deal.

Other items are included to determine the duration of the individual relationships (ranging from less than 6 months to more than 5 years), the frequency of contact (ranging from daily, weekly, to once a year or less), and loss (number of persons no longer available to the individual and the amount of support lost).

Phase I testing for the NSSQ includes establishing reliability (test–retest and internal consistency) and beginning to establish validity (response bias, concurrent validity, and content validity). The test–retest reliability for each of the functional items (affect, affirmation, and aid) and network property items ranged from 0.85 to 0.92. Analysis for internal consistency resulted in 0.89 or above for each of the three functional properties of social support. Correlations among the three network property items ranged from 0.88 to 0.96 and for the three loss items from 0.54 to 0.68.

Testing was performed to determine the degree to which the NSSQ coincides with a known measure of social support, Social Support Questionnaire.[23] Although the two instruments define their component subscales differently, there are rough parallels between tangible support and aid, informational support and affirmation, and emotional support and affect. Moderate levels of concurrent validity were found (range 0.31 to 0.56 for the subscales).

Phase II testing consists of a series of three studies to provide a normative database and to continue to test reliability and validity.[18] Evidence for construct validity was demonstrated with selected Fundamental Interpersonal Relations Orientation (FIRO-B)[51] constructs. Two interpersonal constructs, need for inclusion and need for affection, were significantly corre-lated with NSSQ subscales and composite variables demonstrating convergence, whereas the interpersonal construct of need for control was not significantly correlated with the NSSQ subscales demonstrating divergence. Small to moderate correlations indicate that a person's interpersonal needs for inclusion and affection are related to their self-report of the amount of social support available to them.

The NSSQ was administered to female graduate students ($n = 44$) on entry into gradu-ate school and 7 months later. The correlations between the first testing and the 7-month follow-up for the subscales and variables ranged from 0.58 to 0.78, which represents a moderately high degree of stability over time although lower than the 1-week test–retest correlations, which ranged from 0.85 to 0.92. The NSSQ was sensitive to changes in the composition of the network over time.

Another study was conducted with female graduate students ($n = 55$) to test concurrent validity with the PRQ[19] and to test the predictive validity of the NSSQ in relation to the stress-buffering role of social support described in the literature. Medium levels of association (0.35 to 0.41) between the functional components of the NSSQ and the PRQ were found, and lower, yet significant, levels of association between most of the network properties of the NSSQ and the PRQ were established. The NSSQ subscale, Number Listed in the Network, was not significantly related to the PRQ, a fact that reflects the difference in format between the two instruments. The PRQ is based on global evaluations of support, whereas the NSSQ is based on ratings for previously listed network members. Descriptions of the development and testing of the NSSQ are reported in more detail.[17,18]

The NSSQ measures the perceived social support but, unlike the PRQ, does not assess the extent of satisfaction with the support perceived to be available. A normative database from employed adults to use for comparison of findings from other studies has been reported for the NSSQ,[18] and detailed scoring instructions are available.

▪ SOCIAL SUPPORT QUESTIONNAIRE (SSQ)

Another measure of social support, the Social Support Questionnaire (SSQ) has been devel-oped and tested by Sarason et al.[22] Scores for the perceived number of social supports and satisfaction with the social support available are obtained using the SSQ. Sarason et al.[22] have reported on the psychometric properties of the SSQ, including correlations of the SSQ with personality, adjustment, and life change measures. The SSQ consists of 27 items, each of which asks the respondent to list the people on whom they can rely for the set of circum-stances described and to indicate the degree of satisfaction they have with the support provided. Examples of items are:

Whom do you really count on to be dependable when you need help?

Whom can you really count on to listen to you when you need to talk?

Whom could you really count on to help you out in a crisis situation, even though they would have to go out of their way?[22]

One of the options allows the respondent to answer "no one," but then the degree of satisfaction with the support is still rated (ranging 1–6 points from "very satisfied" to "very dissatisfied"). Correlations of items with total score ranged from 0.48 to 0.72; for the satisfac-tion scores the coefficient alpha was reported as 0.94. The test–retest (4-week interval) correlations for satisfaction and for the number listed were 0.83 and 0.90, respectively. The authors report the SSQ to have stability and high internal consistency among the items,[22] and correlations of the SSQ with scores on other instruments measuring personality indices of well-being and self-esteem are provided.

• INVENTORY OF SOCIALLY SUPPORTIVE BEHAVIORS (ISSB)

Barrera et al.[20] developed a 40-item instrument that measures the frequency with which the respondents were the recipients of supportive actions. The authors have reported test–retest (0.88) and internal consistency (coefficients alpha = 0.93 and 0.94) reliability for this Inventory of Socially Supportive Behaviors (ISSB).[20] The inventory assesses help received from natural support systems. Scores on the ISSB were significantly correlated with size of the network and perceived support of the family. (The subjects for the initial testing were college students.) Social support was conceptualized to include both tangible and intangible forms of assistance, such as provision of goods and services as well as guidance. Each of the 40 items are rated by the respondent on a 5-point scale according to the frequency (ranging from 1, not at all; 2, once or twice; . . . 5, about every day) with which they occurred during the preceding month. Examples of the items are:

> Was right there with you (physically) in a stressful situation.
>
> Did some activity together to help you get your mind off things.
>
> Expressed esteem or respect for a competency or personal quality of yours.
>
> Helped you understand why you didn't do something well.
>
> Told you that she/he feels very close to you.

An important feature of the ISSB is that it can be used to assess the respondents' perceptions of the helping transactions actually received within a specified time period. The ISSB has been subjected to a principal components factor analysis.[52] The investigators concluded that it was appropriate to use the ISSB total score as a global measure of social support. They, however, also retained and rotated four components that were found frequently in the literature to describe types of social support; these are emotional support, tangible/material support, and two kinds of cognitive support (informational and feedback). They concluded that the socializing dimension (having companionship for engaging in a variety of activities) of social support is not measured well by the ISSB.

• ARIZONA SOCIAL SUPPORT INTERVIEW SCHEDULE (ASSIS)

Another instrument, the Arizona Social Support Interview Schedule (ASSIS), was used by Barrera et al.[20] to determine if the frequency of the socially supportive interactions measured by the ISSB were positively related to the network number as measured by the ASSIS. The ASSIS has six questions that correspond to six categories of social support: material aid, physical assistance, intimate interaction, guidance, feedback, and positive social interaction. Respondents indicate the people who are perceived to be available to provide the type of support specified and who of those people actually provided that specific support during the past month.[20] Thus, the ASSIS can be used to assess the size of the network perceived to be available to provide specific types of support as well as the size of the network that provided actual specific types of support in the past 30 days. The ISSB scores were correlated moderately yet significantly with the social support network size of those available and those actually providing supportive functions.

• SOCIAL SUPPORT QUESTIONNAIRE

Schaefer et al.[23] developed and used another instrument, the Social Support Questionnaire. It is a two-part questionnaire. Nine situations are presented in part one as a measure of tangible support; in part two, the respondent lists network members by specific categories, such as spouse, friends, work or school associates, and so forth, and then is asked to rate the people listed for one question about informational support and for four questions about emotional support. Test–retest (over a 9-month interval) reliability is reported as being 0.56 for tangible support and 0.68 for emotional support. Internal consistency for informational and emotional support was 0.81 and for tangible support 0.31. An example of an item from part one is:

> When you are working around the house and find that you need something to finish the job (like a cup of sugar or some nails), what do you usually do about it? a) Borrow from someone? From whom? List the initials of the person(s) and check the category (relative, friend, work associate, neighbor or other) or b) Make a quick trip to the store? or c) Other, please specify.

Another item is:

> Often people rely on the judgment of someone they know in making important decisions about their lives. Is there anyone whose opinion you consider seriously in making important decisions about your family?

They again list the individual(s) by initials and check the appropriate relational category. The informational question in part two is:

> How much did this person give you information, suggestions and guidance over the last month that you found helpful?

One of the emotional items is:

> How much does this person boost your spirits when you feel low?

For part two questions, the ratings range from 1, not at all; 2, slightly; . . . 5, extremely. The conceptualization and health-related functions of social support are described by Schaefer et al.[23] The Schaefer et al.[23] Social Support Questionnaire and the Brandt and Weinert[19] PRQ have been administered concurrently with the NSSQ, and the findings are reported.[17,18]

• PERCEIVED SOCIAL SUPPORT FROM FRIENDS (PSS-Fr)
AND FROM FAMILY (PSS-Fa)

Procidano and Heller[21] developed measures of Perceived Social Support from Friends (PSS-Fr) and from Family (PSS-Fa). The authors report that these were separate valid constructs distinct from network. These represent two different source of support categories and tap different dimensions of social relationships. Each of the measures has 20 items; a "yes," "no," or "don't know" response is given for each item. The internal consistency (Cronbach coefficient alpha) is 0.88 and 0.90 for the PSS-Fr and PSS-Fa, respectively. Factor analysis indicated a single factor for each scale. Validity and reliability testing was performed using undergraduate college students. Scores on the PSS-Fr were related more closely to social competence than were scores on the PSS-Fa. Subjects with high PSS-Fr scores had significantly lower scores on trait anxiety than had those with low PSS-Fr scores.

Examples of items from the PSS-Fr are:

Most other people are closer to their friends than I am.

There is a friend I could go to if I were just feeling down, without feeling funny about it later.

My friends come to me for emotional support.

My friends are good at helping me solve problems.

Examples of items from the PSS-Fa are:

I get good ideas about how to do things or make things from my family.

My family enjoys hearing about what I think.

I rely on my family for emotional support.

When I confide in members of my family, it makes me uncomfortable.

I don't have a relationship with a member of my family that is as close as other people's relationships with family members.

The items include receiving of supportive behaviors and a few that tap the notion of reciprocity, that is, the individual provides support to network members.

There are other instruments that may tap some dimension of social support, but they are not included because the central focus of these other instruments is not the measurement of social support. For example, a Family Environment Scale (FES) developed by Moos[49] has been used to obtain subjective assessments of the respondents' family social environment. It contains subscales and has 90 true–false statements. Although the specific focus of this instrument is not social support, it may capture some aspects of the context necessary for social support.

With the current surge of interest in social support, additional measures will be created and existing instruments will be revised and refined. In selecting an instrument for purposes of clinical assessment or to measure a variable for research, similar criteria need to be used in the selection process. There are some major considerations. The primary question is, does the instrument purport to measure the phenomenon or variable of interest, does it tap the major dimensions of interest to you? Are the clinical, theoretical and empirical premises/bases from which the conceptualizations of the instrument items were derived explicit and congruent with your clinical or research focus? If it is of interest to measure a variable, such as social support, over time, it is important to determine if the instrument is a sufficiently sensitive measure for changes to be detected. For additional information about selecting a measure, refer to Chapter 1.

SUMMARY

Social support is one component of the human context of the individual's social environment. Early work has suggested that social support plays a role in mediating the effects of stressful life events, in protecting health, and in buffering against stressful circumstances or crises. Conceptualizations and measurement of social support remain varied, and several instruments designed to measure one or more dimension of social support are available and have published validity and reliability data. The final selection of an instrument must be based on the congruency between what variable(s) you want to measure and what dimension(s) an instrument has been designed to assess.

REFERENCES

1. Wortman, C.B. Social support and the cancer patient. Conceptual and methodological issues. *Cancer,* 1984, *53*[Suppl.]:2339.
2. House, J.S., & Kahn, R.L. Measures and concepts of social support. In S. Cohen & L. Syme (Eds.), *Social support and health.* New York: Academic Press, 1985, p. 83.
3. Bloom, J.R. Social support systems and cancer: A conceptual view. In J. Cohen, J.W. Culler, & L.R. Martin (Eds.), *Psychosocial aspects of cancer.* New York: Raven Press, 1982, p. 129.
4. Lindsey, A.M., Norbeck, J.S., Carrieri, V.L., & Perry, E. Social support and health outcomes in postmastectomy women: A review. *Cancer Nurs,* 1981, *4*(5):377.
5. Bruhn, J.G., & Philips. B.U. Measuring social support: A synthesis of current approaches. *J Behav Med,* 1984, *7*(2):151.
6. Murawski, B.J., Penman, D., & Schmitt, M. Social support in health and illness: The concept and its measurement. *Cancer Nurs,* 1978, *1*(5):365.
7. Maxwell, M.B. The use of social networks to help cancer patients maximize support. *Cancer Nurs,* 1982, *5*(4):275.
8. Norbeck, J.S. Social support: A model for clinical research and application. *Adv Nurs Sci,* 1981, *3*(4):43.
9. Rundall, T.G., & Evashwick, C. Social networks and help-seeking among the elderly. *Res Aging,* 1982, *4*(2):205.
10. Berkman, B., Stolberg, C., Calhoun, J., et al. Elderly cancer patients: Factors predictive of risk for institutionalization. *J Psychosoc Oncol,* 1983, *1*(1):85.
11. Berkman, L.F., & Syme, S.L. Social networks, host resistance and mortality: A year follow-up study of Alameda county residents. *Am J Epidemiol,* 1979, *109*(2):186.
12. Blazer, D.G. Social support and mortality in an elderly community population. *Am J Epidemiol,* 1982, *115*(5):684.
13. Lindsey, A.M., Ahmed, N., & Dodd, M. Social support network and quality as perceived by Egyptian cancer patients. *Cancer Nurs,* 1985, *8*(1):37.
14. Tilden, V.P. The relation of life stress and social support to emotional disequilibrium during pregnancy. *Res Nurs Health,* 1983, *6*(4):167.
15. Diamond, M. Social support and adaptation to chronic illness: The case of maintenance hemodialysis. *Res Nurs Health,* 1979, *2*(3):101.
16. Hubbard, P., Muhlenkamp, A.F., & Brown, N. The relationship between social support and self-care practices. *Nurs Res,* 1984, *33*(5):266.
17. Norbeck, J.S., Lindsey, A.M., & Carrieri, V.L. The development of an instrument to measure social support. *Nurs Res,* 1981, *30*(5):264.
18. Norbeck, J.S., Lindsey, A.M., & Carrieri, V.L. Further development of the Norbeck social support questionnaire: Normative data and validity testing. *Nurs Res,* 1983, *32*(1):4.
19. Brandt, P.A., & Weinert, C. The PRQ—A social support measure. *Nurs Res,* 1981, *30*(5):277.

20. Barrera, M., Sandler, I.N., & Ramsay, T.B. Preliminary development of a scale of social support: Studies on college students. *Am J Community Psychol,* 1981, *9*(4):435.
21. Procidano, M.E., & Heller, K. Measures of perceived social support from friends and from family: Three validations studies. *Am J Community Psychol,* 1983, *11*(1):1.
22. Sarason, I.G., Levine, H.M., Basham, R.B., & Sarason, R. Assessing social support: The social support questionnaire. J Pers Soc Psychol, 1983, *44*(1):127.
23. Schaefer, C., Coyne, J.C., & Lazarus, R. The health-related functions of social support. *J Behav Med,* 1981, *4*(4):381.
24. Cobb, S. Social support as a moderator of life stress. *Psychosom Med,* 1976, *38*(5):300.
25. Kaplan, B.H., Cassel, J.C., & Gore, S. Social support and health. *Med Care,* 1977, *15*[Suppl 5]:47.
26. Dean, A., & Lin, N. The stress buffering role of social support. *J Nerv Ment Dis,* 1977, *165*(6):403.
27. Kahn, R., & Antonucci, T. Convoys over the life course: Attachment, roles and social support. In P.B. Baltes & O. Brim (Eds.), *Life-span development and behavior* (Vol. 3). New York: Academic Press, 1981, p. 253.
28. Broadhead, W.E., Kaplan, B.H., James, S.A., et al. The epidemiologic evidence for a relationship between social support and health. *Am J Epidemiol,* 1983, *117*(5):521.
29. Nuckolls, J.B., Cassel, J., & Kaplan. B.H. Psychosocial assets, life crisis and the prognosis of pregnancy. *Am J Epidemiol,* 1972, *95*(5):431.
30. Lin, N., Simeone, R., Ensel, W., & Kuo, W. Social support, stressful life events and illness: A model and an empirical test. *J Health Soc Behav,* 1979, *20*(2):108.
31. Pilisuk, M., & Froland, C. Kinship, social networks, social support and health. *Soc Sci Med,* 1978, *12*(B):273.
32. Cohen, F. Personality, stress and the development of physical illness. In G.C. Stone, F. Cohen, & N.E. Adler (Eds.), *Health psychology.* San Francisco: Jossey-Bass, 1979, p. 77.
33. Cassel, J. The contribution of the social environment to host resistance. *Am J Epidemiol,* 1976, *104*(2):107.
34. Heller, K. The effects of social support: Prevention and treatment implications. In A.P. Goldstein & F.H. Kanfer (Eds.), *Maximizing treatment gains: Transfer enhancement in psychotherapy.* New York: Academic Press, 1979, p. 353.
35. Croog, S.H., Lipson, A., & Levine, S. Help patterns in severe illness: The roles of kin network, non-family resources and institutions. *J Marriage Family,* 1972, *34*:32.
36. Cobb, S. Social support and health through the life course. In H.I. McCubbin, A.E. Cauble, & J.M. Patterson (Eds.), *Family stress, coping and social support.* Springfield, IL: Chas. C Thomas, 1982, p. 189.
37. Caplan, G. *Support systems and community mental health.* New York: Behavioral Publications, 1974.
38. Caplan, G. The family as a support system. In G. Caplan & M. Killilea (Eds.), *Support systems and mutual help: Multidisciplinary explorations.* New York: Grune & Stratton, 1976, p. 19.
39. Lowenthal, M.F., & Haven, C. Interaction and adaptation: Intimacy as a critical variable. *Am Sociol Rev,* 1968, *33*(1):20.
40. Miller, P.M., & Ingham, J.G. Friends, confidants and symptoms. *Soc Psychiatry,* 1976, *11*:51.
41. Conner, K.A., Powers, E.A., & Bultera, G.L. Social interaction and life satisfaction: An empirical assessment of late-life patterns. *J Gerontol,* 1979, *34*:116.
42. Weiss, R. The provision of social relationships. In Z. Rubin (Ed.), *Doing unto others.* Englewood Cliffs, NJ: Prentice Hall, 1974, p. 17.
43. House, J.S. *Work stress and social support.* Reading, MA: Addison-Wesley, 1981.
44. Kahn, R.L. Aging and social support. In M.W. Riley (Ed.), *Aging from birth to death: Interdisciplinary perspectives.* Boulder, CO: Westview Press for American Association for the Advancement of Science, 1979, p. 77.
45. Caplan, G. The family as a support system. In H.I. McCubbin, A.E. Cauble, & J.M. Patterson (Eds.), *Family stress, coping and social support.* Springfield, IL: Chas. C Thomas, 1982, p. 200.
46. Mitchell, R.E., & Trickett, E.J. Social networks as mediators of social support: An analysis of the effects and determinants of social networks. *Community Ment Health J* 1980, *16*(1):27.
47. Barnes, J. *Social networks* (Vol. 26). Reading, MA: Addison-Wesley, Modular Pub., 1972, p. 1.

48. Lindsey, A.M. Social support: Selection of a measurement instrument. *Oncol Nurs Forum,* 1984, *11*(2):88.
49. Moos, R.H. *Evaluating treatment environments: A social ecological approach.* New York: Wiley, 1974.
50. Moos, R.H. *Evaluating educational environments: Procedures, measures, findings, and policy implications.* San Francisco: Jossey-Bass, 1979.
51. Schultz, W. *FIRO awareness scales manual.* Palo Alto, CA: Consulting Psychologists Press, 1978.
52. Stokes, J.P., & Wilson, D.G. The inventory of socially supportive behaviors: Dimensionality, prediction and gender differences. *Am J Community Psychol* 1984, *12*:53.

CHAPTER 7

Measuring Coping

Jo Ann Wegmann, R.N., Ph.D.

Coping is a concept that has received much attention in the literature and has been investigated by a variety of disciplines and avenues of study. Early work in coping as a response to stress includes empirical studies by Angell,[1] Koos,[2] and Hill.[3] Stress within families has been investigated, and interest in this area has continued to develop through systematic research. As a result of this systematic research, there are available currently examples of research strategies, methods, and reliable and valid instruments for the study of coping.[4]

There are multiple, often overlapping definitions of coping. For purposes of this chapter, coping is defined as the cognitive and behavioral strategies used to master conditions of harm, threat, or challenge when a normal or routine response is not available.[1,5] As such, coping involves two separate frameworks, as identified by Lazarus,[5] psychologic and sociologic. According to Lazarus,[5] the psychologic taxonomy of coping includes direct action and palliative modes. Direct actions relate to physiologic responses to stress and become evident with threatening changes in one's social or physical environment. Palliative coping encompasses thoughts or actions designed to relieve the emotional impact of stress. Unlike direct actions, palliative coping does not alter threatening or damaging events but serves to make the person feel better.

Sociologic coping behaviors rely on the resources of individuals or groups, such as families. Early research into families identified the importance of family resources, such as cohesion and adaptability, directed at maintaining family organization and functioning during stressful events.[3] Such coping tendencies are closely related to aspects of social support discussed elsewhere in this book (e.g., Chapter 4).

Many instruments exist that measure various aspects of coping, including physiologic and psychologic responses. Singer's paper[6] identifies 14 such instruments, acknowledging that there is no shortage of scales for studying coping. Indeed, coping and stress have been popular topics of other disciplines, such as psychiatry, social work, and psychology.

INSTRUMENTS TO MEASURE COPING

A comprehensive list of data collection techniques or instruments used to measure coping would be extensive, with much duplication among tools. The purpose of this chapter is to identify instruments used recently for research into coping. Sources include family sociology, psychology, psychiatry, and nursing. All instruments described here have been designed to measure the effect of adequate coping behaviors on some outcome and appear to be suitable for many nursing studies.

Typically, coping processes have been evaluated for two reasons: validation or confirmation of a particular theory and evaluation of a patient with a diagnostic clinical instrument.[6] It also is valuable to investigate coping strategies of both individuals and families to assess for inappropriate or inadequate coping patterns, which may have a subsequent impact on health outcomes.

In identifying instruments for the study of coping, it is valuable first to explore broader issues of research into this phenomenon. Because coping represents responses to stressors, the astute investigator must be aware of the sensitive nature of such research, as well as the ethical areas inherent in these types of exploration. Brailey[8] identifies three research issues in the study of coping strategies:

1. The necessity of obtaining an accurate picture of routine coping strategies of individuals
2. The delineation of functions of coping, in order to determine the effectiveness of coping
3. The determination of appropriate measurements of coping efficacy

In her paper, Brailey describes four methods of data collection or types of instruments used in the study of coping (Table 7–1). It is relevant to discuss these here and to identify possible weaknesses with each method.

Direct observation of the subject while he or she is coping with normal events is the first method described by Brailey. This typically involves a longitudinal study, with the risks of effect of observer on responses. Another means of data collection involves the use of vignettes of stressful situations, from which subject responses are obtained. This may provide information about coping strategies, but Brailey cautions that vignettes may not represent realistic situations.

A third data collection technique seeks responses of how subjects usually cope with general stressors. Such instruments typically provide a list of coping responses, rated by the subject on a Likert-type scale. Many instruments that measure coping are designed in this format, yet Brailey cautions that there may be discrepancies between what subjects say they do and what they actually do in specific situations.

The fourth data collection method discussed by Brailey involves the use of real events

---

**TABLE 7–1. FOUR METHODS OF DATA
COLLECTION IN STUDYING COPING BEHAVIORS
OF HEALTHY INDIVIDUALS**

1. Director observation during normal events
2. Responses to stressful events
3. Usual responses to general sources of stress
4. Coping responses to actual stressful events

From Brailey. Nurs Papers Perspect Nurs, 1984, 16(1):5.

from subjects' own lives and asks them to describe coping strategies they used. Although this use of real life events appears advantageous, a potential problem with self-report is selective distortion; thus this method of data collection is used infrequently.

Obviously, the investigator may encounter difficulties using these data collection methods. Singer[6] elaborates somewhat on Brailey's descriptions.[8] This psychologist identifies two types of coping studies. According to Singer, one strategy in coping research assumes a theoretical position on how people function. From such a position, one may identify categories or descriptors for coping behaviors. Scales and other measuring instruments may then be developed based on identified categories. Examples of studies that arise from a theoretical position include comparisons of the relative successes of people in one category of coping style with those in another. The second type of study described by Singer examines the particular stress or stresses, such as illness or bereavement. Examples of such studies include inferential studies about patterns of reactions and functional adaptation to common stressors.

The instruments designed to measure coping that are described here are organized into two broad categories: those related to family sociology research and those derived from studies of health care outcomes. In discussing specific instruments, attempts are made to address the methods of data collection described by Brailey,[8] as well as the two types of coping studies identified by Singer.[6] Issues of reliability and validity are addressed for each instrument. The specific instruments discussed are listed in Table 7–2.

Family Sociology

Early attempts at defining and measuring coping came directly from research into families and family management of stress. Much of the recent literature on coping is found in sociologic sources. McCubbin et al.[9] explore recent investigations into family stress and coping in a decade review of these topics. These authors identify that the study of family coping has depended on many cognitive psychologic theories and sociologic sources. Coping strategies are described in terms of both the individual and the family by Olson et al.[10]

▪ TWO-PART COPING ASSESSMENT SCALE

Sidle et al. developed a structured, easily scorable assessment scale of coping strategies.[11] Their two-part coping scale includes three problem situations for which the subject lists possible approaches, or strategies, and a list of ten strategies for coping with the situation. In the second part of this scale, the subject responds on a 7-point scale the likelihood of his or her using each of the ten strategies. The authors conclude that both free response and ratings are important, since they may elicit different sources of information about coping strategies. The validity and reliability of this scale are not addressed. This study represents an early attempt to develop a pencil and paper measure to elicit information about less socially approved ways of coping and is the groundwork on which more recent instruments have been developed. This tool illustrates the data collection method of the use of vignettes.[8]

▪ PARENTAL COPING SCALE

Hurwitz et al.[12] sought a tool for assessing parent–child relationship patterns in families with juvenile delinquents. Five areas of parental coping are assessed through interviews of both parents, together and separately. These areas are rated immediately after the interviews

TABLE 7–2. A SUMMARY LIST OF INSTRUMENTS USED IN RESEARCH INTO COPING

Tool	Reliability Information	Validity Information	Population
Two-part Coping Assessment Scale (Sidle et al.[11])	No	No	Adults
Parental Coping Scale (Hurwitz et al.[12])	Yes	Yes	Parents
FILE[14]	Yes	Yes	Parents
A-FILE[15]	Yes	Yes	Adolescents and parents
F-COPES[16]	Yes	Yes	Adults
Richmond/Hopkins Family Coping Index[17]	Yes	No	Public health personnel
CPI[18]	No	No	Parents
Health Attitude Scale[19]	No	No	Adults
Patient Attitudes of Chronic Illness (Kinsmon, et al.[20])	No	No	Adults
Chronicity Impact and Coping Instrument[21]	Yes	No	Parents
Goldstein Coper-Avoider Sentence Completion Test[22]	No	No	Adults
Preoperative Coping Scale (Sime[23])	No	No	Adults
Coping Inventory[24]	Yes	No	Handicapped children
Coping Strategy Questionnaire[25]	Yes	No	Adults with low back pain
Respiratory Illness Opinion Survey[26]	Yes	No	Adults
Response to Illness Questionnaire[27]	Yes	No	Long-term hemodialysis adults
Bedsworth and Molen[28] Semistructured Interview	No	No	Spouses of patients with myocardial infarction
Coping Strategies Scale[29]	No	No	Chronically ill adults
Cancer Inventory of Problem Situations[30]	No	Yes	Adults
Jalowiec Coping Scale[31]	Yes	Yes	Adults

with 4-point scores ranging from "very constructive" to "very destructive." This type of data collection is representative of the fourth method of study described by Brailey,[8] that of having subjects identify coping responses used in relation to specific events or situations. Hurwitz et al.[12] state that reliability for the scoring of the interviews has been achieved at the 0.05 level of significance as determined by Chi-square analysis. They describe validity as being achieved through the differentiation of constructive from destructive parental coping mechanisms.

▪ FAMILY INVENTORIES

Olson et al.,[13] at the University of Minnesota Department of Family Social Science, have developed a series of instruments called Family Inventories. These inventories consist of nine instruments that measure various aspects of family life, adaptability, cohesion, and coping. Three instruments in particular were developed as part of the Family Stress and Coping Project.

▪ FAMILY INVENTORY OF LIFE EVENTS AND CHANGES (FILE)

The scale was developed as an index of family stress and is designed to record the normative and nonnormative life events and changes experienced by a family unit.[14] FILE consists of 72 items, grouped into nine scales, with a high raw score indicating low stress and a lower raw score indicating high stress. One of the scales is labeled "losses," and an example of an item from this scale is:

A parent/spouse died.

Responses are recorded as "yes" or "no," and a total score is obtained. The authors suggest that the total scale score be used rather than the separate subscales, since the subscale scores are not as empirically stable.

Reliability for FILE is reported in terms of Cronbach coefficient alpha. As reported by the authors, the overall scale reliability is 0.81, with the subscale scores varying from 0.73 to 0.30. This supports the use of the total scale score, rather than scoring by individual subscales. Validity of this instrument was determined by discriminant analyses between low conflict and high conflict families ($p < .01$).

▪ ADOLESCENT-FAMILY INVENTORY OF LIFE EVENTS AND CHANGES (A-FILE)

A-FILE[15] is a 50-item self-report instrument designed to record normative and nonnormative life events and changes as perceived by an adolescent during the previous 12 months of family life. This instrument measures family life changes and records events experienced by any member of the family. The instrument is comprised of six conceptual dimensions, including transitions. An example of a statement from this dimension is:

Parent started school.

Subjects respond "yes" (coded as 0) or "no" (coded as 1) to each statement. A high score implies low stress.

The total scale alpha reliabilities for this instrument are 0.83 and 0.80, as determined by two different samples. Validity assessments were made by correlating the dimensions with two outcome measures, adolescent substance use and adolescent health locus of control ($p < .01$). A suggested future use of this instrument is in research of adolescents diagnosed with chronic or catastrophic illnesses.

▪ FAMILY COPING STRATEGIES (F-COPES)

This instrument[16] was created to identify effective problem-solving approaches and behaviors used by families in response to problems or difficulties. F-COPES is a 29-item self-report instrument that consists of five conceptual scales. Each item is answered on a Likert-type scale, with answers ranging from "strongly disagree" to "strongly agree." One of the dimensions of F-COPES is seeking spiritual support, and an example of a statement from this dimension is:

Attending church services.

Because of the interval level of data, scores can be obtained, and parametric statistical analyses can be performed on the results. Scores can be obtained for each dimension, and a total score also can be obtained. Reliability for F-COPES was determined by Cronbach coefficient alpha (0.86 and 0.87, for two samples) and test–retest.

▪ RICHMOND/HOPKINS FAMILY COPING INDEX

Choi et al.[17] revised the instructions for the Richmond/Hopkins Family Coping Index, first reported in 1963, and determined that the accuracy and consistency of this instrument could be enhanced. This instrument measures nine domains of family coping, including emotional competence and family living patterns. It is completed by public health personnel during observations of actual family settings. Scores of the nine subscales range from 1 to 5 ("never" to "always"), and the rater is asked to assess how a family is coping in each of the domains. Interrater reliability was established with the modified instructions for use by Cronbach coefficient alpha (0.97). The authors state that the results of improving this scale support its continued use.

▪ CALIFORNIA PSYCHOLOGICAL INVENTORY (CPI)

Kupst and Schulman[18] used the California Psychological Inventory (CPI) subscales to measure personal adjustment in families that include a child with leukemia. These are five self-reported scales completed by the parents, including work and leisure within the overall functioning family unit.

▪ HEALTH ATTITUDE SCALE

Miller et al.[19] studied coping as adherence to medical regimen within five areas, in a group of cardiac patients. Their Health Attitude Scale is a self-report, 7-point bipolar scale that appears to be suitable for measuring coping in a variety of illnesses.

▪ PATIENT ATTITUDES OF CHRONIC ILLNESS

Kinsman et al.[20] investigated patient attitudes of chronic illness in six areas. This 109-item survey is a self-report instrument, with choices of "agree" or "disagree." Areas investigated include optimism, locus of control, and attitudes toward hospitalization.

Health-Related Outcomes and Nursing Sources of Coping Instruments

Health-related outcomes have been addressed in family studies of coping, and specific instruments to determine such outcomes have been developed. The areas explored include measurement of adaptation in specific illnesses and determining coping strategies of patients and families confronting long-term disease problems.

▪ CHRONICITY IMPACT AND COPING INSTRUMENT: PARENT QUESTIONNAIRE (CICI:PQ)

Hymovich[21] reports on the Chronicity Impact and Coping Instrument: Parent Questionnaire (CICI:PQ). This instrument was developed to determine the impact of a child's chronic illness on parents and how parents cope with that impact. The author describes the results of three tests and the three phases of the instrument itself.

The current format of the CICI:PQ contains 167 items divided into six sections, including your child, yourself, your spouse, brothers and sisters hospitalization, and other. This is a self-report instrument completed by parents. There are 60 stressor items, 61 coping items, and 9 value/attitude/belief items. Other items of this tool seek demographic information.

Hymovich reports that internal consistency reliability was determined for each of the three revisions of this instrument. The current version of the CICI:PQ has a Hoyt coefficient of reliability of 0.95, which the author cautions may be artificially inflated. She states further that test–retest reliability still needs to be determined. Although this is a relatively new instrument for measuring coping within families, its true value lies in its ability to determine the current impact and coping status of parents of chronically ill children in order to predict the outcome of intervention with these families.

▪ GOLDSTEIN COPER-AVOIDER SENTENCE COMPLETION TEST (SCT)

Cohen and Lazarus investigated the relationship between the mode of coping with preoperative stress and recovery from surgery.[22] Among the instruments they used to gather information was the Goldstein Coper-Avoider Sentence Completion Test (SCT). This test consists of a series of sentence completion stems, and responses are scored by the investigator for either avoidance or coping. An example of one of the items is:

My greatest fear is. . . .

The authors acknowledge that there may be differences in responses between the sexes, and no information is offered on the reliability and validity of this instrument. Nevertheless, it appears that this is an easily administered test, developed to elicit predictive information about individuals' coping styles before a threatening event. As such, it offers potential value to nursing research.

▪ PREOPERATIVE COPING SCALE

Another study of surgical patients used a preoperative coping scale to assess the extent to which patients desired and sought information about impending surgery.[23] This scale consists of 15 items that deal with such topics as location and size of incision, length of the operation, expected amount of pain, and type of postoperative treatment. Sime[23] reports that quantitative data were derived by assigning a plus or minus to each item and summing across items. Thus, the possible range of scores is −15 to 15, with extreme minus scores representing limited information seeking and extreme positive scores indicating extensive information seeking.

Very little other information is available about the preoperative coping scale. For example, validity and reliability are not addressed in Sime's paper.[23] Yet, this too appears to be a likely instrument for future development in nursing research.

▪ COPING INVENTORY

Zeitlin[24] reports a study with a coping instrument that also may be amenable to nursing research. She used the Coping Inventory, an observation instrument, to assess 48 kinds of coping behaviors of handicapped children. This instrument is used to identify educational and therapeutic planning and is divided into two categories, self and environment. Items are scored on a scale of 1 to 5, where 1 indicates no or very minimal evidence of competency, and 5 indicates effective behavior.

Interobserver reliability of the Coping Inventory ranged from 0.78 to 0.99 in Zeitlin's test. Split-half reliability is reported between a group of nonhandicapped children and a sample of handicapped children.

▪ COPING STRATEGY QUESTIONNAIRE

The Coping Strategy Questionnaire[25] was used to assess cognitive and behavioral pain-coping mechanisms in a sample of chronic low back pain patients. This self-report questionnaire consists of six cognitive coping strategies (e.g., thinking of things that serve to distract one away from the pain) and two behavioral coping strategies (engaging in active behaviors that divert one's attention away from the pain) when the subject feels pain. Items are scored on a 7-point scale, and the respondent indicates how often he or she uses that particular strategy on feeling pain, where 0 = never, 3 = sometimes, and 6 = always.

This questionnaire was found to be internally reliable, with alpha coefficients of 0.71. The authors discuss the predictive value of this questionnaire when working with people experiencing chronic pain. The value of an instrument like this to nursing research in a variety of settings is evident.

▪ RESPIRATORY ILLNESS OPINION SURVEY (RIOS)

Another area of chronic illness that warrants further investigation is respiratory illness. Kinsman et al.[26] report on the Respiratory Illness Opinion Survey (RIOS) as a measure of patient attitudes toward chronic respiratory illness and hospitalization. This instrument consists of 78 items to which the subject responds on a scale of 1 to 5 (1 = strongly agree, 5 = strongly disagree). Six subscales are measured by this tool, including psychologic stigma:

A breathing problem makes me feel foolish.

An example of one item in the subscale, Negative Staff Regard, is the statement:

This hospital is like a prison.

Internal consistency reliabilities are reported as 0.80 and 0.70, and test–retest reliabilities ranged from 0.64 to 0.79.

• RESPONSE TO ILLNESS QUESTIONNAIRE (RIQ)

Pritchard[27] reports on the development of the Response to Illness Questionnaire (RIQ), a 34-item, self-report survey designed to measure aspects of illness behavior. This instrument was administered to two groups of patients undergoing long-term hemodialysis. The actual instrument is not fully described in this brief report,[27] but the temporal reliability was tested. Weighted kappa-values ranged from 0.22 to 0.89. The author concludes that the RIQ has a substantial level of temporal reliability and suggests that this is a valuable instrument for further use in studies of illness behavior.

• BEDSWORTH AND MOLEN'S SEMISTRUCTURED INTERVIEW

To measure the psychologic stress of spouses of myocardial infarction patients immediately after admission to a coronary care unit, Bedsworth and Molen[28] developed a semistructured interview. Four open-ended questions were used to identify perceived threats and perceived coping strategies. These authors identified 45 actual coping strategies and the total actions taken against the preceived threats of a specific group of spouses.

Little information about this semistructured interview is available, yet it appears to be similar to the second method of data collection described by Brailey,[8] that of obtaining subjects' responses to vignettes of stressful situations. Bedsworth and Molen[28] do not address issues of validity or reliability, and indeed, one problem with this type of data collection is the potential for selective distortion by the respondent. Nevertheless, identification of actual coping behaviors used by spouses provides valuable information and suggests possible directions for future research.

• COPING STRATEGIES SCALE

Miller and Nygran[29] used the Coping Strategies Scale developed by Weisman and Worden[30] to seek descriptive information to evaluate the effects of an education program on the adaptability of chronically ill persons to live with their diseases. This scale was designed to categorize behaviors used by people to cope with concerns and problems. It consists of 15 broad types of behavior frequently observed when a person tries to cope with a specific problem. Miller and Nygren[29] state that efforts to classify how individuals cope are awkward and that the Coping Strategies Scale represents a commendable, yet incomplete, attempt to classify and objectify raw data.

▪ CANCER INVENTORY OF PROBLEM SITUATIONS

Heinrich and Schag[31] developed an instrument to document day-to-day physical and psychosocial problems confronted by cancer patients. The Cancer Inventory of Problem Situations is a self-report test that takes approximately 20 minutes to complete. It consists of 131 problem statements with a fine-point rating scale with responses ranging from "not at all" to "very much." The problem statements are grouped into 27 categories. The instrument evaluates the patient's previous month and how each statement applied to him or her during that time. Content and face validity of this instrument have been established.

▪ JALOWIEC COPING SCALE

The Jalowiec Coping Scale is a 40-item self-report psychometric instrument developed in 1979 by a registered nurse doctoral student at the University of Illinois, Chicago Medical Center. This instrument assesses either general coping behavior or situation-specific coping.[31] The Jalowiec Coping Scale yields 15 problem-oriented and 25 affective-oriented coping strategies. Subjects rate each item on a 5-point scale (1 = never; 5 = almost always). Examples of affective-oriented responses are:

> Worry
> Cry
> Work off tension with physical activity or exercise

Examples of problem-oriented responses are:

> Try to maintain some control over the situation
> Accept the situation as it is

The Jalowiec Coping Scale has been assessed for stability and homogeneity reliability. Test–retest reliability has been determined by several nurse researchers, as reported by Jalowiec et al.[32] In one such report, stability was determined using 28 subjects from the general population and retesting after 2 weeks. Spearman rank ordering of the test–retest data yielded significant ($p < .001$) coefficients of 0.79 for total coping scores, 0.85 for problem-oriented scores, and 0.85 for affective-oriented scores.

Homogeneity, or internal consistency reliability, of this instrument was determined by Cronbach coefficient alpha. Homogeneity also has been determined by several authors.[32] Data were collected from 141 subjects, as reported by Jalowiec and Powers.[33] A coefficient alpha of 0.85 was obtained, which indicates overall homogeneity of the content of this scale.

Construct validity of the Jalowiec Coping Scale has been determined by factor analysis.[31] The data from the 141 subjects mentioned previously were analyzed using the Statistical Package for the Social Sciences (SPSS) program for factor analysis. The authors conclude that, after exploring the multidimensionality of coping behavior, conceptualization of the coping scale items is reasonably adequate according to a four-factor solution.

As more sound instruments become available for measuring coping, it is hoped that reports will include thorough information about these important aspects of instrument and utilization.

SUMMARY

Both theory testing and clinical instrument development are considered to be important elements in measuring coping. As the concept of coping is better defined and as coping behaviors are studied more systematically, other properties of coping may emerge.[7]

This chapter has identified 20 instruments of varying designs for use in the measurement of coping. Self-report scales using Likert-type responses usually facilitate data collection and are amenable to a variety of analytic tests. Not addressed in this chapter are other, more qualitative methods of data collection, including interviews, patient narrative reports, some forms of participant observation, and grounded theory. The reader is encouraged to consider such methods for research into coping, since it is possible to gather much rich, descriptive data through qualitative methods.

Instruments used to measure coping are varied and are derived from many disciplines. As this concept is further understood and empirically measured, its value as a moderator variable in health outcomes should become better documented. Coping represents an area that is ripe for further nursing research, and it is anticipated that this summary of instruments which measure coping will be expanded upon and refined by future nurse researchers.

REFERENCES

1. Angell, R.C. *The family encounters the depression.* New York: Scribners, 1936.
2. Koos, E.L. *Families in trouble.* New York: King's Crown Press, 1946.
3. Hill, R. *Families under stress.* Norwalk, CT: Greenwood Press, 1949.
4. McCubbin, H.I., Cauble, A.E., & Patterson, J. (Eds.). *Family stress, coping, and social support.* Springfield, IL: Chas. C Thomas, 1982.
5. Lazarus, R. *Psychological stress and the coping process.* New York: McGraw-Hill, 1966.
6. Singer, J.E. Some issues in the study of coping. Proceedings of ACS Workshop on Methodologies in Behavioral Psychological Cancer Research, April 1983. *Cancer [Suppl],* 1984, *53*:2303.
7. Wegmann, J.A. Instruments that measure coping. *Oncol Nurs Forum,* 1984, *11*(4):119.
8. Brailey, L.J. Issues in coping research. *Nurs Papers Perspect Nurs,* 1984, *16*(1):5.
9. McCubbin. H.I., Joy, C.B., Cauble, A.E., et al. Family stress and coping: A decade review. *J Marriage Family,* 1980, *42*:855.
10. Olson, D.H.J., McCubbin, H.I., et al. *Families: What makes them work.* Beverly Hills, CA: Sage Publications, 1983.
11. Sidle, A., Moos, R., Adams, J., & Cady, P. Development of a coping scale. *Arch Gen Psychiatr,* 1969, *20*(2):226.
12. Hurwitz, J., Kaplan, D., & Kaiser, E. Designing an instrument to assess parental coping mechanisms, *Soc Casework,* 1962, *43*(10):527.
13. Olson, D.H., McCubbin, H.I., Barnes, H., et al. *Family inventories.* St. Paul, MN: Family Social Science, University of Minnesota, 1982.
14. McCubbin, H.I., Patterson. J.M., & Wilson, M. FILE—Family Inventory of Life Events and Changes. In D.H. Olson, H.I. McCubbin, H. Barnes, et al. (Eds.), *Family inventories.* St. Paul, MN: Family Social Science, University of Minnesota, 1982, p. 69.
15. McCubbin, H.I., Patterson, J.M., Bauman, E., & Harris, L.H., A-FILE—Adolescent Family Inventory of Life Events and Changes. In D.H. Olson, H.I. McCubbin, H. Barnes, et al. (Eds.), *Family inventories.* St. Paul, MN: Family Social Sciences, University of Minnesota, 1982, p. 89.
16. McCubbin, H.I., Larsen, A.S., & Olson, D.H. F-COPES—Family Coping Strategies. In D.H. Olson, H.I. McCubbin, H. Barnes, et al. (Eds.), *Family inventories.* St. Paul, MN: Family Social Science, University of Minnesota, 1982, p. 101.

17. Choi, R., Josten, L., & Christensen, M. (1983). Health-specific coping index for noninstitutional care. *Am J Public Health,* 1983, *73*(11):1275.
18. Kupst, M.J., & Schulman, J.L. The CPI subscales as predictors of parental coping with childhood leukemia. *J Clin Psychol,* 1981, *37*(2):386.
19. Miller, P., Wikoff, R., et al. Development of a health attitude scale. *Nurs Res,* 1982, *31*(3):132.
20. Kinsman, R.A., Jones, N.F., et al. Patient variables supporting chronic illness. *J Nerv Ment Dis,* 1976, *163*(2):159.
21. Hymovich, D. Development of the Chronicity Impact and Coping Instrument: Parent Questionnaire (CICI:PQ) *Nurs Res,* 1984, *33*(4):218.
22. Cohen, F., & Lazarus, R. Active coping processes, coping dispositions, and recovery from surgery. *Psychosom Med,* 1973, *35*(5):375.
23. Sime, A.M. Relationship of preoperative fear, type of coping, and information received about surgery to recovery from surgery. *J Personality Soc Psychol,* 1976, *34*(4):716.
24. Zeitlin, S. Assessing coping behavior. *Am Orthopsychiatr Assoc J,* 1980, *50*(1):139.
25. Rosentiel, A., & Keefe, F. The use of coping strategies in chronic low back pain patients: Relationship to patient characteristics and current adjustment. *Pain,* (1983), *17*(1):33.
26. Kinsman, R., Jones, N., Matus, I., & Schum, R. A scale for measuring attitudes toward respiratory illness and hospitalization. *J Nerv Ment Dis,* 1976, *163*(3):159.
27. Pritchard, M. Temporal reliability of a questionnaire measuring psychological response to illness. *J Psychosom Res,* 1981, *25*:63.
28. Bedsworth, J., & Molen, M. Psychological stress in spouses of patients with myocardial infarction. *Heart Lung,* 1982, *11*(4):450.
29. Miller, M., & Nygren, C. Living with cancer—Coping behaviors. *Cancer Nurs,* 1978, *1*(4):297.
30. Weisman, A.D., & Worden, J.W. The existential plight in cancer: Significance of the first 100 days. *Int J Psychiatry Med,* 1976–77, *7*:1.
31. Heinrich, R., & Schag, C. Living with cancer: The Cancer Inventory of Problem Situations. *J Clin Psychol,* 1984, *40*(4):972.
32. Jalowiec, A., Murphy. S., & Powers, M. Psychometric assessment of the Jalowiec Coping Scale. *Nurs Res,* 1984, *33*(3):157.
33. Jalowiec, A., & Powers, M. Stress and coping in hypertensive and emergency room patients. *Nurs Res,* 1981, *30*(1):10.

CHAPTER 8

Measuring Hope

Martha H. Stoner, R.N.-C., Ph.D., A.N.P.

Hope—a subtle, if not unconscious, expectation regarding an abstract but positive aspect of the future—has been identified as an important factor influencing the quality and perhaps the quantity of life for people who have cancer. Nurses and other health care professionals have recognized an empirical relationship between the apparent loss of hope and eventual deterioration and death of patients with life-threatening illnesses.[1-5] Nurses who work with cancer patients have become interested in the influence of hope and hopelessness on patients' abilities to cope with the uncertainty associated with a cancer diagnosis.[6-11] Included in the nursing literature are descriptions of interventions designed to maintain and instill hope in patients.[12-17] These interventions seem to be based on intuition rather than on rationale supported by research. However, the number of investigations of hope, including attempts to measure this concept, have increased in recent years.[18-30] Hopelessness, frequently considered the polar opposite of hope, has also been measured and researched.[31-32]

Hope is recognized as a concept of importance to nurses and to the patients for whom they care. Types of patients for whom hope is a particularly important concept include people awaiting surgery and those with cancer, end-stage renal disease, multiple sclerosis, and spinal cord injuries. Selected instruments available for the measurement of hope are described. Because hope is such a complex, abstract phenomenon, a review of the theoretical foundation of the concept is presented.

THEORETICAL DESCRIPTION OF HOPE

Hope, thought of as wishful thinking or desire, frequently has been discredited as an impure mode of thought. An exception to this rejection of hope as unworthy of consideration is found in the works of philosopher Gabriel Marcel.[33-35] Marcel described hope as being unconditional in that it transcends all particular objects and is more concerned with a person as a being. Central to Marcel's view of hope was its association with captivity and despair and the need to be delivered from some present condition or state. Although hope was described as an inner sense, Marcel believed that there must be an interaction between one who gives and one who receives hope. This intersubjectivity, or bond of love between self and others, is essential to hope as a mysterious but important inner force for human survival.

Lynch also rejected the commonly held view of hope as something vague and even negative.[36] Hope was described as something very definite and positive. Hope is an interior sense that needs a response from outside and has meaning only as it relates to others, an act of collaboration or mutuality. Another similarity Lynch shared with Marcel is the placement of hope in a framework of captivity, a need to imagine a way out of difficulty.

Stotland's definition of hope is not unlike that of Lynch in that hope is seen as a shorthand term for an exception greater than zero of achieving a goal.[37] Hope is the perceived probability of success, a conviction that the desired goal is truly obtainable. Much of Stotland's analysis was devoted to understanding hope as a psychodynamic force in relation to other factors, such as motivation, achievement, and goal attainment.

In summary, these philosophical and behavioral science perspectives of hope contribute to greater understanding of an abstract phenomenon important to nursing. In addition, they provide a conceptual framework for the development of measures of hope.

MEASUREMENT OF HOPE

▪ GOTTSCHALK-GLESER HOPE SCALE

A measure of hope developed by Gottschalk is composed of a set of predetermined weighted categories indicating positive or negative levels of hope.[21–23] The method of quantifying hope, one of several scales within the Gottschalk-Gleser Scales, used typescripts of 5-minute tape-recorded speech samples elicited from subjects in response to purposely ambiguous instructions to talk about any interesting or dramatic personal life experience.[21] An example of a positive category is any reference to self or others getting or receiving help, advice, support, sustenance, confidence, or esteem from others or self. In contrast, an example of a negative weight category was assigned to references to not being or not wanting to be or not seeking to be the recipient of good fortune, good luck, or God's favor or blessing.

Gottschalk reported acceptable construct validity for his Hope Scale and used it in a number of studies. In one study of radiation therapy patients, Gottschalk reported that pretreatment hope scores correlated significantly with duration of survival.[21] In a study of the emotional impact of surgery, Gottschalk and Hoigaard found that women having mastectomies had significantly higher hope scores compared with healthy subjects.[23] The authors concluded that the high hope scores were associated with the use of denial as a coping mechanism. A concern about the use of this instrument relates to measurement of multiple and diverse affects, such as hope, anxiety, and hostility, using the same speech sample.

▪ ERICKSON, POST, AND PAIGE HOPE SCALE

An instrument developed by Erickson, Post, and Paige[20] is a 20-item, self-report instrument based on Stotland's theoretical constructs of hope,[37] that is, the importance of future-oriented goals and the probability of attaining those goals. The goals were focused but not situation specific in an attempt to reflect goals common to American society. Examples of goals are:

To have enough money for basic needs
To see my children turn out well
To have good bodily health

Subjects rate each goal on a 7-point scale of importance and then indicate the 0 to 100 percent probability of attaining those same goals. Erickson et al. reported test–retest reliabilities of 0.79 and 0.78, (p = .001) for importance and probability scales, respectively, when adminis-tered 1 week apart to undergraduate students. In a group of hospitalized psychiatric patients, these researchers found that psychopathology was associated with lower estimates of per-ceived probability of goal attainment, and that effective psychotherapy increased the perceived probability of goal attainment, presumably indicating greater levels of hope.

NURSING INVESTIGATIONS OF HOPE

Nurses have begun to conduct systematic investigations of hope in an attempt to understand better and to use this concept in research and in clinical practice.

▪ PHENOMENOLOGIC APPROACH

In an effort to explicate the concept, Stanley used an existential phenomenologic approach in a study of hope.[26] Her purpose was to isolate discrete descriptive elements common to the experience of hope in healthy young adults, not to measure levels of hope. Junior and senior college students (n = 100) were asked to describe how they felt when they experienced hope in a situation.

The phenomenologic analysis identified the following elements common to experiencing hope:

1. Expectation of a significant future outcome
2. Being "confident" of outcome
3. Taking "action" to effect outcome
4. Experiencing "comfortable feelings"
5. Experiencing "uncomfortable feelings"
6. Having "interpersonal relatedness"
7. Having a quality of "transcendence"

These common elements were synthesized into a general structure of hope as follows:

The lived experience of hope is a confident expectation of a significant future outcome. accompanied by a quality of transcendence and interpersonal relatedness and in which action to effect the outcome in initiated (p. 165).[26]

▪ RELATION OF LOVE, MUTUALITY, FREEDOM, AND NEWNESS TO HOPE

Thompson investigated the relationship of love, mutuality, freedom, and newness with the perception of hope in ten cancer patients.[30] The method used was a field study with indepth interviews, responses to scale items, and observation of behavior. The purpose of the study was to identify and describe variables. Content analysis identified themes that were coded according to an index of hope developed by Thompson.

• TIME OPINION SURVEY

Raleigh investigated hope as it was manifested in physically ill adults within the theoretical framework of Rogers' unitary man.[25] She interviewed 45 people who had chronic illnesses and 45 people who had a life-threatening form of cancer. The purpose of the study was to identify and describe attributes of hope as manifested in the physically ill adult, to describe what these people believed to be factors that influenced their hope, and to explore possible relationships among types of illness, degree of hope, personal control, and length of illness. To accomplish her purpose, Raleigh designed a Time Opinion Survey as the measure of hope. Raleigh is continuing to work on the measurement problems related to the Time Opinion Survey.

• SPHERES AND DIMENSIONS OF HOPE

In a study of hope in elderly persons with cancer, Dufault used participant observation with a sample of 22 women and 13 men between the ages of 65 and 89.[18,19] She reported that her findings support hope as multidimensional and process oriented. Dufault defined hope as "a multi-dimensional dynamic life force characterized by confident yet uncertain anticipation of realistically possible and personally significant desirable future good having implications for action and for interpersonal relatedness" (p. 1821B).[18] Dufault identified two related but distinct spheres of hope. Generalized hope included a general sense that future nonspecific developments would be beneficial. The second sphere, particularized hope, concerned the confident expectation of a specific future goal or personally significant future good for self. All subjects spoke of the behavior of significant others as a source of hope.

• THE CONTINUUM OF HOPE

McGee developed a model of hope in which hope and hopelessness represent opposite ends of a continuum.[24] At one extreme is the unjustifiably or totally hopeful person who may be immobilized by feelings of invulnerability. At the other extreme is the unrealistically hopeless person who gives up to what is perceived as inevitable. The desirable balance in this model is achieved by what McGee labels the realistic copers, those people who have a positive outlook on life while accepting areas of actual hopelessness in life.

• STONER HOPE SCALE (SHS)

The Stoner Hope Scale (SHS) was developed in an attempt to meet the need for a valid and reliable measure of hope.[27,28] A preliminary form of the SHS adhered closely in both form and content to the scale developed by Erickson et al.[20] However, problems in the use of this form of the SHS were encountered when it was used in a pilot study with ten cancer patients.

As a result of the pilot study experience, the SHS was modified. Stotland's conceptualization of hope as the importance and probability of attainment of future-oriented goals was retained. However, the theoretical framework from Lynch and Marcel recognizing hope as an interior sense requiring interaction with external resources had not been adequately reflected. To strengthen this aspect of the scale, the generic and specific categories of hope were replaced by three domains of hope representing spheres of involvement. The domains and the goals within them were identified in consultation with nurse clinicians in oncology and psychiatry. Intrapersonal, interpersonal, and global hope were designated as the three domains of hope.

Intrapersonal hope is defined as the domain of hope founded on interior resources and beliefs. Although it may be influenced by external stimuli, intrapersonal hope arises from within the person and is not dependent on transaction with another being. An example of an item within the intrapersonal domains is:

To overcome fears that I have.

Interpersonal hope is the domain of hope in which the sphere of involvement extends beyond the self and is definitely dependent on transactions with external resources. Thus, interpersonal hope occurs or exists because of the connection between individuals. An example of a goal in the interpersonal hope domain is:

To have people seek me out as a friend.

Global hope is the category of hope that refers to the broad scope of issues and concerns important to people in a general sense. Global hope goes beyond the person and interpersonal relationships to the sphere of involvement, including hope for the human race, the world, and beyond. An example of a goal in the global hope domain is:

To see an end to the threat of nuclear war.

The response sets for both the importance and probability sections used a 4-point Likert-type scale. Scoring the SHS was based on Stotland's conceptualization of hope including both importance and probability as parameters. For each item, the importance score was multiplied by the personality score. These products were then summed to yield subscale (intrapersonal, interpersonal, and global) as well as a total hope score. To estimate content validity, three expert judges, all with postgraduate nursing education, independently placed goals into domains, with nearly 100 percent agreement.[27]

• BECK HOPELESSNESS SCALE (BHS)

Concurrent validity of the SHS was assessed through the use of the Beck Hopelessness Scale (BHS) as a criterion measure.[31,32] The BHS was designed to measure hopelessness and provides a measure of the construct hope in the opposite direction. The BHS has a relatively high degree of internal consistency with a KR-20 reliability coefficient of 0.93 reported by Beck et al.[31] for a sample of 294 suicide attempters. The demonstrated negative relationship ($r = -0.47$, $p = 0.001$) between the SHS and the BHS indicates moderate concurrent validity for the SHS.

Reliability measures for the SHS were computed through the Cronbach coefficient alpha test of internal consistency and canonical factor analysis.[38,39,40] With a sample of 58 cancer patients, the SHS had a high degree of internal consistency as evidenced by a Cronbach alpha coefficient of 0.93. Item-to-total correlations ranged from 0.37 to 0.65, with a mean interitem correlation of 0.53. When the SHS was subjected to canonical factor analysis in which the number of factors was limited to one, all 30 of the items loaded positively on the first factor, with only four items weighted more heavily on another factor. This suggests that all of the items were measuring a single construct presumed to be hope. The computed reliability coefficient omega for the SHS was 0.94.

• NOWOTNY HOPE SCALE (NHS)

The original Nowotny Hope Scale (NHS) was composed of 47 items within six subscales based on dimensions of hope identified from the literature.[29] The dimensions were (1) orients to future, (2) includes active involvement, (3) comes from within, (4) is possible, (5) relates to or involves others or a higher being, and (6) relates to meaningful outcomes to individuals. Sample items are:

> In the future I plan to accomplish many things.
> I have difficulty in setting goals.

In a methodologic study, Nowotny asked 306 adults, both well and ill, to think of a significant life event that they considered stressful. Subjects then responded to the objective statements using a scaled response of "strongly agree," "agree," "disagree," and "strongly disagree."

Internal consistency reliability was demonstrated by a Cronbach coefficient alpha of 0.897. A negative correlation coefficient of 0.471 ($p = 0.001$) between the NHS and the BHS indicates moderate concurrent validity.

Factor analysis extracted six factors for the 29-item NHS. These new subscales were (1) confidence, (2) relates to others, (3) future is possible, (4) religious faith, (5) active involvement, and (6) comes from within. Some of the original dimensions were retained, whereas others were renamed.

SUMMARY

Many of the articles on hope in the nursing literature are anecdotal descriptions of hope as an important clinical phenomenon. Hope is recognized as a powerful force in the survival of patients confronted by life-threatening and chronic illnesses. Although hope remains poorly understood, nurses are frequently encouraged to instill, inspire, and maintain hope as a therapeutic intervention with patients.

Because hope is a complex, abstract phenomenon, this review of instruments to measure hope includes a discussion of the theoretical analysis from the perspective of philosophy and the behavioral sciences. Themes common to most of the discussion of hope, including theoretical, clinical, and measurement issues, are (1) a future orientation, (2) an expectation of attainment of important goals, and (3) recognition of hope as an interior sense that is dependent on interaction with others. Additional research is needed to refine and further evaluate the existing instruments for research purposes and to evaluate the feasibility of their use as clinical evaluation tools.

REFERENCES

1. Engel, G. A life setting conducive to illness: The giving-up given-up complex. *Bull Menninger Clin*, 1986, *32*(2):324.
2. Hyland, J. Death by giving up. *Bull Menninger Clin*, 1978, *42*(4):339.

3. Richter, C.P. On the phenomenon of sudden death in animals and man. *Psychosom Med,* 1957, *19*(3):191.
4. Stewart, W.K. Hopelessness following illness in middle age. *Psychosomatics* 1977, *18*(2):29.
5. Vaux, K.L. *Will to live, will to die.* Minneapolis, MN: Augsburgh Publishing House, 1978.
6. Allen, A. Psychosocial factors in cancer. *Am Fam Physician,* 1981, *23*:197.
7. Buehler, J.A. What contributes to hope in the cancer patient? *Am J Nurs,* 1975, *75*(9):1353.
8. Lange, S.P. Hope. In C.E. Carlson, & B. Blackwell (Eds.), *Behavioral concepts and nursing intervention* (2nd ed.). Philadelphia: Lippincott, 1978, p. 171.
9. Miller, J.F. Inspiring hope. *Am J Nurs,* 1985, *85*(1):22.
10. Roberts, S.L. *Behavioral concepts and nursing throughout the life span.* Englewood Cliffs, NJ: Prentice Hall, 1978.
11. Walsi, E. Hope, a basic nursing concept. *Conference on Teaching Psychiatric Nursing in Baccalaureate Programs,* Atlanta, GA: Southern Regional Educational Board, 1967.
12. Barckley, V. A visiting nurse specializes in cancer. *Am J Nurs,* 1970, *70*(8):1680.
13. Dubree, M., & Vogelpohl, R. When hope dies: So might the patient. *Am J Nurs,* 1980, *80*(6):1046.
14. Laney, M.L. Hope as a healer. *Nurs Outlook,* 1969, *17*(1):45.
15. Limandri, B.J., & Boyle, D.W. Instilling hope. *Am J Nurs,* 1978, *78*(1):79.
16. Taylor, P.B., & Gideon, M.D. Holding out hope to your dying patient. *Nursing 82,* 1982, *82*(2):268.
17. Vaillot, N.C. Hope, the restoration of being. *Am J Nurs,* 1970, *70*(2):268.
18. Dufault, K.J. Hope of elderly persons with cancer (Doctoral dissertation, Case Western Reserve University). *Dissertation Abstracts International,* 1981, *42*(05):1820-1b University Microfilms No. 8118642).
19. Dufault, K.J., & Martocchio, B. Hope: Its spheres and dimensions. *Nurs Clin of North Am,* 1985, *20*(2):379.
20. Erickson, R.C., Post, R.D., & Paige, A.B. Hope as a psychiatric variable. *J Clin Psychol,* 1975, *31*:324.
21. Gottschalk, L.A. A hope scale applicable to verbal samples. *Arch Gen Psychiatry,* 1974, *30*:779.
22. Gottschalk, L.A., Lolas, F., & Viney, L.L. (Eds.). *Content analysis of verbal behavior: Significance in clinical medicine and psychiatry.* New York: Springer-Verlag, 1986.
23. Gottschalk, L.A., & Hoigaard, J. Emotional impact of mastectomy. In L.A. Gottschalk, F. Lolas, & L.L. Viney (Eds.), *Content analysis of verbal behavior: Significance in clinical medicine and psychiatry.* New York: Springer-Verlag, 1986, p. 171.
24. McGee, R.F. Hope: A factor influencing crisis resolution. *Adv Nurs Sci,* 1984, *6*(4):34.
25. Raleigh, E.D. An investigation of hope as manifested in the physically ill adult (Doctoral dissertation, Wayne State University). *Dissertation Abstracts International,* 1980, *41*(04):1313B (University Microfilms No. 8022786).
26. Stanley, A.T. The lived experience of hope: The isolation of discrete descriptive elements common to the experience of hope in healthy young adults (Doctoral dissertation, The Catholic University of America). *Dissertation Abstracts International,* 1978, *39*(03):1212B (University Microfilms No. 7816899).
27. Stoner, M.J.H. Hope and cancer patients (Doctoral dissertation, The University of Colorado). *Dissertation Abstracts International,* 1982, *44*(1):115B (University Microfilms No. 8312243).
28. Stoner, M.H., & Kaempfer, S.H. Recalled life expectancy information, phase of illness and hope in cancer patients. *Res Nurs Health,* 1985, *8*(3):269.
29. Nowotny, M.L. Measurement of hope as exhibited by a general adult population after a stressful event (Doctoral dissertation, Texas Woman's University). 1986.
30. Thompson, M. *An investigation of the relationship of love, mutuality, freedom, and newness with the perception of hope in patients with the diagnosis of cancer.* Unpublished thesis, California State University, 1980.
31. Beck, A.T., Lester, D., Trexler, L., & Weisman, A. The measurement of pessimism: The hopelessness scale. *J Consult Clin Psychol,* 1974, *42*:861.
32. Durham, T.W. Norms, reliability, and item analysis of the hopelessness scale in general psychiatric, forensic psychiatric, and college populations. *J Clin Psychol,* 1982, *38*(3):597.
33. Marcel, G. *Homo viator.* (E. Crawford, trans.). San Francisco, CA: Harper and Row, 1962.

34. Marcel, G. *The mystery of being: Vol. II: Faith and reality.* South Bend, IN: Regnery/Gateway, 1951.
35. Marcel, G. Desire and hope. In N. Lawrence, & D. O'Connor (Eds.), *Readings in existential phenomenology.* Englewood Cliffs, NJ: Prentice-Hall, 1967, p. 277.
36. Lynch, W.F. *Images of hope.* Baltimore, MD: Helicon, 1965.
37. Stotland, E. *The psychology of hope.* San Francisco, CA: Jossey-Bass, 1969.
38. Mitchell, S.K. Interobserver agreement, reliability, and generalizability of data collected in observational studies. *Psychol Bull,* 1979, *86*:376.
39. Anastasi, A. *Psychological testing (4th ed.).* New York: Macmillan, 1970.
40. Allen, M.P. Construction of composite measures by canonical-factor-regression method. In H.L. Costner (Ed.), *Sociological methodology.* San Francisco, CA: Jossey-Bass, 1974, p. 51.

CHAPTER 9

Measuring Aspects of Spirituality

Jan M. Ellerhorst-Ryan, R.N., M.S.N., C.S.

The nursing profession has long taken pride in its holistic approach to care, which recognizes the needs of the total person. In light of nursing's focus on the total person, the noticeable absence of the spiritual dimension in nursing theory and research is cause for concern. Perhaps nurses consider matters of spirituality too personal for nursing involvement. Perhaps they believe that spiritual needs are better met by the clergy. In some cases, the client's spiritual needs may be mistaken for psychosocial needs.[1]

Nursing professionals who are truly committed to viewing humans in a holistic manner must broaden their focus to include the client's spiritual concerns. In summarizing a study of clients' spiritual needs, Highfield and Cason stated, "We cannot abdicate our responsibility for treating a person's spiritual needs to the chaplain, any more than we can abdicate our responsibility for man's physical needs to the physician, or his psychosocial needs to the psychologist and social worker" (p. 191).[1] Spirituality must become more than the sum of the client's religious preference, religious beliefs, and religious practices.

The 1971 White House Conference on Aging defined the spiritual dimension as pertaining to "man's inner resources, especially . . . the central philosophy of life, which guides a person's conduct, the supernatural and non-material dimensions of human nature" (p. 3).[2] It encompasses humans' need to find satisfactory answers to questions about the meaning of life, illness, and death.

The Third National Conference on Classification of Nursing Diagnoses (1978) recognized the importance of spirituality by including "spiritual concerns," "spiritual distress," and "spiritual despair" in the list of approved nursing diagnoses. In 1980, the Fourth National Conference combined these three categories into one, "spiritual distress," which they defined as "a disruption in the life principle which pervades a person's entire being and which integrates and transcends one's biological and psychosocial nature" (p. 332).[3] This definition, although a beginning, is vague and does not, therefore, lend itself easily to research.

An investigation of the spiritual dimension is hampered by the frequent use of overlapping terms (spirituality, spiritual distress, spiritual needs, spiritual concerns) with no consensus on definition. Most research dealing with spirituality has focused on religiosity. Moberg and Bruske,[4] in comparing religiosity and spiritual well-being, associate the former with institutional goals and behaviors. Measures of religious practice are not always reliable indicators of spirituality.

Spirituality, on the other hand, encompasses but is not limited to religiosity. Spirituality relates to the "totality of man's inner resources, the ultimate concerns around which all other values are focused, the central philosophy of life that guides conduct, and the meaning-giving center of human life which influences all individual and social behavior" (p. 2).[5] Spirituality concepts are applicable to persons who are religious, nonreligious, or antireligious. For this reason, investigations of spirituality issues are more likely to produce meaningful information to nurses. Researchers should remember that a religious component and a psychosocial component are involved in spiritual concerns. Both should be addressed in a tool designed to assess aspects of spirituality.

The concept of "God" is one that does not easily conform to a universal definition. It is, therefore, important that the researcher consider ways to elicit information about the subject's perception of God. Traditional views of God characterize Him as the ultimate Deity. For others, particularly those who are nonreligious or antireligious, God may be whatever they value most, the focal point of life—work, family, community service, or other aspect. In view of the significant influence that the Judeo-Christian philosophy has had on the development of Western culture, the instruments discussed most often reflect that perspective. Applicability to people who have other religious orientations are included for several of the instruments presented.

SPIRITUAL NEEDS

Before selecting a measurement tool, the researcher must define "spiritual needs" in measurable terms. This, in itself, is not an easy task. The 1971 White House Conference on Aging acknowledged the multidimensional nature of spiritual concerns, which they defined as "the human need to deal with sociocultural deprivations, anxieties and fears, death and dying, personality integration, self-image, personal dignity, social alienation, and philosophy of life" (p. 351).[6]

Hess and Stoll, two nurses who are well known for their interest in spiritual concerns of patients, have defined spiritual needs as factors necessary to establish and maintain a relationship with God, however "God" is defined by the individual.[7,8] These factors include forgiveness, love and relatedness, hope, and meaning and purpose in life. The Fifth National Conference on Nursing Diagnoses supported the approach taken by Hess and Stoll by incorporating these spiritual needs into the "spiritual distress" diagnostic category.[9] Research instruments for investigating an individual spiritual need are discussed in other chapters of this book.

An interview schedule using open-ended questions may be a more useful tool for studies that are qualitative rather than quantitative in nature. The interview tools described here can be used in populations that include people with diverse religious beliefs and orientations.

▪ HESS' SPIRITUAL NEEDS SURVEY

Hess' Spiritual Needs Survey was designed for use in hospitals or extended care facilities but could be modified easily for use in other settings.[10] The survey consists of five questions that focus on the patient's awareness of his or her spiritual needs and efforts to address them:

Were you aware of having a spiritual need at any time during your hospitalization?

With whom did you discuss this need?

• STOLL'S GUIDELINES FOR SPIRITUAL ASSESSEMENT

Although Stoll's Guidelines for Spiritual Assessment were not designed for use as a research tool, they have been used in conjunction with other measurement scales to evaluate the ability of hospitalized patients to have their spiritual needs met.[8,11,12] Stoll's Guidelines include 13 questions addressing the person's concept of God, sources of hope and strength, religious practices, and the relationship between spiritual beliefs and health. Sample items include:

To whom do you turn when you need help?

Has being sick made any difference in your feelings toward God? toward yourself? toward others?[11]

Fish and Shelly[13] modified Stoll's Guidelines to reorganize the questions into four categories: understanding a person's beliefs about and involvement with God and religious practice, determining the extent to which a person's religious practices serve as a resource for faith and life, assessing whether resources for hope and strength are founded on reality, and extending an opportunity to accept spiritual help. Excluding the fourth category, which is an invitation for intervention by the interviewer, the remaining three categories contain a total of 11 open-ended questions.

• SPIRITUAL NEEDS OF PATIENTS QUESTIONNAIRE

Martin et al.[14] used an interview schedule and a two-part questionnaire in their study of spiritual needs. The Spiritual Needs of Patients Questionnaire, administered first, is comprised of ten statements about spiritual care to which the subject indicates degree of agreement or disagreement on a 5-point Likert scale. Examples of items in the questionnaire include:

Nurses are too busy to help patients with their spiritual needs.

A nurse who sits down and listens is helping me spiritually.

Statements chosen were representative of those reported in a 1969 Nursing Christian Fellowship study of the spiritual needs of patients.[13]

The second part of Martin's questionnaire consists of two items. The first asks the participant to rank seven spiritual needs in order of importance, such as:

Relief from fear of death

Knowledge of God's presence

The second item lists eight possible nursing interventions, including:

Pray with a patient

Show kindness, concern and cheerfulness when giving care

Participants check those items that they believe are appropriate spiritual interventions for nurses.

The interview schedule contains six questions, five from Hess' Spiritual Needs Survey plus:

How do you think nurses might help patients meet spiritual needs?

SPIRITUAL WELL-BEING

An alternative approach to assessing spiritual needs is the evaluation of spiritual well-being, which has been defined by the National Interfaith Coalition on Aging as "the affirmation of life in a relationship with God, self, community and environment that nurtures and celebrates wholeness" (p. 331).[15] The universality of spiritual well-being was summarized by Moberg:

> A central concern of the Christian faith, if not also of Islam, Judaism, Hinduism, and Buddhism, is to enhance the spiritual well-being of people. Although the semantics and theology of this concern vary from one group to another, it is located at the very core of many religious goals. It also is central to the ultimate values of Soviet Marxism, which hopes to shape "the new man" who combines "spiritual richness" with "moral purity" (p. 351).[6]

▪ SPIRITUAL WELL-BEING SCALE

The Spiritual Well-Being Scale, a 20-item Likert-type tool authored by Ellison and Paloutzian, reflects the belief that spiritual well-being involves a vertical and a horizontal dimension. The vertical dimension refers to the sense of well-being in the relationship with God, and the horizontal dimension refers to sense of purpose in and satisfaction with life.[15,16] These two dimensions can be addressed separately using one of the two subscales that comprise the Spiritual Well-Being Scale. The Religious Well-Being subscale measures the vertical component, and the Existential Well-Being sub-scale focuses on the horizontal. For example, the statement "I have a personally meaningful relationship with God" refers to religious well-being. "I believe that there is some purpose for my life" refers to existential well-being.[15] Responses to each item range from "strongly agree" to "strongly disagree."

Factor analysis of the Spiritual Well-Being Scale using the Varimax rotation was performed on data obtained from 206 students at three colleges having a religious orientation. The items clustered together as expected, with existential items loading into two subfactors, life direction and life satisfaction.[15,16]

The scale was then administered to 100 student volunteers at the University of Idaho. Test–retest reliability coefficients were 0.93 (spiritual well-being), 0.96 (religious well-being), and 0.86 (existential well-being). Internal consistency was evaluated using coefficient alpha, yielding 0.89 (spiritual well-being), 0.87 (religious well-being), and 0.78 (existential well-being).[15]

Examination of item content supports the face validity of the scale. In addition, the Spiritual Well-Being Scale scores have correlated in predicted ways with other theoretically related measures, including the Purpose in Life Test and Intrinsic Religious Orientation.[15]

The authors of the Spiritual Well-Being Scale acknowledge that the tool arises from the Judeo-Christian perception of religious well-being in which God is conceived in personal terms. However, they note that "it is . . . possible that those from eastern religions such as Hinduism and Buddhism may be able to use the scale if they can meaningfully interpret the statements about relationship with " (p. 333). [15]

• MOBERG'S INDEXES OF SPIRITUAL WELL-BEING (SWB)

Moberg's Indexes of Spiritual Well-Being (SWB) are a 45-item questionnaire that include a variety of factors that may influence spiritual well-being: social attitudes, self-perceptions, theological orientation, activities serving others in charitable, political, and religious contexts, and religious beliefs, opinions, experiences, preferences, and affiliation. [6] Seven indexes identified through factor analysis include Christian faith, self-satisfaction, personal piety, subjective spiritual well-being, optimism, religious cynicism, and elitism.

Answer categories for most items range from "strongly agree" to "strongly disagree." Items in the personal piety index differ in that they require a response that indicates how frequently the subject participates in a particular activity. Examples from this tool include:

My faith helps me to make decisions. (Christian faith)

How often do you pray privately? (personal piety)

Organized religion has hindered or harmed my own spiritual well-being more than it has helped. (religious cynicism)[6]

The Indexes of Spiritual Well-Being are believed to have face validity, since the items were based on information gained through multiple earlier studies performed by Moberg. Preliminary data support criterion validity of the indexes. When scores for evangelical Christians were compared with those of other Christians, differences were in the expected direction. Likewise, scores for Christians were higher than scores for people professing to be agnostics or atheists. [6] Additional testing with other criterion groups is needed to establish further the tool's validity. Further analysis of the validity of the Indexes has demonstrated coefficients ranging from 0.60 to 0.86 when scores were correlated with the Spiritual Well-Being Scale.

Moberg's Indexes of Spiritual Well-Being represent a major attempt to demonstrate the multifaceted nature of spiritual well-being. However, the Indexes have two characteristics that may limit their usefulness in nursing research. The tool in its present form is somewhat lengthy and, therefore, may not be practical for use with certain patient populations, such as those with extensive disease who would tire easily. The Indexes are also specific to Christianity and could not be used in their present form with patients of Jewish or Eastern orientations.

SPIRITUAL COPING

The importance of religious faith is often overlooked by nurses when routinely assessing how a person copes with disease. Investigation of spiritual coping may appear, at the surface, to document the performance of religious activities. Spiritual coping actually looks beyond the actual behavior to the meaning or significance the behavior holds for the participant.

▪ PATIENT SPIRITUAL COPING INTERVIEW

The Patient Spiritual Coping Interview was developed by McCorkle and Benoliel[17] and adapted for use in a one-time interview format by Sodestrom and Martin.[18] This semistructured interview contains 30 items that investigate relationship with God or a "higher being," use of spiritual behaviors or resource persons, expressions of spiritual needs, and perception of the nurse's role in spiritual care.[18] Questions include:

> Do you ever watch religious TV or listen to religious radio?

> Have you spoken about your spiritual thoughts or concerns to someone?

> How do you think nurses can assist you with your spiritual needs?

Content validity of the interview was established by its consistency with the current literature. The interview schedule was reviewed by a panel of expert judges, three in oncology nursing research and two in theology, who agreed that the items included were adequate and appropriate. Reliability was inferred by the assumption that subjects are reliable sources of information pertaining to the use of spiritual coping strategies.[18]

▪ INTRINSIC RELIGIOUS MOTIVATION SCALE

The importance of spirituality in a person's life can be evaluated by the Intrinsic Religious Motivation Scale developed by Hoge.[19] An intrinsically motivated person is one whose most central and ultimate motive in life can be found in his or her religious faith. The extrinsically motivated person views his or her religion as subservient to other aspects of life, such as money or social status.[20] The scale consists of ten statements to which the participant answers "yes" or "no." "One should seek God's guidance when making every important decision" indicates intrinsic motivation. "It doesn't matter what I believe as long as I lead a moral life" is consistent with extrinsic motivation.[19]

The Intrinsic Religious Motivation Scale was administered to 42 adult Protestants, 21 of whom were judged by their ministers as intrinsically motivated and 21 judged as extrinsically motivated. The initial scale included 30 items. The final scale is composed of the 10 items having highest validity, reliability, item-to-item correlations, and item-to-scale correlations. All 10 items correlated with the ministers' opinions in the direction predicted beyond 0.03 level of significance. The reliability of the scale, measured by the KR 20, was 0.901. Item-to-item correlations ranged from 0.132 to 0.716, with 22 of 45 item-to-item correlations greater than 0.5.[19]

The shorter version of the Intrinsic Religious Motivation Scale may be easier to use when compared to the Patient Spiritual Coping Interview. However, the Intrinsic Religious Motivation Scale fails to identify specific behaviors that provide a source of comfort or strength to the subject. Another potential problem with the Intrinsic Religious Motivation Scale lies in the classification of items. Seven of the items are indicative of intrinsic motivation, whereas only three reflect external motivation. The author has acknowledged this limitation and suggests deletion of the intrinsic item, "My faith sometimes restricts my actions." With this change, the Kuder-Richardson score becomes 0.902.[19]

SPIRITUAL NEEDS OF CHILDREN

The potential difficulties in obtaining spiritual data from children were well summarized by Shelly:

> If sound assessment is crucial to caring for adults, it is even more important in the pediatric setting. Children, especially young children, have a limited ability to communicate, particularly about abstract concepts (p. 88).[21]

A study of adolescents reported by Elkind[22] used only two questions:

When do you feel closest to God?

Have you ever had a particular experience when you felt especially close to God?

Responses from 144 ninth grade students to these items indicated differences between males and females and between honor students and average students, with $p < 0.05$. Differences were also noted between Protestants, Catholics, and Jews. However, the uncertainty about exact numbers in each denomination precluded statistical analysis.

A Nurses Christian Fellowship task force developed a seven-question assessment tool to obtain information about the spiritual needs of children:

How do you feel when you're in trouble?

Do you know who God is?

What is He like?[21]

Additional information can be obtained from young children by asking them to draw pictures of God and themselves with or without significant others. Using this technique requires special skill in interpretation in order to obtain meaningful data.

NURSES AND SPIRITUAL NEEDS OF PATIENTS

Several tools are available to measure nurses' awareness of and appropriate interventions for spiritual needs.

• CHADWICK'S QUESTIONNAIRE

Chadwick devised a seven-item multiple-choice questionnaire to investigate "awareness and preparedness of nurses to meet spiritual needs."[23] Sample questions include:

How long has it been since you last recognized a spiritual need in your patients?

Have you ever read the Bible or prayed with a patient?

• NURSE INTERVIEW

Sodestrom and Martinson devised a Nurse Interview schedule to correspond to the one discussed for patients. Seventeen items were selected from the patient interview and modified to evaluate nurses' awareness of the spiritual strategies used by patients in coping with disease.[18] Nurse participants answer "yes," "no," or "don't know" to such questions as:

Do you know if your patient has spoken to a clergyman?

Do you know if he or she has read the Bible?

Does your patient make reference to guilt feelings related to God?

Reliability and validity for the Nurse Interview are based on the same data as the Patient Spiritual Coping Interview.

• HIGHFIELD-CASON QUESTIONNAIRE

Highfield and Cason developed a 49-item questionnaire for their study of nurses' ability to identify behaviors and conditions expressive of spiritual health or spiritual need.[1] Nurse participants are instructed to note whether the behavior or condition described is related to either the spiritual or psychosocial dimension. They are also to rate on a scale of 1 to 5 how frequently each behavior or condition is noted in their patients. Finally, participants are to note each item considered to be a patient problem.

The items contained in the Highfield-Cason Questionnaire were identified from the nursing and pastoral care literature and were submitted to a review panel of theology and psychology experts. Although many items in the questionnaire are legitimately a part of the spiritual domain (e.g., "expresses resentment toward God," "expresses despair"), several are less clear (e.g., "expresses fear of tests and diagnosis," "is unable to pursue creative outlets"). The less specific items could easily represent a psychosocial problem rather than or in addition to a spiritual problem. This ambiguity needs to be addressed by researchers who use the Highfield-Cason Questionnaire.

SUMMARY

Nursing research related to spiritual issues has been hampered by a variety of factors, including discomfort among nurses who believe that spirituality and spiritual needs are a private matter, difficulty in distinguishing psychosocial needs from spiritual needs, lack of valid and reliable measurement tools that address spiritual concerns, and confusion about differences between spiritual concerns and religiosity.

The tools described here represent a heightened awareness of different aspects of spirituality. The development of new measures and further refinement of tools currently available will enable us to expand our understanding of this underresearched area.

REFERENCES

1. Highfield, M., & Cason, C. Spiritual needs of patients—Are they being recognized? *Cancer Nurs,* 1983, *6*(3):187.
2. Moberg, D. Spiritual well-being: Background and issues. Washington, DC: White House Conference on Aging, 1971.
3. Kim, M., & Moritz, D. *Classification of nursing diagnoses: Proceedings of the Third and Fourth National Conferences.* New York: McGraw-Hill, 1980.
4. Moberg, D., & Brusek, P. Spiritual well-being: A neglected subject in quality of life research. *Soc Indicators Res,* 1978, *5*(3):303.
5. Moberg, D.O. Development of social indicators of spiritual well-being for quality of life research. In D.O. Moberg (Ed.), *Spiritual well-being: Sociological perspectives.* Washington, DC: University Press of America, 1979, p. 1.
6. Moberg, D.O. Subjective measures of spiritual well-being. *Rev Relig Res,* 1984, *25*(4):351.
7. Stallwood, J. Spiritual dimensions of nursing practice. In I. Beland & J. Passos (Eds.), *Clinical nursing.* New York: Macmillan, 1975.
8. Stoll, R. Guidelines for spiritual assessment. *Am J Nurs,* 1979, *79*(9):1574.
9. Kim, M., McFarland, G., & McLane, A. *Classifications of nursing diagnoses: Proceedings of the Fifth National Conference.* St. Louis, MO: Mosby, 1984.
10. Hess, J.S. Spiritual needs survey. In S. Fish & J.A. Shelly (Eds.), *Spiritual care: The nurse's role.* Downers Grove, IL: Intervarsity Press, 1983, p. 157.
11. Stoll, R. Spiritual assessment: A nursing perspective. Presented at Spirituality in Nursing Workshop. Marquette University, Milwaukee, WI, August 1984.
12. Fordyce, E. An investigation of television's potential for meeting the spiritual needs of hospitalized persons (Doctoral dissertation, Catholic University of America, 1981). *Dissertation Abstracts International,* 1982.
13. Fish, S., & Shelly, J.A. *Spiritual care: The nurse's role* Downers Grove, IL: Intervarsity Press, 1983.
14. Martin, C., Burrows, C., & Pomilio, J. Spiritual needs of patients study. In S. Fish & J.A. Shelly (Eds.), *Spiritual Care: The Nurse's Role.* Downers Grove, IL: Intervarsity Press, 1983, p. 160.
15. Ellison, C.W. Spiritual well-being: Conceptualization and measurement. *Journal of Psychology and Theology,* 1983, *11*(4):330.
16. Paloutzian, R., & Ellison, C.W. Loneliness, spiritual well-being, and the quality of life. In A. Peplau & D. Perlman (Eds.), *Loneliness: A sourcebook of current theory, research, and therapy.* New York: Wiley, 1982, p. 224.
17. McCorkle, R., & Benoliel, J.Q. *Manual of data collection instruments.* Unpublished manual, University of Washington, 1981.
18. Sodestrom, K.E., & Martinson, I. Oncology patients' and professional nurses' identification of spiritual coping strategies. *Oncol Nurs Forum,* (in press).
19. Hoge, D.R. Validated intrinsic religious motivation scale. *J Scientific Study Religion,* 1972, *11*(4):369.
20. Soderstrom, D., & Wright, E.W. Religious orientation and meaning in life. *J Clin Psychology,* 1977, *33*(1):65.
21. Shelly, J.A. *Spiritual needs of children.* Downers Grove, IL: Intervarsity Press, 1982.
22. Elkind, D., & Elkind, S. Varieties of religious experience in young adolescents. *J Scientific Study Religion,* 1962, *2*(1):102.
23. Chadwick, R. Awareness and preparedness of nurses to meet spiritual needs. In S. Fish & J.A. Shelly (Eds.), *Spiritual care: The nurse's role.* Downers Grove, IL: Intervarsity Press, 1983, p. 177.

CHAPTER *10*

Measuring Information-Seeking Behaviors

Caroline Bagley-Burnett, R.N., M.S.N.

Information is a key to understanding the problems, challenges, and frustrations with which an individual is faced throughout his or her lifespan. Information is essential in decision making and is considered by many to be a means of coping with and reducing stress.[1-7] For these reasons, it is important for nurses (1) to understand the concept of information seeking, (2) to possess a knowledge of the behaviors exhibited by people seeking information, (3) to develop the skills necessary to assess the amount and type of information desired by people, and (4) to recognize the contextual and situational variables that influence a person's desire for information.

The purposes of this chapter are to present relevant background on the concept of information seeking as found in both the consumer and health care literature, to describe the development of instruments used to measure aspects of information seeking, to evaluate the utility of these instruments for their ability to fulfill their designed purpose, and to discuss the relevance of the concept of information seeking and the described instruments to nursing practice.

A review of the consumer and health care literature reveals that the concept of information seeking is both complex and poorly understood. Research in this area can be found as early as the 1920s in the consumer literature, when studies that focused on consumer prepurchase information-seeking activities were described as a component of marketing theory. After that, the literature is sparse until the 1960s when one finds studies that address the prepurchase activities of people purchasing both durable and nondurable goods.[8,9]

Reference to information-seeking activities within the health care literature is not found until the 1960s, and these accounts are predominantly clinical anecdotes.[1] Gradually, however, more studies have been conducted addressing the many facets of information-seeking activities for consumers of health care, and, of the few studies in this area, four have been conducted by nurses.[1,3,10,11]

CONSUMER INFORMATION-SEEKING BEHAVIOR

In the last 20 years, there has been a dramatic increase in interest concerning consumer prepurchase behavior. There are several reasons for this increased interest. Manufacturers, retailers, and advertisers benefit from data on consumer prepurchase behavior, which enables them to better target the interests of people and results in increased product sales. Both the consumer's and women's movements have played a role in the desire for information and also in researchers' interest in what motivates people to seek information. Legislators, health care professionals, and policy makers have shown increased interest in information-seeking prepurchase behavior, possibly reflecting the interests of their constituencies. Nationally, laws have been enacted that mandate informed consent and the inclusion of patient package inserts in such drugs as oral contraceptives and estrogens. Fourteen states require the development of a booklet that describes the treatment options for breast cancer. Health insurance companies often reimburse for health education and frequently prorate insurance rates accordingly. Organizations, for example, the American Cancer Society and the National Cancer Institute, and many drug companies have developed their own information sources for use by consumers. Finally, changes in the economic climate, including income and levels of employment, periods of high inflation, skyrocketing medical costs, reduced provider payments, and cutbacks in federal funding, have contributed to increased preference for more information.

As a result of these changes, consumers have better access to information necessary to make decisions concerning health care. Physicians and nurses are more likely to offer explanations about diagnosis, treatments, side effects, and expected outcomes. Consumers tend to ask more questions and to seek information from several sources. Studies have shown that sources of information include physicians, nurses, pharmacists, such media as television, radio, newspaper, and magazines, and to a lesser degree family and friends.[12] However, a discrepancy still exists between what consumers say they want to know and how much information physicians believe they want to know. Faden et al. reported that physicians consistently underestimate the amount of information people want about treatments and their side effects, and studies performed with patients receiving patient package inserts show similar results.[13]

Although the results of such studies tend to demonstrate a desire on the part of consumers for more information, caution must be applied in generalizing these findings and in forming assumptions, such as: more information is better; all people desire complete information; and more information reduces stress and enhances the ability to cope with this stress. Although these assumptions may well be true, research is needed that focuses on how much information a person wants and what variables alter the amount desired. For example, do such variables as age, sex, race, and psychosocial, cultural, economic, and educational background play a role in determining what type, how much, and when an individual wants information? What factors, such as previous illness, experiences with the health care system, or significant others with similar problems, influence information-seeking activities?

The problem today, then, is not so much the availability of information as the identification of the type of information the person wants, how much and under what circumstances he or she wants this information, and what role, if any, the mentioned variables play.

Little has been written on theories of information-seeking behaviors. Lazarus' theory of stress and coping is often used as the conceptional framework when studying the concept of information-seeking activities. He maintains that having knowledge is a means of reducing stress and thereby enhancing coping.[7] It seems logical that if people can actively seek information, they may enhance their ability to cope with a particular situation.

Information has been conceptualized as a form of cognitive control because it often results in the interpretation of an aversive event so that the threat is lessened.[14] Search is conceptualized as an interpersonal process with the primary sources of information being others to whom one has direct access or can be referred.[1] This process contains six steps: (1) a stimulus, (2) goal setting, (3) a decision regarding whether to seek information actively, (4) search behavior, (5) information acquisition and codifications, (6) decision regarding the adequacy of the information acquired, and (7) outcomes.[1]

Information seeking is conceptualized by Hopkins as a process that occurs throughout a series of related stressful episodes and is characterized by the polar extremes of avoidance and hypervigilance. It is defined as a coping strategy of varying levels of intensity measured as a quantitative score on the Information Preference Questionnaire.[3]

Research in the area of information-seeking activities is needed, (IPQ), and instruments that are designed to assess behaviors exhibited by people in this process must be developed.

REVIEW OF THE CONSUMER LITERATURE

Initially, since little was known about people's activities prior to purchase, most studies were exploratory, descriptive, and retrospective in nature. The data were generally gathered by survey or interview. Recent studies have failed to develop standardized instruments, which raises questions about their validity and reliability. Sampling presents another problem, since factors relating to the representativeness of the samples were often ignored. Therefore, care must be taken when analyzing the data, correlating variables, or generalizing from the results.

Several problems that exist must be recognized and accepted as limitations if one plans to extrapolate data from this literature. The first problem deals with methodology. Most of the studies are retrospective, with time having passed between consumer purchase and when the survey took place, thus arousing doubts about the validity of the studies. The second problem is one of instrumentation. This raises questions about the validity and reliability of the results. A third problem is in the method employed for data analysis. Earlier studies tended to yield only frequency scores and few, if any, described correlations between variables of search or contextual variables related to the people's purchase decision. Recognizing the limitations of the analyses used and the seminal state of this work, one can still extrapolate much data on which to build models of consumer prepurchase information-seeking activities.

Based on earlier research, the following variables have been identified as significant factors in consumer prepurchase search:

- The number of shopping trips before purchase
- The number of prepurchase visits to the store of purchase
- The time spent at a shopping center
- The time spent in the decision process
- The number of brands examined
- The number of price ranges considered
- The number of kinds of sources of information used
- The extent to which buyers sought information on product characteristics, cost, and services[8]

Newman and Lockman listed the determinants of external search; these include previous purchase history, demographic background, buyer personality, perceived risk, and perceived costs of the search.[8] Kiel and Layton identified three dimensions of consumer information seeking: a source of information dimension, a brand dimension, and a time dimension.[9] The source of information dimension includes retailer search, media search, and interpersonal search. The categories described represent the collation of those variables relevant when addressing consumer prepurchase information seeking. The variables described by Newman and Lockman can be classified according to the dimensions proposed by Kiel and Layton, adding a contextual category as described by Newman and Lockman[8,9]:

Sources of information dimension
- Number and kinds of sources of information used
- Extent to which buyers sought information on product characteristics, cost, and services

Time dimension
- Number of shopping trips made before purchase
- Number of prepurchase visits to the store of purchase
- Time spent at a shopping center
- Time spent in the decision process

Brand dimension
- Number of brands examined
- Number of price ranges considered

Contextual dimension
- Previous purchase history (including product knowledge)
- Demographic background
- Buyer personality
- Perceived risk
- Perceived costs of search
- Need factors related to product (e.g., hedonistic, basic to life, emergency)

A voluminous literature addresses prepurchase information-seeking activities of individuals. This research falls into several categories designed to address one or more of the dimensions described. The studies can be categorized as (1) retrospective surveys, (2) a combination of observation and survey methods (which have the potential advantage of combining retrospective and current occurrences), and (3) the use of hypothetical purchase decisions which subjects are required to make based on situations designed for the study.[8,9,15-17] Each method has strengths and limitations that must be critically weighed before adapting them for use in research designed to identify information-seeking behavior of people making health care decisions.

Despite problems associated with retrospective studies, a factor in their favor, in this instance, is that actual reference is made to real life situations to which a person has had to respond. Observational studies attempt to eliminate some of the problems of the retrospective design, since by their very nature, they record an event as it is occurring. One must be aware of the potential ethical issues that arise, however, if the participant is unaware that he is being observed, and the researcher must be aware of the potential halo effects from this type of method. It is obvious that a major limitation of this approach in the health care setting concerns the lack of availability of subjects during the information-seeking process. The use of hypothetical examples of choice, as described in the information display board method,[16,17] provides more structure in the decision process than is found in real life situations. In addition, the element of risk or stress conveyed by making a choice is somewhat less than one would be faced with in real life.

As a result of the research conducted on consumer prepurchase information-seeking behavior, a body of knowledge has been accumulated that has conceptual relevance to research conducted in the health care field. For example, the works of Payne[16] and Englander and Tyszka[17] have used the information display board method. This method consists of an information display matrix that has rows listing alternatives and columns describing the attributes of each alternative.[17] They found that people proceeded in either an intradimensional or interdimensional manner, that is, when faced with several alternatives and the choice of characteristics within each alternative, the person might choose to exhaust all characteristics with one alternative (intradimensional) or might choose to explore all the alternatives (interdimensional) before investigating characteristics within each alternative. Unfortunately, the authors did not identify individual characteristics of people or contextual variables that might be predictive of the type of approach chosen. However, they did find that people, when faced with many alternatives, tended to limit the intradimensional search component, thus sacrificing some depth of knowledge about an alternative, to seek more limited information on the large number of alternatives. Conversely, when faced with only two alternatives, people tended to extend the depth of search. When faced with many alternatives, people attempted to eliminate or collapse the categories to decrease the total number of options to be evaluated. The apparent purpose is to both decrease the complexity of the task and decrease the strain or tension experienced in the evaluation process.

Conceptually, this approach is extremely relevant to research conducted on information-seeking behaviors used by consumers of health care. Nurses can apply these findings in their contacts with patients during health teaching, at the time of diagnosis as well as throughout the treatment phase. In addition, these findings provide stimulation for generation of hypotheses for further research.

INSTRUMENTS USED TO MEASURE INFORMATION-SEEKING ACTIVITIES IN HEALTH CARE

Within the health care literature a number of factors have been identified that are thought to play a role in an individual's search for information. One of these relates specifically to an individual's health locus of control.

• HEALTH LOCUS OF CONTROL (HLC) SCALE

Wallston et al. developed and validated the Health Locus of Control (HLC) Scale.[5] The scale is a measure of expectation regarding locus of control developed for the prediction of health-related behavior. Development of the scale evolved from perceived deficiencies in the Rotter Internal-External (I-E) Locus of Control Scale, which was thought to be unsuccessful in predicting behavior in the health area. The HLC was developed under the assumption that a health locus of control scale would provide more sensitive predictions of the relationship between internality and health behaviors.[5]

The development of this scale has relevance to instruments designed to measure information-seeking behaviors. By determining a person's locus of control, Wallston et al. hypothesized that one could gain information on his or her need for exposure to more information.

TABLE 10–1. SELECTED ITEMS FROM THE HEALTH LOCUS OF CONTROL SCALE

Item	Direction
1. If I take care of myself, I can avoid illness.	I
2. Whenever I get sick, it is because of something I've done or not done.	I
3. Good health is largely a matter of good fortune.	E
4. No matter what I do, if I am going to get sick I will get sick.	E
5. Most people do not realize the extent to which their illnesses are controlled by accidental happenings.	E
6. I can only do what my doctor tells me to do.	E
7. There are so many strange diseases around that you can never know how or when you might pick one up.	E
8. When I feel ill, I know it is because I have not been getting the proper exercise or eating right.	I
9. People who never get sick are just plain lucky.	E
10. People's ill health results from their own carelessness.	I
11. I am directly responsible for my health.	I

I, internally worded statements; E, externally worded statements.
From Wallston, Kaplan, Maides. J Consult Clin Psychol, *1976,44(4):580.*

The authors conducted two studies using the HLC that were designed to test two hypotheses, one of which is relevant to information seeking. The hypothesis was designed to "test the proposition that subjects who held internal locus of control beliefs and who also highly valued health would choose to expose themselves to more information about a given health condition, hypertension, than internals who valued health less or than externals regardless of the value they placed on health" (p. 582).[5] They concluded that health-related information-seeking behavior is a joint function of an internal health-related locus of control belief and holding health in high value.[5] Consistent with other authors, they recognized that the entire area of information seeking in relation to health is a complex entity. These authors have contributed to the body of knowledge in this area by identifying individual factors, that is, internality and externality, as they relate to search. In addition, they found that it is not just these two factors that determine the extent of search but also the value the person places on health. The specific goal of the search and the content of the information being sought also have a role in the process. The contribution of this scale broadens what is known about the process of search by including individual behavioral variables as integral components. Selected items from the scale can be found in Table 10–1.

An indepth discussion of the concept of locus of control is presented in Chapter 16.

▪ LENZ ANALYTICAL MODEL OF AN INFORMATION SEARCH EPISODE

Lenz developed a model (Fig. 10–1) that "represents the analytically distinct steps hypothesized to comprise a search episode, the flow of events which precede the initial voluntary contact (or attempted contact) with a health service provider" (p. 182).[1]

As can be seen, there are several decision points along the continuum. It is assumed that the person desires a health-related service or, at the least, information about health resources that may be used at a later time. Search then commences, varying in length and extent.

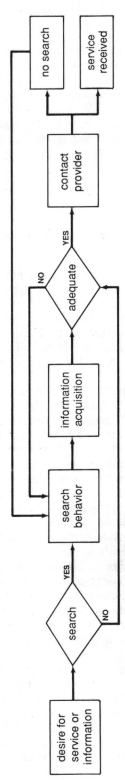

Figure 10—1. Lenz model. *(From Lenz. In Bowens , Clinical nursing research: Its strategies and findings. II, 1979. p. 183. Courtesy of Sigma Theta Tau.)*

Information continues to accrue until the person has acquired sufficient data according to some predetermined criterion. The person then decides whether to use the information immediately, store it for future use, or continue the search if the information acquired is insufficient. It was hypothesized that the individual will follow this sequence of events each time a new search is undertaken.

According to Lenz, the model serves as a basis for describing the search process and for generating hypotheses that predict the relationships among variables in a step with one or more variables in subsequent steps. The purpose of the study was to answer the following questions:

- How do newcomers seek and acquire information about local health services?
- To what extent does their search behavior relate to the information they acquire and the service they receive?
- What role do nurses and other health professionals play as consultants to newcomers in their information search? (p. 182)[18]

The study sample was people who had moved to a community from a distance of at least 20 miles within 8 to 12 months of the study. Retrospective household interviews were conducted using a semistructured interview technique. A stratified random sample of 129 households was used. The interview focused on (1) ascertaining from whom the household members had received health services since the move, (2) a description of the search process undertaken before receiving services, and (3) ascertaining information about search activities that did not result in use of services. Lenz and others have recognized the retrospective character of the study as a major drawback.

The results of the survey are consistent with the Lenz model of search behavior. Associations between identified variables of the search episodes are all highly significant using either the Cramer's V, Pearson product moment correlation coefficient, or Kendall's tau. Some of the variables that are strongly associated include the type of stimulus and the extent of search (Cramer's V $= 0.40$, $p < 0.001$), the time allotted and the extent of search (Kendall's tau $= 0.16$, $p < 0.001$), the extent of search and the amount of information acquired (Pearson product moment correlation coefficient $= 0.32$, $p < 0.001$), and the amount of information acquired and level of satisfaction (Kendall's tau $= -0.09$, $p < 0.003$).

Lenz's results are consistent with other findings about search reported in the consumer literature. An interesting finding of significance to nurses is that subjects in this study (newcomers to a community) began their search before the actual need for services. This finding may be a result of the sample characteristics: high socioeconomic status, more than 50 percent of the heads of households were professionals, owners, managers, or proprietors, more than 89 percent were headed by people younger than 45 years of age, and 60 percent of the households included children. The findings might be related to some unknown behavioral attributes, such as internal versus external locus of control. Finally, some combination of factors may be at work here. This information is important if one desires to use this model to design health-related information sources that would target groups appropriately and efficiently.

The Lenz model is an interesting and useful conceptualization of the information search process. Her initial research has identified that people carry out the search process in an organized fashion that approximates the proposed model. Further research is needed to validate this approach in other settings and with other samples. The identification of both demographic and psychosocial behavioral attributes that contribute to the search process is needed in order to determine variation in search patterns within groups. Development of an instrument to measure these variables derived from the model appears to be a reasonable next step in this research. This model has the potential of being applied in many settings and with a diverse population for the purpose of providing health education and illness prevention.

▪ MILLER BEHAVIORAL STYLE SCALE (MBSS)

It is well known that people cope with life experiences in a variety of ways. For example, denial is frequently used when an individual is faced with an aversive situation. The use of a defense mechanism (e.g., denial) is protective and provides the person with time to adjust to the stressful situations with which he or she is faced. Past experiences, previous defense mechanisms used, and outcomes all determine how a person will cope with a new situation. As stated previously, information is frequently viewed as an effective means of coping. It is believed that the more information a person has, the more his coping ability is enhanced, thereby reducing stress. Until recently, the assumptions related to more-is-better have been accepted as an underlying philosophy that guides approaches to information dissemination to patients and families. Little attention has been given to individual preferences for or capabilities to assimilate information.

As can be seen from earlier instruments designed to assess information preferences and prepurchase search activities, more attention was paid to the manner in which a consumer proceeded with a search than with specific behaviors unique to the individual. This has changed in recent years. Recognition of the complexity of this concept has forced researchers to address not only information-seeking activities but also the psychologic and behavioral profile of consumers to better meet their needs.

Miller and Grant described the development of a scale designed to classify people in terms of their preference for monitoring or blunting in a stressful situation.[19] Monitoring involves being alert for and sensitized to the negative aspects of the event. Blunting, on the other hand, involves distraction from and cognitive avoidance of objective sources of danger.[4] Miller et al. have conducted considerable research designed to determine when an individual employs a certain coping style and when and if it is stress reducing. They have demonstrated that the effectiveness with which people cope with stressful situations is determined by their coping style and by the fit of their preferred strategy to the specific properties of the situations.[4]

These research findings are derived from the Miller Behavioral Style Scale (MBSS), an instrument designed to measure informational preferences. Specifically, the scale describes four situations that have the potential to be stress producing for a person. Each situation has eight statements that describe different ways in which the individual might deal with it. Four of the statements are considered to be of the monitoring or information-seeking type, and four are of the blunting or information-avoiding type. One vignette is:

> Vividly imagine that you are on an airplane. Thirty minutes from your destination the plane unexpectedly goes into a nose dive and then suddenly levels off. The pilot announces that everything is okay, although the rest of the ride may be rough. You are not, however, convinced that all is well.

One monitoring response is, "I would listen carefully to the engines for unusual noises and would watch the crew to see if their behavior was out of the ordinary." A blunting response would be, "I would watch the end of the movie even if I had seen it before."

This scale has been shown to predict preference for information versus distraction in response to threatening situations.[4] Chorney et al. have used the instrument in an experimental setting to determine how monitors and blunters perform on a cold pressor task. A sample of 92 male undergraduate psychology students volunteered for this study. Monitors performed better when the experimental strategy encouraged monitoring, and blunters did better when the situation was compatible with blunting. Their results confirm those of other studies that report the importance of matching an individual's cognitive strategies with his or her coping styles. They conclude that the MBSS "appears to provide a useful, straightforward measure of an important coping style, one which here and elsewhere has been shown to predict performance differences in stress situations" (p. 7).[20]

Miller has used the MBSS with people faced with a short-term aversive stimulus, for example, a gynecologic examination, and those faced with a chronic disease, such as cancer or hypertension. She found that monitors in certain situations might actually do worse i.e., exhibit more stress than those who detract themselves. A possible explanation for this is related to the quantity of information received by this group. Possibly, teaching a monitor some blunting behaviors, for example, distractions, might lessen stress and enhance coping. Further research in a variety of settings is needed.

The utility of this instrument for nursing practice is unknown. Because of the design of the instrument, that is, the use of vignettes, administration is lengthy and might be a factor in the clinical setting. Also, the use of hypothetical situations may not accurately reflect people's behaviors in stressful situations. The subjective nature of the responses may yield data that are not easily quantifiable. A strength of the MBSS is that it yields data on the process used by people under stress. Knowing whether individuals want information, how much, and under what circumstances is critical information for nurses to have.

▪ INFORMATION STYLES QUESTIONNAIRE (ISQ)

Cassileth et al. developed the Information Styles Questionnaire (ISQ).[6] This instrument is a self-report tool designed to ascertain the preferences of cancer patients for information about their disease and their desire to participate actively in their treatment. The questionnaire has six sections; five contain individual questions designed to obtain general data about desire for information and preference for involvement in self-care. For example, one question has the person choose from five possible response options that describe their preference for information. These options range from 1 (no more details than needed) to 5 (as many details as possible). Another question asks the person if he or she desires other information; if the answer is "yes," the person is asked to explain. The patient is asked to choose from the following statements that which best describes their point of view:

> I prefer to leave decisions about my medical care and treatment up to my doctor.

> I prefer to participate in decisions about my medical care and treatment.

An additional question asks the person to select one of the following statements:

> I only want the information needed to care for myself.

> I want additional information only if it is good news.

> I want as much information as possible, good or bad.

The sixth section contains a list of 12 items designed to elicit the specific types of information needed as "absolutely need," "would like to have," or "do you want" the information. A sample of the statements used to elicit specific information follows:

> What all the possible side effects are.

What treatment will accomplish.

Whether or not it is cancer.

What the likelihood of cure is.

The instrument was pilot-tested on 50 people, and the items "were shown to use wording that patients found meaningful and comprehensible and were able to discriminate among patients' viewpoints" (p. 832).[6] The issues of instrument validity and reliability were not addressed. In addition, no specific information is given describing the development of the instrument or the rationale for item choice.

The ISQ has been used subsequently with 256 cancer patients from a major urban medical center[6] and 109 cancer patients from a small community hospital. Fitzpatrick compared the frequencies of information styles and participation preferences between his sample[21] and that of Cassileth et al.[6] Generally, the results appear similar in both groups; however, no statistical tests were performed to determine if significant differences existed between the responses of the two groups.[21] Since the issues of validity and reliability of the instrument were not addressed, it would have been useful to compare the two groups.

Fitzpatrick stated that the results of his research essentially replicate those of Cassileth et al. This is significant, since Cassileth et al. stated that a potential source of bias was the setting from which the patients came. Unfortunately, no detailed demographic comparison is made between the two groups. Such a comparison might have provided some clues about the magnitude of the bias if any exists. Fitzpatrick indicated that demographic variables may, in fact, account for some of the differences that occurred. The issues of the validity and reliability of the ISQ must be addressed, and the instrument should be compared with other scales to determine its discriminant validity. Further use of the ISQ with other samples, comparing specific demographic, psychologic, and sociologic variables, will contribute to establishing the instrument's reliability.

The ISQ appears to be a comprehensive instrument designed to elicit many aspects of information preferences. Its clinical utility for nursing practice lies in its structure, which can be used relatively easily, and with the information that is generated. Nurses need to know about patient preferences for information and their desire to participate in decision making in order to design appropriate nursing interventions. Information obtained from this instrument is consistent with the concepts inherent in a self-care theoretical framework, such as Orem's, thereby enhancing its appropriateness for nursing practice.

▪ KRANTZ HEALTH OPINION SURVEY (HOS)

Krantz et al. developed the Krantz Health Opinion Survey (HOS), which has two subscales, one measuring information preference and the second measuring the degree of behavioral involvement.[22] The original instrument consisted of 40 items that addressed the issues of how informed a person wants to be and how active a role he or she desires to play in his or her health care. The five items addressed are:

- Beliefs in the efficiency and benefits of self-care
- Frequency of information seeking and questioning of physicians and nurses
- Beliefs about the benefits or disadvantages of making one's own medical decisions
- Attitudes toward use of a physician versus oneself as a health care provider
- Frequency of self-diagnosis

Krantz et al. reported that extensive testing was undertaken to determine the instrument's validity and reliability. The initial 40-item instrument was pilot-tested on 200 undergraduate students, after which 14 items were eliminated because they had a correlation of less than 0.20 with the total score or because they had a narrow distribution of response alternatives.[18] The remaining 26 items were retested with a sample of 159 undergraduates. Factor analysis was used to identify components of the instrument and yielded the two subscales. The Information Subscale (I-Scale) contains 7 items measuring desire to ask questions and wanting to be informed about medical decisions. The following are examples of the statements found on the I-Scale:

- I usually don't ask the doctor or nurse many questions about what they're doing during a medical examination.
- I'd rather have doctors and nurses make the decisions about what's best than for them to give me a whole lot of choices.
- Instead of waiting for them to tell me, I usually ask the doctor or nurse immediately after an examination about my health.
- I usually wait for the doctor or nurse to tell me the results of a medical examination rather than asking them immediately (p. 980).[22]

The Behavior Involvement Subscale (B-Scale) contains 9 items that measure attitudes toward self-treatment and active behavioral involvement of patients with their care. The following are examples of the statements found on the B-Scale:

- Except for serious illness, it's generally better to take care of your own health than to seek professional help.
- It is better to rely on the judgment of doctors (who are the experts) than to rely on "common sense" in taking care of your own body.
- Clinics and hospitals are good places to go for help, since it's best for medical experts to take responsibility for health care.
- Learning how to cure some of your illness without contacting a physician may create more harm than good.
- Recovery is usually quicker under the care of a doctor or nurse than when patients take care of themselves. (p. 980).[22]

The scale then yields a total score, which is a composite of the two subscales, and individual I-Scale and B-Scale scores. The binary, agree–disagree format was designed so that high scores represent positive attitudes toward self-directed or informed treatment (p. 980).[22]

Discriminant validity was established by administering the HOS in conjunction with the Crowne-Marlowe Social Desirability Scale and the Health LOC Scale to a sample of 100 male and 100 female undergraduates. A second sample consisting of 38 undergraduates received the HOS and the Minnesota Multiphasic Personality Inventory (MMPI) Hypochondriac Scale. A third sample ($n = 87$) received the HOS and the Ullman Repression-Sensitization (R-S) Scale. A fourth sample ($n = 80$) received the HOS two times during a 7-week interval to determine test–retest reliability.[22]

Application of the KR 20 test strongly confirmed the reliability of the HOS Scale and its component subscales (KR = 0.77). The authors remark that females in general tended to score higher than males on all parts of the HOS Scale. The authors do not discuss the positive significance of this finding.

The B-Scale and I-Scale were not correlated significantly with one another. The HOS and the Wallston Health Locus of Control Scale had a correlation of 0.31, and the correlations were 0.26 and 0.23 for the B-Scale and I-Scale, respectively. The authors suggest that these low correlations indicate that the two subscales are probably measuring relatively independent processes. The HOS does not show significant correlations with the R-S, the MMPI, and the Crowne-Marlowe Social Desirability Scale.

Additional studies were conducted for the purpose of establishing predictive, construct, and discriminant validity of the HOS. For these studies, Krantz et al. chose groups representing extremes in preferences for different approaches to health-related services. This approach provided the investigators with a relatively heterogeneous population. The HOS was administered to a sample of 149 students, including 56 randomly selected residents of a college residence hall, 81 students reporting to a college infirmary for routine treatment of minor illnesses, and 12 students enrolled in a medical self-help course at the same school.[18] It was predicted that the criterion group, those students attending a medical self-help course, would score higher on the behavioral involvement, information, and total scores of the HOS, since their involvement in such a course was believed to demonstrate greater interest in obtaining information about health.

The scores of the self-help and clinic samples were compared to those of the residence hall students using one-way analyses of variance and Dunnett's t-tests. One-tailed tests were used, since directional predictions were specified. The total HOS scores and the B-Scale scores were higher for the self-help group than for the residence hall group, significant at the $p < 0.005$ level. The clinic users did not differ on the total HOS score or the I-Scale but were significantly lower on the B-Scale, $p < 0.05$. Krantz et al. established discriminant validity of the instrument in its ability to predict correctly the differences between the criterion group of high self-care students and the general population and in the fact that the low B-Scale scores were correlated with high use of clinic facilities.

The authors reported on three studies designed to establish reliability and validity of the HOS Scale. They noted that the scale is predictive of behaviors that relate to seeking routine medical care for minor illnesses that require short-term interventions. It has not been established if the instrument is valid or reliable in predicting illness-seeking behavior in long-term chronic or traumatic illness. Results of these studies suggest that people who prefer to be more active in their own health care are more likely to care for themselves when faced with a minor illness than to seek care from a physician.

Further testing is required to ensure the validity and predictive potential of the HOS. Since the initial design of the HOS, it has been used in several other settings. Auerbach et al. used the scale with 40 patients scheduled for dental surgery.[23] The study attempted to provide construct validation data for the I-Scale of the HOS. The study subjects were asked to complete several measures in conjunction with the HOS (e.g., Rotter Internal Locus of Control Scale and Corah Dental Anxiety Scale). The results demonstrated that the HOS subscales are positively correlated with the total HOS scales (I-Scale $= 0.73$, $p = 0.0001$; B-Scale $= 0.63$, $p = 0.0001$), but the subscales are not related to each other or to other scales. These results are consistent with those described by Krantz et al.[22]

The appeal of the Krantz HOS instrument is its brevity, ease of scoring, and bidimensional approach in identifying a person's desire for information and the relevant behavioral components. Nurses could use this instrument in a variety of settings and with different populations as part of an initial assessment. The resultant data could be used to plan appropriate nursing interventions targeted to individual needs.

A possible limitation of this scale, recognized by the authors, is that items on the scale are related to routine aspects of medical care; the instrument has not been used in situations where the illness is traumatic, severe, or chronic. The authors recommend that, in future use of the scale, revisions may be necessary to clarify meanings and eliminate redundancy.[22]

▪ MESSERLI QUESTIONNAIRE

Messerli et al. conducted a study designed to determine if women with breast cancer received sufficient information about all aspects of their therapy and, if not, what information did they need.[10] The sample included women who had a masectomy for breast cancer within the past 5 years, and surgeons who treated breast cancer.

The study assumed that the discovery of a lump precipitated a crisis and that providing information served to lessen the crisis. Messerli et al. developed a questionnaire to obtain data about the resources women and surgeons relied on for information about breast cancer. The questionnaire was designed with the help of women with breast cancer and surgeons. It was then pretested on a sample from each group.

The questionnaire designed to be administered to women with breast cancer focused on:

What information was provided on breast cancer and its treatment
What information they would like to have had
Sociodemographic information

The surgeons were asked questions concerning:

What type and how much information they provided to patients
The number of mastectomies performed in the past 5 years
Demographic data

These questionnaires were mailed to 180 women and 182 surgeons. The response rate was 34 percent and 51 percent, respectively.

Although the authors stated that the instrument was pilot-tested on a sample of women and physicians, they did not indicate the size of the sample or whether revisions were made in the questionnaire as a result of the pilot. Since the study was exploratory, issues of instrument validity and reliability were not addressed. Although it is true that in exploratory studies formal instruments are rarely used and one tends to rely on observation of events with narrative notes, it is important to establish the reliability of the sources from which the data are derived and by whom they are interpreted. If, however, one is actually conducting a survey, the reliability of the instrument becomes more important.[24] Neither of these issues is clearly addressed in this study. The specific questions asked of each group are not described, even though the results of the rankings of resources by each group are presented. Further research in this area is necessary to confirm these results and to address the issues related to instrumentation.

▪ INFORMATION PREFERENCE QUESTIONNAIRE (IPQ)

Hopkins developed the Information Preference Questionnaire (IPQ), a quantitative measure of information seeking.[3] To establish face validity and clarity, the IPQ was given to a nurse educator, an oncologist, and three patients. As a result of their responses, minor revisions were made in the questionnaire. The IPQ was then pilot-tested on 38 women who were receiving chemotherapy for breast cancer. Test–retest reliability was high at 0.92 ($n = 30$). The internal consistency of the IPQ was tested by calculation of Chronbach coefficient alpha ($r = 0.88$; $n = 38$). The author attempted to establish criterion-related validity by correlating IPQ scores with test scores from the Chemotherapy Knowledge Questionnaire (CKQ).[11] Hopkins hypothesized that subjects who had a high degree of information seeking would score

ID NUMBER:_____   DATE:_____

DIRECTIONS: A number of statements which people have used to describe themselves as they receive chemotherapy are given below. Read each statement and check (✔) the box to the right which best indicates how much you agree or disagree with the statement.

	STRONGLY AGREE	AGREE	UNCERTAIN	DISAGREE	STRONGLY DISAGREE
1. I tend to ask my doctor a lot of questions about my chemotherapy and how it is going.					
2. It's a good idea to get information and advice about chemotherapy from as many people as possible.					
3. I read everything I can about chemotherapy and why I am getting it.					
4. I believe in asking plenty of questions about my chemotherapy so I know what to expect before it even happens.					
5. I can never get too much information about my diagnosis and chemotherapy treatment.					
6. It is better to take each day as it comes than to ask a lot of questions ahead of time about my chemotherapy treatment.					
7. I know practically everything there is to know about my chemotherapy and why I receive it.					
8. I dislike getting advice about how to manage my chemotherapy treatments.					
9. Family members, friends, and people at work can be good sources of information about dealing with chemotherapy.					
10. There is no point in asking a lot of questions about my chemotherapy, since people will tell me what I need to know.					
11. Chemotherapy either works or it doesn't work, so there is no point in asking questions about it.					
12. I listen carefully when people give me advice or information related to my chemotherapy.					
13. I prefer not to know very much about my diagnosis and my chemotherapy treatment.					
14. It is better not to know ahead of time all of the details about chemotherapy.					

Figure 10-2. Information Preference Questionnaire. (From Hopkins. Information seeking and adaptational outcomes in women receiving chemotherapy for breast cancer. Ca Nurs, 1986, 9(5):256.)

high on a test of their knowledge of chemotherapy. Pearson product moment correlations of the CPQ with means of the IPQ revealed no relationship.

Although the author gives no reason for the lack of correlation, several explanations are possible. First, a time lag may have existed between the diagnosis and explanation of chemotherapy and the administration of the IPQ and CKQ. Second, the CPQ measures retention of information about chemotherapy, which is significantly different from desiring information. Factors, such as anxiety and stress, that may motivate information seeking might impede information retention. Third, the scores reported for the CPQ are not high, and it is not clear what that means. It may be related to the method of information dissemination, the timing of the education, the variables within the sample itself, or a combination of factors. The lack of correlation between these instruments may be related to intervening variables, and if one corrected for mood or time since diagnosis or education, a more significant correlation might emerge.

The IPQ has since been used with a convenience sample of 58 women with primary or recurrent breast cancer. Several hypotheses were tested in this study. Of particular interest is the hypothesis that "a statistically significant negative relationship exists between information-seeking as measured by the IPQ and chronological age." The results indicate that older people tend to demonstrate less information seeking than younger subjects (-0.30 correlation; $p < 0.11$). This is consistent with the generational trend found by the work of Cassileth et al.[6] and with the fact that the older patients in Fitzpatrick's study[21] tended to be information avoiders. This consistent finding in three studies encourages exploration of what other factors besides age are at work. In addition, it yields some preliminary data upon which nursing interventions can be structured for a subgroup of people requiring health care.

An alternative hypothesis—that the intensity of information seeking is positively associated with higher levels of education—was not confirmed. ($r = 0.0419$, $p < 0.381$).[21] Cassileth et al.'s sample found a strong association, indicating that better educated people wanted more information. Two possible explanations are offered for this discrepancy. One is that educational level was not clearly defined by either study, and the other is that the two instruments may not be comparable.

Hopkins, noting the limitations of her study, recommends that tests be conducted on the IPQ in order to establish construct and criterion-related validity. She suggests that perhaps discriminant analysis could be conducted with the IPQ, the ISQ, and the HOS. Further testing of the IPQ with different populations and larger samples and additional use of the Dodd and Mood Chemotherapy Knowledge Questionnaire (CKQ) are recommended.

As with the HOS, the IPQ can be administered with ease. In addition, its brevity, quantitative nature, and ease of scoring are positive factors that enhance the instrument's utility in a variety of clinical settings (Fig. 10–2). A limitation is that the instrument is specifically designed to be used with people receiving chemotherapy, although this may, in fact, be advantageous. Because of its narrow focus, more specific nursing interventions could be designed that target the needs of a well-defined group.

SUMMARY

A review of the literature on consumer and health care information-seeking activities and instruments developed to measure this concept reveals that the type and amount of information desired by consumers varies with the individual and that accurate means of assessing information-seeking behavior styles are critical. Dimensions of the search process reported in the consumer literature—informational, time, and contextual—are conceptually relevant to information-seeking activities within the health care system. The information dimension is the amount of information that an individual has and will determine the amount of time and energy invested in search activities to solve the present problem. Those people who have extensive health care experience are more likely to limit their search than are people who are facing an illness for the first time. The time dimension includes the amount of time a person spends in identifying health care resources, the number of visits to health care institutions for evaluations and tests, and the time spent in the actual decision process. The contextual dimension includes an individual's previous experience with the health care system, demographic background, perceived risks, benefits, and costs of the search process, and need factors related to the critical nature of the problem.

The relevance of this to nursing is apparent. Nurses are involved in all aspects of health care and have the opportunity to obtain knowledge about individuals' coping styles and information-seeking activities in order to tailor nursing interventions. Instruments, such as those presented in this chapter, provide a method for an organized, consistent manner for identifying clusters of behavioral factors about individuals and their search activities. From this will emerge more complete profiles of patients with similar problems, potentially facilitating more efficient targeting of patient needs.

Future research should be directed at additional use of these instruments, combining their use with other valid and reliable scales, and collaborating with other researchers to increase the knowledge in this area.

REFERENCES

1. Lenz, E.R. Information seeking: A component of client decisions and health behavior. *Adv Nurs Sci* 1984, *6*(3):59.
2. Janis, I.L., & Mann, L. *Decision making: A psychological analysis of conflict, choice and commitment.* New York: The Free Press, 1977.
3. Hopkins, M.B. Information seeking and adaptational outcomes in women receiving chemotherapy for breast cancer. *Ca Nurs,* 1986, *9*(5):256.
4. Miller, S.M., Leinbach, A.L., Brody, D.S. Coping styles in hypertensives: Nature and consequences. *J Consult Clin Psychol.* 1987, in press.
5. Wallston, K.A., Kaplan, G.D., & Maides, S.A. Development and validation of the health locus of control (HLC) scale. *J Consult Clin Psychol,* 1976, *44*(4):580.
6. Cassileth, B.R., Zupkis, R.V., Sutton-Smith, K., & March, V. Information and participation preferences among cancer patients. *Ann Intern Med,* 1980, *92*(6):832.
7. Lazarus, R.S. *Psychological stress and the coping process.* New York: McGraw-Hill, 1966.
8. Newman, J.W., & Lockman, B.D. Measuring prepurchase information seeking. *J Consumer Res,* 1975, *2*(3):216.
9. Kiel, G.C., & Layton, R.A. Dimensions of consumer information seeking behavior. *J Market Res,* 1981, *18*:233
10. Messerli, M.L., Garamendi, C., & Romano, J. Breast cancer: Information as a technique of crisis intervention. *Am J Orthopsychiatry,* 1980, *50*(4):728.
11. Dodd, M.J., & Mood, D.W. Chemotherapy: Helping patients to know the drugs they are receiving and their possible side effects. *Cancer Nurs,* 1981, *4*(4):311.
12. Fleckenstein, L., Joubert, P., Lawrence, R., et al. Oral contraceptive patient information: A questionnaire study of attitudes, knowledge and preferred information sources. *JAMA,* 1976, *235*(13):1331.
13. Faden, R.R., Lewis, C., Becke, C., et al. Disclosure standards and informed consent. *J Health Polit Policy Law,* 1981, *6*(2):255.

14. Mills, R.T., & Krantz, D.S. Information, choice, and reactions to stress: A field experiment in a blood bank with laboratory analogue. *J Pers Soc Psychol,* 1979, *37*(4):608.
15. Claxton, J.D., Fry, J.N., & Portis, B. A taxonomy of prepurchase information gathering patterns. *J Consumer Res,* 1974, *1*:35.
16. Payne, J.W. Task complexity and contingent processing in decision making: An information search and protocol analysis. *Organizational Behav Hum Performance,* 1976, *16*:366.
17. Englander, T., & Tyszka, T. Information seeking in open decision situations. *Acta Psychol,* 1980, *45*:169.
18. Lenz, E.R. Newcomers' search for information about health services. In E. Bowens (Ed.), *Clinical nursing research: Its strategies and findings. II.* Indianapolis: Sigma Theta Tau, 1979, p. 182.
19. Miller. S.M., & Grant, R.P. The blunting hypothesis: A view of predictability and human stress. In P. Sjoden, S. Bates, W. Dockens (Eds.), *Trends in behavior therapy.* New York: Academic Press, 1979.
20. Chorney, R.L., Efran, J.S., Ascher, L.M., & Lukens, M.D. The performance of monitors and blunters on a cold pressor task. Presentation: Eastern Psychological Association, 1982.
21. Fitzpatrick, R.J. Emotional distress, locus of control, and information preferences among cancer patients. Unpublished doctoral dissertation, University of Tennessee, Knoxville, 1983.
22. Krantz, D.S., Baum, A., & Wideman, M.V. Assessment of preferences for self-treatment and information in health care. *J Pers Soc Psychol,* 1980, *39*(5):977.
23. Auerbach, S.M., Martelli, M.F., & Mercuri, L.G. Anxiety, information, interpersonal impacts and adjustment to a stressful health care situation. *J Pers Soc Psychol,* 1983, *44*(6):1284.
24. Diers, D. *Research in nursing practice.* Philadelphia: Lippincott, 1979.

BIBLIOGRAPHY

Booth, A., & Babchuk, N. Seeking health care from new resources. *J Health Soc Behav,* 1972, *13*(1):90.
Cook, T.D., & Campbell, D.T. *Quasi-experimentation design and analysis issues for field settings.* Boston: Houghton Mifflin, 1979.
Dabbs, J.M., & Kirscht, J.P. Internal control and the taking of influenza shots. *Psychol Rep,* 1971, *28*(3):959.
Davis, W.L., & Phares, E.J. Internal-external control as a determinant of information-seeking in a social influence situation. *J Pers,* 1967, *35*(4):547.
Derdiarian, A.K. Informational needs of recently diagnosed cancer patients. *Nurs Res,* 1986, *35*(5):276.
DeVito, A.J., Bogdanowicz, J., & Reznikoff, M. Actual and intended health-related information seeking and health locus of control. *J Pers Assess,* 1982, *46*(1):63.
Dodd, M. Preference for information in patients with cancer receiving radiation therapy (Abstr). American Cancer Society's Annual Nurse Research Day, Hawaii, 1985.
Hopkins, M.B. Information-seeking and adaptional outcomes in women receiving chemotherapy for breast cancer. *Cancer Nurs,* 1986, *9*(5):256.
Lanzetta, J.T., & Driscoll, J.M. Preference for information about an uncertain but unavoidable outcome. *J Pers Soc Psychol,* 1966, *3*(1):96.
Locander, W.B., & Hermann, P.W. The effect of self-confidence and anxiety of information seeking in consumer risk reduction. *J Market Res,* 1979, *16*:268.
Midgley, D.F. Patterns of interpersonal information seeking for the purchase of a symbolic product. *J Market Res,* 1983, *20*:74.
Miller, S.M. When is a little knowledge a dangerous thing? Coping with stressful events by monitoring versus blunting. In S. Levine & H. Ursin (Eds.), *Coping and health.* Proceedings of a NATO Conference. New York: Plenum Press, 1980.
Phares, E.J. Differential utilization of information as a function of internal-external control. *J Pers,* 1968, *36*(4):649.
Polit, D.F., & Hungler, B.P. *Nursing research: Principles and methods.* Philadelphia: Lippincott, 1978.
Schaninger, C.M., & Sciglimpaglia, D. The influence of cognitive personality traits and demographics on consumer information acquisition. *J Consumer Res,* 1981, *8*(2):208.

Sime, A.M. Relationship of preoperative fear, type of coping, and information received about surgery to recovery from surgery. *J Pers Soc Psychol,* 1976, *34*(4):716.

Wallston, K.A., Maides, S., & Wallston, B.S. Health-related information seeking as a function of health-related locus control and health value. *J Res Pers,* 1976, *10*(2):215.

Woods, W.A. Psychological dimensions of consumer decision. *J Marketing,* 1960. *24*:15.

CHAPTER *11*

Measuring Self-Care Activities

Marylin J. Dodd, R.N., Ph.D.

Many individuals and families have performed self-care in the past. Today many more health care consumers are taking increased interest in their health and assume greater responsibility for their own care. Among the several reasons for this resurgence of interest, three main reasons can be identified and explained. The first concerns dissatisfaction with current cost-control systems and measures, maldistribution of physicians and medical facilities, and iatrogenic outcomes. The second is the shift from acute to chronic health problems. The third is the gradual change in value and belief systems in which clients desire more control over themselves, their environment, and their social systems, including the health care system.[1-4]

Since the 1960s, health care professionals have incorporated the self-care philosophy into their practice. However, in this era of dwindling community health resources and diagnostic related groups (DRGs), the concept of self-care has taken on a new central and critical importance in the attainment of quality health promotion and illness-related care. People (healthy individuals, patients, and families) simply must now manage more by themselves. The mandate for health care professionals to provide prerequisite information and skills to everyone is clear.

The concept of self-care has a wide range of meanings given the various perspectives from which self-care is viewed in relation to its dependence on or interdependence with the health care system and its professional practitioners. These views range from a conservative ideology,[5-7] with emphasis on minimal dependence on the current health care system, to a less conservative view,[8] in which the health care professional, for example, the nurse, plays a significant role not only in assisting the patient in the acquisition of self-care skills but as a manager of the patient's self-care.

Levin defines self-care as "a process whereby a lay person can function effectively on his own behalf in health promotion and prevention and in disease detection and treatment at the level of the primary health resource in the health care system" (p. 170).[7] It is important to note that Levin's definition implies that self-care is part of the health care system, that is, the patient is presumed to have access to the technology and skills of the health care system.

At an international symposium on self-care, Frye,[5] a leading British proponent of self-care, identified the following self-care roles: health maintenance, disease prevention, self-diagnosis, self-medication and self-treatment, and participation by the patient in professional care. Frye went on to define self-care as:

> a voluntary, self-limited, non-organized, universal, varying complex of behaviors evolved through a mixture of socializing and cognitive experiences . . . an indigenous phenomenon, wholly outside the framework of professional health resources, although obviously influenced by the nature of social institutions of care and the context of economic, social and political structures (p. 10).[5]

Norris, somewhat on the liberal side of the continuum, defines self-care as "those processes that permit people and families to take initiative, to take responsibility, and to function effectively in developing their own potential for health" (p. 486).[2]

Pratt, discussing the role of the family in self-care, attempted to define family self-care by asking and responding to seven key questions[9]:

1. Who does it? The answer is simply oneself. It is acknowledged that activities range from simple to complex and may be performed fully independent of or under the supervision of health care professionals.
2. What form of care? In addition to traditional family activities of personal attention, support, bodily care, and sharing of workload, family self-care could include the use of medical technology and procedures.
3. How is it done? Self-care is carried out by the family by having access to the necessary tools—drugs, diagnostic, therapeutic, and comfort equipment.
4. Where is it done? Self-care activities occur in the home.
5. Who knows how? Since self-care requires knowledge and skill, the implication is that laymen and families would have access to the necessary information and that allocation of health resources would include training that could develop their capabilities for self-care.
6. Who manages the family care? The power to choose options related to health care resides within the family and its members.
7. Who runs the system? It is suggested that family representatives participate in a variety of activities, including the governance of health care agencies, hospital accrediting process, and licensing of professionals. (p. 125)

Orem defines self-care as "the practice of activities that individuals initiate and perform on their own behalf in maintaining life, health, and well-being" (p. 6).[8] She clearly emphasizes the significant role of the nurse in assisting patients to meet their self-care demands when actual or potential deficits exist.

The meaning of self-care as described by some of its proponents is presented here in an attempt to identify similarities in ideology as well as to create an awareness that significant differences exist. Similarities identified include the performance of activities for oneself in relation to matters that affect health. There is recognition that this performance requires both knowledge and skills, ranging from simple to complex, on the part of the one providing self-care. Access to medical technology is considered a part of self-care. Another common belief is the need for client input in setting client goals and program planning and evaluation. A major difference is the extent to which the client performs self-care activities independent of the health care system and its professionals. Inherent in this difference are the issues of control and the extent to which the patient should have unsupervised access to medical technology. The researcher desiring to measure self-care needs to consider these varying definitions and select an instrument congruent with purposes of determining self-care.

What emerges from a review of the literature on self-care is the individual's readiness to learn about a health or disease-related situation,[10,11] knowledge of what to do,[12-16] and possession of the functional ability to perform self-care activities.[17-23] Suggestions on how to assess the individual's readiness to learn, instruments to determine knowledge about the situation, and the psychophysiologic capabilities to initiate self-care are not within the scope of this chapter. The focus of the chapter is a review of tools to measure actual self-care activities.

Orem's conceptualization of self-care as consisting of three categories is useful in organizing this review.[8] According to Orem, self-care is undertaken to meet three types of self-care requisites: universal, developmental, and health-deviation. Universal self-care requisites focus on life processes and the maintenance of human structure and function, for example, sufficient air, water, and food. Developmental self-care requisites focus on human developmental processes and events during various stages of the life cycle and on events that may adversely affect development. Health-deviation self-care requisites arise from disabilities, deviations, or defects in human structure and function and from medical diagnosis and treatment of disease conditions. The greatest preponderance of self-care research and many of the methodologic issues that the researcher must consider have involved health-deviation self-care.

HEALTH-DEVIATION SELF-CARE REQUISITE

Several methodologic problems have plagued research in health-deviation self-care and thwarted the development of the concept. First, the conceptualization in these studies is often nonexistent or inadequately developed, and the operational definition of self-care is rarely given. Second, the measure of self-care activities is limited to only a few interview or questionnaire items[15,24,25] embedded in an instrument that also assesses patients' attitudes, values, knowledge, disease and treatment parameters, and functional (psychomotor) abilities. Third, the interview or questionnaire items[26] and patients' self-reports[27,28] are not described clearly, and their psychometric properties (reliability and validity data) frequently are not reported. Finally, in some studies, self-care activity items can be identified in instruments that have not been developed for the specific measurement of self-care per se.[27]

These methodologic issues are especially grave given the flood of intervention studies designed to enhance self-care activities in arthritic,[15] elderly,[21] hypertensive,[29] cerebral vascular accident,[30] neurologically impaired (e.g., quadriplegic and paraplegic),[31] chronic obstructive pulmonary disease,[32] obese,[33] dental,[34] cancer,[35,36] and ambulatory[37] patients.

The vast majority of these experimental studies have focused on disease outcomes, that is, normal glucose, blood pressure, or cholesterol levels, and have failed to assess systematically the self-care activities patients performed to obtain or not obtain the desired disease and treatment outcomes. Table 11–1 presents a schema of the majority of these pretest and posttest experimental studies.

TABLE 11–1. SCHEMA OF POPULAR RESEARCH DESIGNS IN SELF-CARE INTERVENTION STUDIES

Time 1	Intervention	Unknown	Time 2
Patient's disease parameters are assessed	Usually educational in nature	What self-care patient actually performs	Reassessment of patient's disease parameters

Compliance by patients with treatment protocol is not presented in this chapter. Compliance connotes a passivity of following what another tells one to do, whereas self-care conveys active participation and decision making that may or may not be consistent with the views of health care professionals.[38]

HEALTH-DEVIATION SELF-CARE INSTRUMENTS

▪ KLEIN-BELL ACTIVITIES OF DAILY LIVING (ADL) SCALE

The Klein-Bell Activities of Daily Living (ADL) Scale was developed by Klein and Bell[39] to measure the performance of self-care in ADL. The self-care theory or self-care definition that provided the basis for the study is not provided in the report. However, the investigators provide a useful discussion of the basic qualities for an ADL scale and critique methodologic issues of previous ADL scales. They used empirical analysis to identify critical and easily observable components of ADL behavior of virtually all people, handicapped or able-bodied, and expressed the 170 behavioral items in terms that apply to all people. For example, the item "achieving bathing position" could refer to getting into a bathtub and sitting down, transferring to a bath bench, wheeling into a shower stall, or any similar self-care behavior necessary for bathing.[39] An example from one category (dressing) on the Klein-Bell ADL Scale is:

Shorts/Pants
> Reach shorts to foot
> Get right leg into right leg hole
> Get left leg into left leg hole

Other categories include mobility, elimination, bathing/hygiene, eating, and emergency telephone use.

Klein and Bell contend that the activities that must be observed by health care personnel are among those currently observed in any thorough ADL evaluation. Once these observations have been made, scoring the scale items takes approximately 15 minutes for the initial evaluation and less for subsequent evaluations.

The derivation of the scoring of the scale by ten experienced rehabilitation professionals (occupational therapists, physical therapists, and nurses) is presented in detail.[39] The 170 items on the scale are scored as either "achieved" (behavior is performed without verbal or physical assistance from another person) or "failed" (assistance is needed). A person who independently operates adaptive equipment to perform an ADL gets full credit for achievement of that item, since the use of the equipment increases that person's level of independence. A patient who achieves an item receives all points assigned to that item (weighted by difficulty 1, 2, or 3 points, 3 being the most difficult). "Failed" receives zero points. The total points achieved within each ADL area (e.g., dressing, eating) are added and can be combined to yield an overall ADL independence score.

Interrater reliability initially was obtained by having 20 patients rated independently by two occupational therapists or by two rehabilitation nurses. In all, three pairs of occupational therapists and three pairs of nurses participated. Agreement or disagreement among raters was noted on each item for each patient. Partial agreement is not possible, since the patient is rated as either independent ("achieved") or dependent ("failed") on each item. For all items on all patients, there was a 92 percent agreement between raters. Klein and Bell consider this agreement to be low and explain that these raters were not extensively trained in the use of the scale but simply were introduced to it and asked to complete the items.[39] The validity of the scale was established by contacting 14 patients (spinal cord injuries, cerebral vascular accident, or traumatic head injury) 5 to 10 months after discharge. These patients had been rated on the Klein-Bell ADL Scale just before discharge. Using a structured phone interview, a determination of how many hours per week of assistance (any type) the patient was receiving for ADL activities was made. A significant negative correlation coefficient was obtained between the ADL scale scores at discharge and the number of hours per week of assistance received 5 to 10 months after discharge ($r = -0.86$, $p < 0.01$). The finding indicates that people with low ADL scale scores at discharge can be predicted to require more assistance.

Klein and Bell contend that an accurate measurement tool for ADL self-care functioning has many obvious research and clinical applications. The uses of the tool could include documenting a patient's progress, communicating objective results to patient, family, and medical insurance coverers, and overall program evaluation. Other investigators have used the bathing section of the Klein-Bell ADL Scale[31] to demonstrate whether or not occupational therapy intervention increases bathing independence for disabled people. The ADL scale was found to be useful compared to other scales that were too global to be precise enough to document progress specific to the activity of bathing. The ADL scale breaks down this function into its component parts to allow an accurate evaluation. No further reliability or validity data were provided in the report.

• SELF-CARE BEHAVIOR QUESTIONNAIRE

The Self-Care Behavior Questionnaire was developed by Dodd[36] to measure the self-care activities of cancer patients experiencing side effects of chemotherapy. The self-care theorists Levin and Orem provided the conceptual bases for this tool. Self-care was defined as activities the patient (family or friends) did to alleviate the side effects experienced from chemotherapy.

In the Self-Care Behavior Questionnaire, the patient is asked to report the experienced side effects of chemotherapy and indicate on a 5-point Likert scale how severe the side effect was. The scale ranges from 1 for "barely noticeable" to 5 for "most severe." For each side effect, the patient is asked to indicate the actions taken to alleviate the side effect. The patient's perception of the effectiveness of each self-care behavior is obtained by a second 5-point scale ranging from 1 for "did not help at all" to 5 for "completely alleviated the side effect." In addition, the patients are asked to give the source of information for each self-care behavior they report.

If a patient experiences more than one side effect and initiates self-care behaviors to manage these side effects, a performance score is computed for each self-care behavior. The Self-Care Behavior Performance Score is obtained by dividing accrued points for Self-Care Behavior by the number of side effects reported by the patient. This procedure allows for comparisons between patients who experience more than one side effect. Self-care behavior performance, consisting of initiation of self-care behavior, perception of effectiveness, and decisions based on these two factors, is point-scored on a range of 1 to 5. Patients who initiate and continue self-care behavior they perceive as effective in alleviating a side effect are awarded the highest point score. Patients who do not initiate self-care behavior, who discontinue effective self-care behavior, or who do not initiate a second self-care behavior if the original behavior is low to moderately effective are assigned progressively lower scores. A table depicting this scoring process is available in another report.[40]

The reliability of the Self-Care Behavior Questionnaire was assessed by the test–retest method with the control group. The preintervention and postintervention self-care behavior performance scores did not correlate significantly between interviews conducted 7 to 9 weeks apart; $r = 0.21$, $t_{(11)} = 0.21$, $p = 0.52$. The content validity of the Self-Care Behavior Log was established by two groups of medical oncologists and four oncology clinical nurse specialists. In the analysis of the Self-Care Behavior Questionnaire, the correlations between the average self-care behavior performance scores and the average number of self-care behaviors were significant at the preintervention and postintervention interview; $r = 0.88$ and $r = 0.97$, respectively.[36,41] This finding provides evidence for concurrent validity.

The utility of this questionnaire for other patient populations is obvious. Side effects from different treatments and symptoms of disease could be easily incorporated into the Self-Care Behavior Questionnaire.

▪ SELF-CARE BEHAVIOR LOG

The Self-Care Behavior Log was developed by Dodd to measure the self-care activities of cancer patients experiencing side effects of radiation therapy[41,42] and chemotherapy.[43,44] In an earlier study,[36] in which Dodd developed and tested the Self-Care Behavior Questionnaire, the patients were asked to recall in an interview what self-care activities they had performed. Concerned with the lack of accuracy of the patient's memory, Dodd devised an adaptation of this questionnaire, the Self-Care Behavior Log, in which the patient records the experienced side effects of either radiation therapy or chemotherapy as they occur.

For each side effect experienced, the patient indicates the date of onset of the side effect and, on two 5-point Likert scales, how severe and how distressing the side effect is. The patient also records the activities performed to alleviate the side effect and the date the activities occur. The patient's perception of the effectiveness of each self-care behavior is obtained on a third 5-point Likert scale. Finally, the patient records the source of information for each self-care behavior.

Four ratios have been established to score the quantitative variable of self-care behavior. Details of these scoring ratios are available in another report[41] and are an extension of the scoring methods described with the Self-Care Behavior Questionnaire.

A preventive self-care dimension also is included in the Self-Care Behavior Log.[44] Patients are asked to record the potential side effects that can occur with their chemotherapy, to think about what self-care activity is to be taken to prevent the side effect from occurring, and the date the activity takes place. They are asked to record the source of the idea for the activity. The scoring method for the preventive self-care activity has been limited to frequency counts because of the lack of patient recall of potential side effects and preventive self-care activities for the potential side effects.[44]

There are no reliability or validity data reported for the Self-Care Behavior Log beyond those presented with the Self-Care Behavior Questionnaire. In the two descriptive studies that have used the Self-Care Behavior Log,[41,43,44] no patient difficulties in keeping this self-report have occurred.

The utility of this log for other patient populations is clear. Self-report of signs and symptoms of diseases other than cancer or other treatment side effects could be incorporated easily into the Self-Care Behavior Log.

▪ SELF-OBSERVATION AND REPORT TECHNIQUE (SORT)

The Self-Observation and Report Technique (SORT) was developed by Stephens et al.[45] to measure everyday behaviors of patients with recent spinal injuries, where these behaviors occur, whether aid is provided, and, if so, by whom. A conceptual framework for this tool is not provided. However, a behavior unit is defined as something overtly done by or done to the patient, spans at least 5 minutes, and represents a discrete molar event.

The SORT has patients observe various characteristic units of their own behaviors and report these units chronologically to an interviewer at a specified time period. Patients are given specific guidelines for observing and reporting their own behavioral units and sequences. The *SORT* tool includes 25 categories of behavior, 5 categories of location, and 5 categories of aid. These categories were derived from an independent sample of the activities of disabled and nondisabled adults. The categories of behavior include exercise, transfers, education, extended sitting and lying, and social behaviors. All of these behaviors would be included in a broad definition of self-care. In the study where the SORT tool was tested, an average of approximately 22 minutes was required to obtain and code data on behavior occurring over a 4.5-hour reporting period.[45]

The SORT provides a descriptive chronology of behaviors and differs from more frequently used rating scales and questionnaires in two important ways. First, it records behavior wherever and whenever behavior occurs rather than under test conditions. Second, it provides direct assessments of behavior by recording discrete units of behavior relatively soon after they occur rather than estimating or summarizing performance occurring over longer time periods.

The scoring of the SORT instrument consists of frequency counts of behavioral units, sites where behaviors occur, aid provided, and by whom.

Self-reporting accuracy was assessed by comparing self-reports with data recorded by independent observers. Minute-by-minute comparisons of self-report and independent observations indicated moderate to high levels of agreement. Structural agreement of the reports was assessed in terms of the extent to which the two kinds of reports (self and observer) accounted for a specified time in the same way. Agreement ranged from 77.1 percent to 94.9 percent. Frequency of occurrence agreement was determined by examining SORT reports for their inclusion of behavior units coded by observers without respect to sequence. The agreement ranged from 86.3 percent to 99.7 percent. Weekly measures of performance derived from the two types of reports showed high agreement. Reported accuracy was relatively unaffected by the amount of time between occurrence of a behavior and its report and by the personal importance of various behaviors to the patients. The importance of behavior was measured by the Behavioral Importance Questionnaire, developed by the investigators for the study that tested the SORT tool. It was tested and included as a possible moderating variable of self-report accuracy.

Stephens et al.[45] state that self-reporting offers major advantages over observation, especially when used to monitor patients' behavior over time. The SORT can be used in many kinds of settings. Indices of other factors, such as level of activity, aid, mobility, social participation, and involvement of families, can be derived for different settings and kinds of behavior. Usually it is not practical or possible for an independent observer to follow a patient everywhere. When patients report their own behaviors, patients and investigators can be at separate locations without affecting the data collection. This flexibility makes the SORT particularly valuable in monitoring patients' behavior beyond the period of hospitalization until the resumption of their lives in the community.

UNIVERSAL SELF-CARE REQUISITE

The definition of the universal self-care requisite includes the life processes and the mainte-nance of human structure and function, for example, sufficient air, water, and food. For purposes of this chapter, both prevention and screening activities are incorporated in this definition. These preventive and screening activities include breast self-examination, smoking behaviors, and frequency of annual checkup. Many of the methodologic issues of the research with health-deviation self-care are evident in studies of universal self-care. For example, a conceptual framework for the study and the definition of self-care are often not given, [46–49] measurement of universal self-care activities includes only a few interview or questionnaire items within an instrument,[46–48] and the interview items or self-reports are inadequately described.[47]

UNIVERSAL SELF-CARE INSTRUMENTS

▪ EXERCISE OF SELF-CARE AGENCY SCALE

The Exercise of Self-Care Agency Scale was developed by Kearney and Fleischer.[50] The self-care theory of Orem provides the conceptual basis for this study. Orem's definition of self-care agency as "the power of an individual to engage in estimative (what should be done) and productive (what is actually done) operations essential for self-care" (p. 81),[51] is central to the scale development. The derivation of the 43-item scale and the delineation of four subconstructs that contribute to a person's exercise of self-care agency are described else-where.[50] From these subconstructs, indicants of a person's exercise of self-care agency are considered to be (1) an attitude of responsibility for self, (2) motivation to care for self, (3) the application of knowledge to self-care, (4) the valuing of health priorities, and (5) high self-esteem. Scale items for each indicant are formulated. Hence, the scale measures more than self-care activities. The time required to complete the scale is not given. Examples of items from the Exercise of Self-Care Agency Scale are:

> I eat a balanced diet.
>
> I am a good friend to myself.
>
> Life is a joy.

The authors do not provide information about which item belongs to a particular indicant. Each item on the scale is rated on a 5-point Likert scale, with the respondent indicating whether the item is "very characteristic," "somewhat characteristic," "no opinion," "some-what uncharacteristic," or "very uncharacteristic."

Each item that is positively oriented toward self-care is scored from 0 to 4, according to the participant's response on the Likert scale. A score of 0 is assigned to the response, "very uncharacteristic of me," whereas a score of 4 is assigned to the response, "very charac-teristic of me." Eleven of the items are worded negatively with respect to exercise of self-care; thus the reverse scoring method is assigned to the response, that is, 4 instead of 0, 3 instead of 1, and so on. The maximum score possible on the instrument is 172, indicating a high degree of exercise of self-care agency.

The reliability data for the Exercise of Self-Care Agency Scale were obtained with nursing students using the test–retest (5 weeks) ($r = 0.77$) and students in psychology courses using the split-half (Spearman-Brown) formula ($r = 0.77$) methods. Content validity of the initial instrument was established by having five experts in the self-care concept rate each of the items on its worth as an indicator of exercise of self-care agency. At the suggestion of these raters, 1 of the 44 items was deleted and 1 item was reworded. Two other instruments (Adjective Checklist and Rotter Internal-External Locus of Control Scale) were used in establishing construct validity. There was a low but significant positive correlation of exercise of self-care agency with the Adjective Checklist subscales of self-confidence ($r = 0.23$, $p = 0.05$), achievement ($r = 0.32$, $p < 0.01$), and intraception ($r = 0.26$, $p = 0.05$), whereas a negative significant correlation existed between exercise of self-care agency and abasement ($= 0.35$, $p < 0.01$). These findings support to some extent the claim of construct validity in the Exercise of Self-Care Agency Scale. The findings failed to suggest that locus of control is associated with exercise of self-care agency.

Kearney and Fleischer[50] contend that this scale is global in nature and will allow nurses to document the effectiveness of their care based on the demonstration of clients' increasing their exercise of self-care agency.

▪ BASIC PREVENTIVE HEALTH PRACTICES QUESTIONNAIRE

The Basic Preventive Health Practices Questionnaire was developed by Turnbull[52] to determine the relationship of the practice of six basic preventive health measures with the practice of breast self-examination. The conceptual model used to guide the study and instrument development is not provided. The definition of basic preventive health practices is tasks undertaken to maintain and/or promote a state of positive health by adequate rest, nutrition, exercise, weight maintenance, medical and dental care, and the practice of breast self-examination. The questionnaire includes seven preventive health questions. Examples of the questions are:

I obtain a Pap smear:
    a) at least yearly _____
    b) every 1 to 3 years _____
    c) at intervals of 3 years or more _____

On the average, I obtain sleep nightly which makes me feel:
    a) well rested _____
    b) occasionally rested _____
    c) very often tired _____

To each participant's response, a rating of 3, 2, or 1 is assigned from the most desirable response (3) to the least desirable (1). All individual item ratings are summed to yield a total score.

These psychometric data are not reported. However, findings from the study where this questionnaire was developed and tested reveal that the practice of breast self-examination was related to overall health practices among younger (≤ 35 years) but not among older (> 35 years) respondents. This finding, at best, indicates the sensitivity of the Basic Preventive Health Practices Questionnaire to determine differences between groups by age.

The Basic Preventive Health Practices Questionnaire could be used with other prevention and screening self-care behaviors, for example, dental examination or testicular self-examination. The gender-specific items in the original questionnaire would need to be modified to include male self-care behaviors.

▪ SELF-CARE HEALTH DIARY

The Self-Care Health Diary was developed by Freer[53] to measure any health upsets and activities to manage these upsets. The investigator contends that the health upsets are transient problems, and just as health is not the absence of symptoms, the presence of health problems does not indicate ill health (p. 860).[53] The conceptual model used to develop and test the Self-Care Health Diary is not provided. Self-care is defined as including self-medication, self-referral, and resting. The diary consists of a structured sheet of questions that are answered each evening by the participants. Examples of these questions are:

What kind of a day has it been for you?
(responses are made on a 7-point Likert scale from 1 for poor to 7 for good)

If you recorded any problems yesterday, which, if any, persist today?
(open-ended response)

Did you take any medicine today in addition to your usual medicine? If so what was it for
  and what was its name?
(Yes or No response for first question, then open-ended response for second question)

The diary questions were tested, and some were modified through a series of pilot studies.[53] Subjects are instructed to record health upsets no matter how trivial or transient. By design, the study was restricted to those aspects of self-care practiced in response to perceived upsets in health and recorded in answer to the relevant questions in the diary. This excluded any preventive health measures.

The frequency of reported health upsets and activities (medical and nonmedical self-care responses) to manage these upsets is the scoring method. The diary questions yield both quantitative and qualitative data.

Reliability data are not presented. However, Freer contends that the diary questions are valid in that the participants' reported morbidity and self-referral patterns were very similar to published results from a British diary study that included a comparable sample. Furthermore, the amount and type of self-medication agrees with the extensive literature on the subject.[53]

Considering the lack of specificity for any health upset, the Self-Care Health Diary could be used with many different populations across a variety of settings.

▪ HEALTH-PROMOTING LIFESTYLE PROFILE (HPLP)

The Health-Promoting Lifestyle Profile (HPLP) was developed for use in testing the Health Promotion Model proposed by Pender.[54] It is an instrument to measure health-promoting behavior, conceptualized as a multidimensional pattern of self-initiated actions and perceptions that serve to maintain or enhance the level of wellness, self-actualization, and fulfillment of the individual. The 48-item instrument is a summated behavior rating scale that uses a 4-point response format to measure the frequency of self-reported health-promoting behaviors. The instrument consists of six subscales: self-actualization, health responsibility, exercise, nutrition, interpersonal support, and stress management. The number of items in each of the subscales varies, ranging from 5 items in the exercise subscale to 13 items in the self-actualization subscale. Examples of these are:

Perform stretching exercises at least three times per week
(responses are made on a 4-point Likert scale from 1 for "never" to 4 for "routinely")

Feel I am growing and changing personally in positive directions
(responses are similar to those given in above item)

The HPLP was developed from a 100-item checklist of positive health behaviors designed by Walker et al. as a clinical nursing tool arranged in ten categories.[55] Prior to empirical testing, modifications were made in format to a Likert scale, and 7 items were added. The resulting 107-item instrument was administered to 952 adults recruited from a variety of community settings. Item analysis, factor analysis, and reliability estimates resulted in six factors being identified (current six subscales on the HPLP) and a reduction in the number of items to 48. By design, items related to prevention/detection of specific diseases were deleted because they lacked concept validity. In addition, all items concerned with undesirable health practices or bad habits (e.g., smoking and alcohol use) were eliminated on the basis of item and reliability analysis.

The HPLP is scored by summing the responses to all 48 items; subscale scores may be obtained by summing the responses to subscale items. The authors note that comparison of subscales may be more meaningful if a mean, rather than a sum, of item responses is calculated.[55]

Reliability and validity data have been established in samples of healthy adults.[55] The 48 items of the HPLP were entered into a principal axis factor analysis, with six factors extracted and obliquely rotated. All items loaded on expected factors at a level of 0.35 or higher, and the six factors explained 47.1 percent of the variance in the instrument. Second-order factor analysis of the correlations among the six identified factors extracted a single factor measured by the instrument, which was interpreted as health-promoting lifestyle. The 48-item instrument was found to have high internal consistency (alpha = 0.922). The six subscales were found to have acceptably high internal consistency estimates, with alphas ranging from 0.70 (for stress management) to 0.90 (for self-actualization). To evaluate stability, the instrument was administered twice to a sample of 63 adults at an interval of 2 weeks. Pearson r was 0.93 for the total score and ranged from 0.81 to 0.91 for the subscales.[55]

By design, the HPLP instrument is a measure of health-promoting behavior in healthy adults. It is not intended to be administered to clinical populations with specific diagnosed conditions.

▪ HEALTH DIARY

The Health Diary was developed by Frank-Stromborg[56] for the purpose of measuring health-promoting behaviors in ambulatory cancer patients. Health-promoting behaviors are defined as those actions that are directed toward sustaining or increasing the levels of well-being, self-actualization, and fulfillment of an individual. The Health Diary is based on Pender's Health Promotion Model[54] and the six subscales contained in the HPLP.[55] The Health Diary is a personal record of health-related events that is filled out every day (12 items) for 4 weeks. Each week comprises a separate instrument and is designed so that it can be mailed postage-paid to the investigators at the end of the week. The diary includes four items that have a Likert 7-point scale format and eight open-ended questions to measure what ambulatory cancer patients do to make themselves feel better. Examples of these questions are:

How would you rate your health today?
(responses are made on a 7-point Likert scale from 1 for "poor" to 7 for "excellent")

What specifically did you do today that you feel helped your physical health or decreased
    a physical problem you were having?
(open-ended response)

The Health Diary is being used currently in an ongoing study of ambulatory cancer
patients ($n = 108$).[56] No problems have been reported of the keeping of the diary by the
patients.

Since the Health Diary is primarily qualitative in nature, content analysis of the participants' responses is the appropriate data analysis technique.

Frank-Stromborg and others[57,58] report high levels of reporting, sensitivity to detail,
reduction of memory recall bias and error, and the ability to accurately reflect individual daily
reports of health and health actions as advantages to the diary technique. The qualitative
research issues of interrater reliability of coding and computer analysis of the ethnography
data are not presented in the ongoing project involving ambulatory cancer patients.[56]

Since the Health Diary items are nonspecific to the disease of cancer, the diary could be
used in a variety of clinical populations.

DEVELOPMENTAL SELF-CARE REQUISITE

The definition of developmental self-care requisite includes human developmental processes
and events during various stages of the life cycle and events that may adversely affect
development. This area of self-care has received the least amount of attention by researchers.
Consequently, no published tools to measure developmental self-care can be located. One
dissertation study[59] developed a self-care agency instrument in a sample of healthy adolescents. However, this research did not focus on defining self-care abilities in adolescence as a
developmental phase with certain tasks of self-care to be mastered.

SUMMARY

Self-care as a concept for clinical practice is flourishing. However, the lag often seen between
implementing a change in health care and the systematic research of that change is clearly
evident in the dearth of self-care tools. Obviously, greater effort is needed in this area.
especially in developmental, family and community self-care instruments and empirical
testing.

REFERENCES

1. Green, L.W. Research and demonstration issues in self-care: Measuring the decline of medico-
   centrism. *Health Educ Monogr,* 1977, *5*(2):161.
2. Norris, C. Self-care. *Am J Nurs,* 1979, *79*(3):486.
3. King, C. The self-help/self-care concept. *Nurse Pract,* 1980, *5*(3):34.
4. McCorkle, R. Nurses as advocates for self-care. *Cancer Nurs,* 1983, *6*(1):17.
5. Levin, L., Katz, A., & Holst, E. *Self-care: Lay initiatives in health.* New York: Prodist, 1976.
6. Levin, L. Self-care: An international perspective. *Soc Policy,* 1976, *7*:70.

7. Levin, L. Patient education and self-care: How do they differ? *Nurs Outlook,* 1978, *26:*170.
8. Orem, D. *Nursing: Concepts of practice.* New York: McGraw-Hill, 1980.
9. Pratt, L. Changes in health care ideology in relation to self-care by families. *Health Educ Monogr,* 1977, *5:*121.
10. Facteau, L. Self-care concepts and the care of the hospitalized child. *Nurs Clin North Am,* 1980, *15*(1):145.
11. Steiger, N.J., & Lipson, J.G. *Self-care nursing.* Bowie, MD: Brady, 1985.
12. Fitzgerald, S. Utilizing Orem's self-care nursing model in designing an educational program for the diabetic. *Top Clin Nurs,* 1980, *2*(2):57.
13. Backscheider, J. Self-care requirements, self-care capabilities, and nursing systems in the diabetic nurse management clinic. *Am J Public Health,* 1974, *64*(12):1138.
14. Miller, J.F. Categories of self-care needs of ambulatory patients with diabetes. *J Adv Nurs,* 1982, *7*(1):25.
15. Lorig, K., Laurin, J., & Gines, G.E.S. Arthritis self-management. *Nurs Clin North Am,* 1984, *19*(4):637.
16. Stanaszek, W.F., & McDonald, O.W. Self-care habits and disease-state understanding of diabetic patients. *Am J Hosp Pharm,* 1981, *38*(9):1337.
17. Gotch, P. Incorporating activity into diabetic self-care. *Occup Health Nurs,* 1982, *30*(2):16.
18. Windsor, R., Roseman, J., Gartseff, G., & Kirk, K. Qualitative issues in developing educational diagnostic instruments and assessment procedures for diabetic patients. *Diabetes Care,* 1981, *4*(4):468.
19. Whatley, K., Guthrie, P., & Turner, W.W. Developing a patient assessment and teaching program for right atrial catheters. *J NITA,* 1984, *7:*529.
20. Rameizl, P. CADET, a self-care assessment tool. *Geriatric Nurs,* 1984, *7*(1):43.
21. Karl, C.A. The effect of an exercise program on self-care activities for the institutionalized elderly. *J Gerontol Nurs,* 1982, *8*(5):282.
22. Kuriansky, J., & Gurland, B. The performance test of activities of daily living. *Int J Aging Hum Devel,* 1976, *7*(4):343.
23. Harvey, R.F., Jellinek, H.M. Functional performance assessment: A program approach. *Arch Phys Med Rehabil,* 1981, *62*(9):456.
24. Kubricht, D.W. Therapeutic self-care demands expressed by outpatients receiving external radiation therapy. *Cancer Nurs,* 1984, *7*(1):43.
25. Izzo, M. Assessing the coping abilities of hypertensive patients. *Top Clin Nurs,* 1982, *4*(2):33.
26. Dropkin, M.J. Compliance in postoperative head and neck patients. *Cancer Nurs,* 1979, *2*(5):379.
27. Avery, C.H., March, J., & Brook, R.H. An assessment of the adequacy of self-care by adult asthmatics. *J Community Health,* 1980, *5*(3):167.
28. Berg, A.O. Targeting symptoms for self-care education: A multivariate analysis of physician contact. *Med Care,* 1980, *18*(5):551.
29. Stahl, S.M., Kelley, C.R., Neil, P.J., et al. Effects of home blood pressure measurement on long-term BP control. *Am J Public Health,* 1984, *74*(7):704.
30. Anna, D.J., Hohon, S.A., Ord, L., & Wells, S.R. Implementing Orem's conceptual framework. *J Nurs Admin,* Nov. 1978, *8*(11):entire volume.
31. Shillam, L.L., Beeman, C., & Loshin, P.M. Effect of occupational therapy intervention on bathing independence of disabled persons. *Am J Occup Ther,* 1983, *37*(11):744.
32. Brough, F.K., Schmidt, C.D., Rasmussen, T., & Boyer, M. Comparison of two teaching methods for self-care training for patients with chronic obstructive pulmonary disease. *Patient Couns Health Educ,* 1982, *4*(2):111.
33. Behn, S., & Lane, D.S. A self-teaching weight-control manual: Method for increasing compliance and reducing obesity. *Patient Educ Couns,* 1983, *5*(2):63.
34. Weinstein, P., Fiset, L.O., & Lancaster, B. Assessment of a behavioral approach in long-term plague control using a multiple baseline design: The need for relapse research. *Patient Educ Couns,* 1984, *5*(3):135.
35. Dodd, M.J. Self-care for side effects of cancer chemotherapy: An assessment of nursing interventions. *Cancer Nurs,* 1983, *6*(1):63.

36. Dodd, M.J. Measuring informational intervention for chemotherapy knowledge and self-care behavior. *Res Nurs Health,* 1984, *7*(1):43.
37. Vickery, D.M., Kalmer, H., Lowry, D., et al. Effects of a self-care education program on medical visits. *JAMA,* 1983, *250*(21):2952.
38. Barofsky, I. Compliance, adherence and the therapeutic alliance: Steps in the development of self-care. *Soc Sci Med,* 1978, *12*(5A):369.
39. Klein, R.M., Bell, B. Self-care skills: Behavioral measurement with Klein-Bell ADL scale. *Arch Phys Med Rehabil,* 1982, *63*(7):335.
40. Dodd, M.J. Assessing patient self-care for side effects of cancer chemotherapy. Part 1. *Cancer Nurs,* 1982, *5*(6):447.
41. Dodd, M.J. Patterns of self-care in cancer patients receiving radiation therapy. *Oncol Nurs Forum,* 1984, *10*(3):23.
42. Dodd, M.J. Efficacy of proactive information on self-care in radiation therapy patients. *Heart Lung,* 1987, *16*(5):538.
43. Dodd, M.J. Patterns of self-care in patients with breast cancer. *West J Nurs Res,* in press.
44. Dodd, M.J. Self-care for patients with breast cancer to prevent side effects of chemotherapy. *Public Health Nurs,* 1984, *1*(4):202.
45. Stephens, M.A.P., Norris-Baker, C., & Willems, E.P. Patient behavior monitoring through self-reports. *Arch Phys Med Rehabil,* 1983, *64*(4):167.
46. McCusker, J., & Morrow, G. The relationship of health locus of control to preventive health behaviors and health beliefs. *Patient Counseling Health Educ,* 1979, *1*(1):146.
47. Carstenson, R., & O'Grady, L.F.A. Breast self-examination program for high school students. *Am J Public Health,* 1980, *70*(12):1293.
48. Howe, H. Social factors associated with breast self-examination among high-risk women. *Am J Public Health,* 1981, *71*(3):251.
49. Howe, H. Proficiency in performing breast self-examination. *Patient Counseling Health Educ,* 1980, *2*(4):151.
50. Kearney, B.Y., & Fleischer, B.J. Development of an instrument to measure exercise of self-care agency. *Res Nurs Health,* 1979, *2*(1):25.
51. Nursing Development Conference Group. *Concept formalization in nursing: Process and product.* Boston: Little, Brown, 1973.
52. Turnbull, E.M. Effect of basic preventive health practices and mass media on the practice of breast self-examination. *Nurs Res,* 1978, *27*(2):98.
53. Freer, C.B. Self-care: A health diary study. *Med Care,* 1980, *18*(8):853.
54. Pender, N. *Health promotion in nursing practice.* Norwalk, CT: Appleton-Century-Crofts, 1982.
55. Walker, S.N., Sechrist, K.R., & Pender, N.J. Health-promoting lifestyle profile: Development and psychometric characteristics. *Nurs Res,* 1987, *36*(2):76.
56. Frank-Stromborg, M. Health promotion behaviors in ambulatory cancer patients: Facts or fiction? *Oncol Nurs Forum,* 1986, *13*(4):37.
57. Verbrugge, L.M. Health diaries. *Med Care,* 1980, *18*(2):73.
58. Kosa, J., Alpert, J.J., & Haggerty, R.J. On the reliability of family health information: A comparative study of mother's reports on illness and related behavior. *Soc Sci Med,* 1967, *1*(12):165.
59. Denyes, M.J. Development of an instrument to measure self-care agency in adolescents. University of Michigan, *Dissertation Abstracts International,* 1980, *41*(5):1716B.

CHAPTER 12

Measuring Body Image

Judy M. Diekmann, R.N., Ed.D., O.C.N.

The concept of body image has application in a wide range of disciplines, including medicine, psychology, physical therapy, dentistry, dietetics, and nursing. The importance of body image in our culture is obvious—one only has to note the widespread expenditure of time, effort, and money by people seeking to alter their appearance in order to look like an ideal image they have of themselves.

Life events that result in an alteration of a person's body can have a profound effect on how that person imagines himself or herself and functions in society. Such alterations can be very disrupting and anxiety provoking to the individual. Alteration in the body caused by trauma, surgery, or therapy may result in feelings of depression and lowered self-esteem. Nurses care for patients experiencing a variety of alterations of body image, including changes in body structure and function, deformities, loss of body boundaries, and depersonalization. These changes may be a consequence of surgery, drugs, sensory deprivation, fatigue, stress, immobility, or anesthesia. Assessing the degree of alteration of body image is important in order to plan nursing interventions focused on promoting the reestablishment or maintenance of self-esteem. Nursing care that successfully assists patients to integrate physical changes into self can be a major factor in helping patients to adapt and survive. The quality of life people experience may be inextricably related to how they imagine their bodies.

THE CONCEPT OF BODY IMAGE

The body image concept has been thoroughly researched by several authors, and their publications have become classics on the subject.[1-3] Schilder defined body image as "the picture of our own body which we form in our mind, that is to say, the way in which the body appears to ourselves" (p. 11).[2] Body image is a term that refers to the body as a psychologic experience and focuses on the individual's feelings and attitudes toward his or her own body.[3] It refers to subjective experiences with one's body and the manner in which one has organized life events. Norris believes that it is a "social creation . . . basic to identity and it has been referred to as the somatic ego" (p. 8).[4]

The concept of body image has been approached from different perspectives, including neurologic, somatic, and psychologic characterizations. The definitions include both the direct perception (visual, tactile, proprioceptive) of the body and the attitudes, emotions, and reactions of the individual that contribute to the final perception.[5]

The meaning of the term "body image" differs from the meaning of the term "self-concept." Body image refers to a person's perception of his or her body. Self-concept denotes how one feels about oneself. Sometimes these terms are used interchangeably even though they refer to distinct concepts.

The first written account of body image disturbance was by Ambroise Paré, a seventeenth century surgeon. He, and others who have followed, noted that after a limb amputation, people reported an illusionary feeling of continued presence of the missing limb. The image of the missing limb remained, although the limb ceased to exist.

Neurologists observed that patients with various brain lesions showed a wide range of distorted body ideas. Such patients were unable to distinguish one side of the body from the other, denied the existence of various body parts, denied the incapacitation of various parts, or falsely attributed new body parts to themselves.[6] At present, it is believed that body image disturbances may occur with brain lesions at any level. However, the parietal region of the minor hemisphere commonly is regarded as being of special significance because of the relationship that exists between right parietal disease and disorders of body image.[3]

In the field of psychiatry, many investigators have studied the concept of body image and reported that numerous schizophrenic patients showed almost the same range of distortions of body image as observed in neurologic patients.[7] To substantiate this phenomenon, Fisher and Cleveland reviewed and classified the bizarre body perceptions reported by many schizophrenics.[3] They grouped these distortions into several categories. One prominent cluster of disturbed body attitudes centers around issues of masculinity and femininity. It includes such distortions as feeling that one has the body parts of the opposite sex or that one is half-man, half-woman. A second group of distortions involves feelings of body disintegration and deterioration. Commonly, these involve sensations that some minor part of the body had been destroyed. Another category refers to feelings of depersonalization. People report a sense of unreality about the existence of body parts or the total body. The person experiences his or her own body as if it were alien or belonged to a stranger. The fourth category of distortions proposed by Fisher and Cleveland is a sense of loss of body boundaries. People with this disorder feel that things happening elsewhere and to other people are happening to them.

Researchers are turning increasingly to analysis of the normal individual's body perception as a psychologic phenomenon. They postulate that the normal person's attitude toward his or her body may influence responses in the same way other significant attitudes do. Feelings about the body appear to affect decisions at all levels; even decisions relating to self-survival may be biased by the person's prevailing body image.

Studies of patients with the syndrome of anorexia nervosa support the interrelationship between body image distortions and feelings of inadequacy. The uniqueness of this syndrome is demonstrated by the body image characterization, which includes a negative evaluation of body appearance as well as a tendency to overestimate body size.[8] In addition to studies of people with the syndrome of anorexia nervosa, increasingly more research findings are published that describe the relationship between distorted body image and obesity.[9-13]

Dropkin defines normal body image as a perceptual homeostasis.[14] As an adaptive mechanism, it perpetuates balance among the physiologic, psychologic, and sociocultural components of the body.

ISSUES IN MEASURING THE BODY IMAGE CONCEPT

Although most agree that the concept of body image has a substantial place in health-related disciplines, there is little consensus about the best procedure to measure this phenomenon. Theoretical models of body image, although thought-provoking, have not resulted in realistic methods to measure it. Often the literature is unclear about which disturbances in body image are functions of direct sensoriperceptual deficits and which are distortions in the thought process or distortions in affective experiencing.[9,15]

The most popular measurement techniques of the major dimensions of the body image concept include questionnaires and scales, draw-a-person tests, body image boundary determinations, direct measurement of perceived body size, distortion techniques, and videotape feedback. When administering the instruments and interpreting their results, the assistance of a psychologist or psychiatrist may be helpful. The reader should be cognizant of the fact that many instruments currently available to measure the concept of body image do not have established psychometric properties.

Questionnaires and Scales

In 1898, Hall used a questionnaire to determine the earliest memories children have of their body parts that first attract their attention.[16] Subsequently, Curran and Levine extensively questioned 30 prostitutes and an equal number of nonprostitutes to determine and compare their attitudes toward their body.[17] They used a 96-item questionnaire developed by Schilder in 1935.[2] They asked their subjects such questions as:

What do you think of your own strength, of your beauty, of your health?

How many characteristics of the opposite sex do you have?

What is the most important part of your body?

They concluded that in this population, unattractive respondents tended to deny and minimize their deviations from normal.

▪ BODY FOCUS QUESTIONNAIRE

There is reason to believe that the amount of attention focused by a person on any given sector of his or her body is linked to the intensity of conflict about a particular theme associated with that part.[18] Because of this, Fisher developed a questionnaire to study the manner in which people distribute their attention to various regions of their bodies.[18] The perception of different parts of the body (attention brought to them) may be estimated with the Body Focus Questionnaire.

The format of the questionnaire involves presenting the subject with a series of 108 forced-choice alternatives corresponding to paired body regions and asking the subject to choose one of the two parts that is "at the moment most clear in your awareness." The items are placed within eight scales: back/front, right/left, stomach, mouth, eyes, arms, head, and heart. These were chosen by Fisher as representative focal body parts identified by subjects in previous studies. The subject's score on each scale is the number of times an item on that scale is chosen. In 1978, Bruchon-Schwitzer constructed an adaptation of this questionnaire in French and administered it to 118 subjects.[19] She reported significant test–retest reliability. Since 1979, a succession of articles debating the independence of the Body Focus Questionnaire Scales has been published in *Perceptual and Motor Skills*.[20-25]

▪ GRAY QUESTIONNAIRE TO DETERMINE BODY AFFECT

Gray reported results of a study that examined two aspects of body image: perception and normalcy of weight and affect. She determined the relationship of demographic characteristics (sex, age, race) and actual body weight (underweight, normal weight, overweight) to body image distortion.[26] She developed a short 10-item Questionnaire To Determine Body Affect. In responding to this questionnaire, subjects are asked to indicate on a scale of 1 to 5 whether they "agree" or "disagree" with statements such as:

When I look in the mirror, I feel bad about the food I've recently eaten.

I have often been self-conscious with people I am attracted to because of my body appearance.

The last question is whether subjects consider themselves underweight, average, or overweight, and their classification is used as a criterion for comparing their perception of their body as underweight, normal weight, or overweight to the Metropolitan Life Insurance Company's standards for weight. Because the insurance standards are derived through sampling, the researcher assumed that the study sample would have standards for weight-related appearance that were consistent and that deviations from these standards could be attributed to perception. Reliability and validity have not been reported for this instrument.

In terms of physical attractiveness, I consider my face as:
  a. Very attractive
  b. Moderately attractive
  c. Neither attractive nor unattractive
  d. Moderately unattractive
  e. Very unattractive

The part of my body I like the best is _____

The part of my body I like the least is _____

Consider your life to be a ladder from 1 to 10; 10 represents the best possible happy life; 1 represents the worst possible life. On what rung were you or do you expect to be as a:
  a. Young child _____
  b. Adolescent _____
  c. Adult _____
  d. Middle age _____
  e. The future _____

My social life is:
  a. Very satisfactory
  b. Moderately satisfactory
  c. Neither satisfactory nor unsatisfactory
  d. Moderately unsatisfactory
  e. Very unsatisfactory

I view myself as a:
  a. Very fat person
  b. Moderately fat person
  c. Normal weight person
  d. Moderately thin person
  e. Very thin person

Figure 12–1. Sample Questions from the Self-Attitude Questionnaire. *(Courtesy of Gloria Leon, Ph.D.)*

• SELF-ATTITUDE QUESTIONNAIRE (SAQ)

The Self-Attitude Questionnaire (SAQ) is a self-administered, 40-item, multiple choice instrument.[27] The individual items were developed to obtain information about a person's present attitude toward his or her body, best and least liked body parts, and attitudes about his or her physical and sexual attractiveness. It also elicits information about various kinds of interpersonal activities and attitudes toward food and eating. Psychometric properties have not been reported.

Figure 12–1 shows some sample questions. The SAQ appears to be easily administered and interpreted and would be valuable for research conducted with a variety of subjects who manifest eating disorders.

• BERSCHEID ET AL. QUESTIONNAIRE

In 1972, Berscheid et al. developed a 109-item questionnaire to survey readers of *Psychology Today* about their attitudes toward their bodies.[28] Sixty-two thousand people returned the questionnaire. In completing this instrument, subjects are instructed to judge their satisfaction and dissatisfaction with 24 body parts, using a 4-point scale that extends from "quite or extremely dissatisfied" to "quite or extremely satisfied." The 24 body parts include face, hair, eyes, ears, nose, mouth, teeth, voice, chin, complexion, shoulders, arms, hands, feet, size of abdomen, buttocks, hips, legs and ankles, height, weight, general muscle tone or development, chest/breast, size of sex organs, and appearance of sex organs.[29] The complete instrument is published in *Psychology Today*.[28] No reliability or validity data have been reported for this instrument.

• BODY CATHEXIS SCALES

In 1953, Secord and Jourard developed two scales to measure body cathexis.[30] Body cathexis is defined as the degree of self-reported satisfaction with aspects of one's own body.[31] The first scale was a 46-item Body Cathexis Scale (Appendix I). The second scale was constructed to determine self-cathexis or general self-satisfaction (Appendix II). In devising the instruments, Secord and Jourard assumed that body esteem could be expressed as a single score based on the sum of the individual's responses to the items. Mayer and Eisenberg reported split-half reliability of $r = 0.81$ for the two scales.[32] They also reported that the items of the 46-item scale have "high face validity" for what they measure. They suggested that the scales are a valid measure of body perception and satisfaction.

In 1984, Hammond and O'Rourke conducted a study with 398 subjects to further investigate the psychometric properties of the Body Cathexis Scale using a 51-item version. They reported that the instrument had a "tight internal structure" with unidimensional properties. They recommend the instrument for researching the role of body feelings in self-concept and personality.[33]

• SECORD AND JOURARD MODIFIED BODY CATHEXIS QUESTIONNAIRE

In 1955, Jourard and Secord modified their scale in the Secord and Jourard Modified Body Cathexis Questionnaire to include 12 body parts (Table 12–1). Each body part is rated by the subject on a 7-point scale ranging from 1, "strong positive feeling," to 7, "strong negative

**TABLE 12–1. SECORD AND
JOURARD MODIFIED BODY
CATHEXIS QUESTIONNAIRE**

Height	Ankles
Bust	Feet
Hips	Nose length
Thighs	Shoulder width
Calves	Neck length

From Jourard, Secord. J Abnormal Soc
Psychol, *1955, 50:243.*

feeling."[31] The total score of all 12 body parts is divided by 12 to give the final score, which can range from 1 to 7. Fawcett and Frye reported an internal consistency of 0.74 for all 12 scale items, using Cronbach coefficient alpha.[34]

• BODY ESTEEM SCALE

In 1984, Franzoi and Shields reported a new Body Esteem Scale they had developed.[35] Their scale is composed of 23 original Body Cathexis Scale items from Secord and Jourard and 13 new items.[35] Factor analysis of their scale revealed that body esteem is a multidimensional construct that differs for males and females. Factor analysis resulted in clusters of variables that made it possible to identify concepts of body esteem. For males, the body esteem dimensions dealt with physical attractiveness, upper body strength, and physical condition. For females, the dimensions dealt with sexual attractiveness, weight concern, and physical condition. Measures of internal consistency using Cronbach coefficient alpha ranged from 0.78 to 0.87.

To establish convergent validity (i.e., measuring the same trait with a different method), Franzoi and Shields correlated scores from their three subscales with scores from the Rosenberg Self-Esteem Scale, which provides a general measure of self-esteem.[36] A high score on the Rosenberg Self-Esteem Scale indicates positive self-esteem, and a low score indicates negative self-esteem. With the exception of the females' weight concern factor, the results supported a moderate correlation between general self-esteem and each of the three body esteem subscales.

Franzoi and Shields also tested their instrument for discriminant validity (i.e., a procedure for providing a statistical basis for distinguishing between two or more groups of subjects) for both female and male subscales. The results of the statistical analysis indicated that the subscales significantly discriminated the groups. Discriminant function analysis with a Wilkes lambda stepwise selection method indicated that only the "weight concern subscale" discriminates anorexic females from nonanorexic females (lambda = 0.86, $p < 0.001$, canonical correlation = 0.37). Using the same means of analysis for the data from the male subjects, they determined that only the upper body subscale significantly differentiated male weightlifters from nonweightlifters (lambda = 0.90, $p < 0.01$, canonical correlation = 0.34).

• SECORD HOMONYM TEST

The Secord Homonym Test is a word association procedure that is used to probe unconscious body attitudes.[37] The technique involves eliciting associations to a recited list of 100 homonyms. These homonyms have meanings pertaining to either body parts or body processes or common nonbody meanings. The words "colon," "graft," and "tablet" are illustrations. Examples of homonym body responses might be "colon–intestine," "graft–skin," "tablet–aspirin," whereas three nonbody responses might be "colon–comma," "graft–police," and "tablet–paper." The test also includes some stimulus words that are not homonyms but that also elicit body responses, for example, "acid," which could yield the body responses "burn" or "sour" or the nonbody responses "base" or "sulfuric." The word list is read at a pace that ensures relatively spontaneous rather than considered response. The score is the number of body reference responses given. The number of body responses on the homonym test is indicative of the degree of importance of the body to the subject.[37] Interrater reliability (0.95), test–retest (0.94), and split-half (0.85) reliability of scores derived from the full word test was very high. There is evidence that the test taps existing levels and changes in unconscious body involvement.[38] The Secord word list presented in Appendix III was adapted by Jupp et al. in 1983.[11]

▪ OTHER SCALES

Two instruments used in studies by Leon et al. also are appropriate for nursing research.[12,13,27,39] Two scales each using 16 bipolar scales were adapted from the scale developed by Osgood et al.[40] One scale is for the concept My Body Right Now (Appendix IV). The other scale is for the concept My Personality Right Now (Appendix V). Seven of the adjective scales are used for both concepts. Reliability and validity data were not reported for these tools.

▪ DRAW-A-PERSON TEST

The Draw-a-Person Test was developed initially by Manchover, based on the belief that an individual's spontaneous drawing of the human figure represents in many ways a projection of his or her own body image.[41] In taking this test, subjects are instructed to draw a figure that looks like themselves. Although some studies[42,43] reported significant relationships between actual body type and the body types of figures drawn, many investigators[3,44,45] cautioned that this method of studying body image, although it may be potentially valuable, has often been used in a "vague impressionistic manner." Fisher and Cleveland noted that there has been limited success in differentiating which aspects of the drawing are linked with body image, which with drawing skill, and which are due to the manner in which the drawing is obtained.[3] It appears that considerable expertise in administering projective tests is required to interpret the drawings.

▪ ASKEVOLD METHOD FOR MEASURING BODY IMAGE

Askevold described a method he discovered to measure a subject's own body image.[46] His instructions are:

> The material to be used is: a roll of wrapping paper for about 100 recordings, two black and one red marking pencils, one angle, a yard-stick and a roll of tape. One piece of wrapping paper—1.5 by 1 m is taped to the wall. The subjects' initials, date, age, height and weight are put in the upper right corner, and in the upper left two lines at right angles, one horizontal and one vertical. The subject is then asked to mark on these lines the length of two corresponding

dimensions seen at a distance of 2 m. This is to measure the subjects' accuracy in determining dimensions generally. The subjects are given one black-marking pencil in each hand placed within reaching distance of the paper and instructed to keep the pencils close to the paper all the time without touching it until asked to do so. This is to avoid a source of error. The subjects are then asked to imagine themselves standing before a mirror and looking at themselves. The investigator stands behind the subjects and with his finger tip he firmly touches the certain body points chosen for marking. The subjects are then asked to make a cross on the paper where they "see" those points in the mirror. The body points chosen are easy to identify correctly anatomically, and are: body height, the acromio-clavicular joints, narrowest waist width and the trochanters of the femoral bones. When the marking is finished, the subjects turn their backs close to the paper; by help of the angle and the red pencil the investigator can mark the correct position of the body points. The difference is measured with the yard stick (pp. 72–73).[46]

Additional studies using this instrument have not been reported in the literature, and there was no information about reliability or validity.

▪ BODY IMAGE BOUNDARY CONCEPT

In 1958, Fisher and Cleveland devised a means of obtaining body image boundary scores, derived from projective responses to Rorschach inkblots.[3] Numerous studies have been based on the index devised to evaluate boundary definiteness. The Body Image Boundary Concept is based on the hypothesis that people may view their bodies as clearly and sharply bounded with a high degree of differentiation from nonself objects, or they may regard their bodies as lacking demarcation from the environment. Translating the concept of body image boundaries into operational scores, Fisher and Cleveland developed the barrier score derived from the content analysis of an inkblot protocol. This score equals the number of responses elicited by an inkblot series that are characterized by an emphasis on the protective, containing, or covering functions of the periphery.[3] It measures an aspect of how individuals experience their body, and it provides data concerning the manner in which individuals conceptualize their private body domain. Some examples of barrier responses include:

Cave with rocky walls

Person covered with a blanket

Mummy wrapped up

Vase

In each of these responses, the boundary is highlighted.

Another boundary measure is the penetration score. This is based on a count of all inkblot responses in which there is an emphasis on the destruction, evasion, or bypassing of the boundary. Responses illustrative of penetration concepts are:

Bullet piercing flesh

X-ray of inside of body

Rotting wood

The higher the penetration score, the less definite the body image boundary is considered to be. Interrater reliability of barrier scores and penetration scores was reported by Datson and

McConnell at 0.84 and 0.79, respectively, using the Pearson product moment correlation.[47] Hartley pointed out that the procedure to obtain the barrier score from the Rorschach was complicated and time consuming.[48] This instrument is best administered in conjunction with professionals trained in administering psychologic tests.

▪ DIRECT MEASUREMENT OF PERCEIVED BODY SIZE

Dillon devised an instrument for the direct measurement of the visually perceived body—height, width, and depth.[49] The device is constructed of wooden beams, two vertical beams forming the sides of a doorway and a short horizontal beam forming the top. The right vertical beam is fixed, whereas the left is movable, and the horizontal distance between these two vertical beams is adjustable by means of a rope and can be set from 0 to 4 feet. The horizontal beam is also movable and can be fixed at a height from 0 to 7½ feet. With this apparatus, subjects are instructed to adjust the beams (from a distance of 6 feet) to form a doorway that they believe they can just fit through. Subjects estimate five vertical dimensions during 10 sessions. If the dimensions are estimated in ascending direction, the order of estimation is height to the knee, height to the hip (top of pelvis), height to the shoulder, height to the mouth, and full height; width of the head (ear to ear), depth of the body, width of the body, and length of the arm (with the arm held horizontally). The vertical dimensions are obtained before the horizontal estimates. The order is reversed when descending estimates are made. Both ascending and descending estimates are made in each session.

In a companion article, Dillion reported that no systematic variation in the error of estimate (estimate minus actual measurement) occurred when subjects were tested, except for the subjects' estimation of knee height, which was greater (15 percent for the average estimate) than all other errors.[50] He also reported test–retest reliability that ranged from 0.85 to 0.95. The coefficients of validity ranged from 0.00 to 0.95; these were significant only for full height, mouth height, and shoulder height ($r = 0.95$). He reported a gradual increase in the degree of both reliability and validity as the height estimates progressed from the knee to full height.

A similar but less awkward apparatus has been designed by Slade and Russel.[51] Their apparatus consists of two lights mounted on a horizontal bar. The lights are attached so that they can be moved to indicate perceived widths of specific regions. Subjects, seated in a darkened room, are asked to estimate the dimensions of various body regions (as well as those of an inanimate object) by adjusting the lights. These data are then compared with the actual dimensions. Perceived widths of specific body regions are expressed as a ratio, the body image perception index:

$$\frac{\text{Perceived size} \times 100}{\text{Real size}}$$

Using this index, a value of 100 corresponds to accurate perception, a value less than 100 shows that physical size is underestimated, and a value greater than 100 shows that physical size is overestimated. Traub and Orbach stressed that these methods were concerned primarily with estimation of "disembodied size" rather than with direct visual perception of one's body.[15] One should also note that both techniques involve recall rather than recognition of size. These researchers also reported that significant intercorrelations between the four indices of body image perception (i.e., face, chest, waist, and hip) suggested both a substantial degree of reliability for the measures and a general factor of body image disorder.

Another device used to measure perceived body space has been described by Fawcett and Frye.[34] This device was initially developed by Schlachter[52] and modified by Fawcett.[53] It consists of a 54-inch square sheet of opaque yellow ochre vinyl upon which are superimposed concentric circles ranging from 11 to 54 inches in diameter.[53] Each circle is 1 inch larger in diameter than the preceding one and is distinguished by a two-digit random number. To determine perceived body space, subjects are instructed to position themselves inside the center circle and to indicate which circle represents the amount of space they believe their bodies occupy. To facilitate understanding, subjects are told to imagine they are encased in a cylinder whose base is one of the circles. The data collecter then records the code number of the circle specified by the subject and later converts it to inches. Fawcett and Frye reported that the device has face validity as a measure of perceived body space. In addition, they reported test–retest reliability coefficients of 0.89 for a 3-hour test–retest period and 0.74 for a 1-week period in a sample of 26 young adults.[34] Nurse researchers could easily employ these instruments in research. Further work to establish psychometric parameters is required.

▪ DISTORTION MIRROR

Studies related to body image are increasingly using mirror images and other self-representations in their endeavor to measure subjects' internalized picture of their body's physical appearance. Traub and Orbach have designed a Distorting Mirror to explore the visual perception of the physical appearance of the body.[15] A special full-length mirror can be adjusted to reflect the body of the observer on a distortion continuum ranging from extremely distorted to completely undistorted. The observer (subject) adjusts his or her reflection until it appears undistorted. As the subject continues to adjust the mirror, the reflection of the body undergoing constant change is seen. The mirror is capable of a wide range of distortions in height, width, and shape of the reflected object. The total effect is described as being equivalent to a kaleidoscope of hundreds of mirrors, each with its own degree of distortion.

Subjects are given the following instructions:

> If you make the proper adjustments, you will end up with an accurate reflection of yourself. However, if you should find that, no matter what you do, the reflection never looks exactly like you, just stop when the reflection looks most like you (p. 61).[15]

When adjustments have been completed, a record is made of the final adjustment. Data consist of two numbers that are deviations from zero distortion. These numbers are obtained from counterdials geared to each motor shaft that reflect the degree of distortion.

Studies employing this technique have drawn attention to the fact that normal subjects are extremely vague about their mirror images, despite infinite experiences of such confrontation. Nevertheless, it has been argued that although the "adjustable body-distorting mirror" has objectivity and face validity rarely achieved in body image studies, its usefulness as a measurement technique can be disputed. Rather than a conception of the body, this test involves a direct perception of it. Some argue that body image involves a recall of the relation of body parts rather than recognition of the mirror image of the body.[6]

▪ BODY-SIZING APPARATUS

Glucksman and Hirsch describe a body-sizing apparatus developed for a study they conducted to determine the response of obese patients to weight reduction.

The apparatus consists of a Hilux 102 variable anamorphic lens with a magnification of 1.0 to 2.0 times and with a regular, fixed-distance, corrector lens supplied by Projection Optics Co., Inc., Rochester, N.Y. Attached to the lens is a 16 mm. Agfa Diamator slide projector. The anamorphic lens is motorized, allowing both subject and experimenter to control it by means of manual devices. A dial, consisting of 10 equal units, is attached to the anamorphic lens, enabling the experimenter to measure the amount of distortion in two directions—obese and thin. The midpoint on this dial corresponds to an undistorted image. Thus, with the dial set at midpoint, a slide placed in the slide projector and projected through the anamorphic lens onto a screen results in an undistorted image. With the dial at other settings, an obese or thin image results. The subject is not allowed to observe the dial (p. 2).[10]

The procedure involves projecting slides of obese and nonobese subjects and systematically distorting them in the direction of either obesity or thinness. Subjects are requested to make the distorted screen images correspond to their body size. In addition, slides of a symmetrical vase are presented. The initial slide shows the vase's true dimensions, and the succeeding images are distorted. Subjects are instructed to correct the screen images to the initial, undistorted one (p. 2).[10]

Results of Gluckman and Hirsch's work indicate that obese subjects increasingly overestimate their own body size during and after weight loss. In contrast, nonobese subjects underestimate their own size during a period of weight maintenance. In the reduced state, obese subjects perceive themselves as if they had lost almost no weight. In addition, they consistently overestimate the size of other objects external to themselves before, during, and after weight loss. In a subsequent study, Garner et al. were in agreement with Glucksman and Hirsch's findings, but only for a small number of superobese subjects.[9] Psychometric properties have not been reported for this technique. Garner et al. pointed out that distorting photograph techniques and direct measure of perceived size may measure different aspects of self-perception. They suggested that the distorting photograph technique may be a more sensitive measure of one's perceptions and feelings about one's overall appearance.[9]

• VIDEOTAPE FEEDBACK

Videotape recordings are used more and more by health professionals because they afford people with an opportunity to scrutinize how they appear to others.[54–59] Techniques, such as videotape playback, have been employed with a wide range of patients to achieve such effects as "overcoming resistance," "evoking insight," "increasing motivation for psychotherapy," and "shocking alcoholics back to reality."[58] The procedure generally involves making a recording of the subject's behavior or a sample of therapeutic interaction. The tape is then played back to the participants and often used as a basis for discussion and further treatment.

Allebeck et al. have described an elaborate television system they developed to assess body image.[5] The reader is directed to their article for an indepth description of the apparatus. In brief, a picture of the subject or external object is displayed on a television monitor. The subject adjusts the size and height/width proportions of the picture. The deviations from correct measures are read directly by means of electrical instruments. Psychometric parameters were not reported.

Griffiths and Gillingham suggested that videotape feedback has effects that are specific and temporary.[59] They also proposed that the model that is postulated to explain and predict the response to videotape confrontation will be complex.

SUMMARY

There are many instruments available to measure the different aspects of body image. It is important to note that body image is a complex construct that cannot be measured with any single instrument. Most likely, multiple instruments will need to be employed. Few studies have been published by nurse researchers that investigate the body image construct.[34,60-63] Nurse researchers are in an excellent position to expand the knowledge about body image across the lifespan in both healthy and ill populations. It is evident that much more work is needed to determine the usefulness, reliability, and validity of each of the instruments described in this chapter. Studies employing a single instrument need to be replicated with various samples to establish psychometric properties.

APPENDIX I. SECORD AND JOURARD BODY CATHEXIS SCALE

Instructions: On the following pages are listed a number of things characteristic of yourself or related to you. You are asked to indicate which things you are satisfied with exactly as they are, which things you worry about and would like to change if it were possible, and which things you have no feelings about one way or the other.

Consider each item and encircle the number (not shown) which best represents your feelings according to the following scale:

1. Have strong feelings and wish change could somehow be made.
2. Don't like, but can put up with.
3. Have no particular feelings one way or the other.
4. Am satisfied.
5. Consider myself fortunate.

hair	width of shoulders
facial complexion	arms
appetite	chest
hands	eyes
distribution of hair over body	digetion
	hips
nose	skin texture
fingers	lips
elimination	legs
wrists	teeth
breathing	forehead
waist	feet
energy level	sleep
back	voice
ears	health
chin	sex activities
exercise	knees
ankles	posture
neck	face
shape of head	weight
body build	sex (male or female)
profile	back view of head
height	trunk
age	

From Secord, Jourard. J Consult Clin Psychol,1953, 17:343.

APPENDIX II. SECORD AND JOURARD SELF-CATHEXIS SCALE

Instructions: You are asked to indicate which things you are satisfied with exactly as they are, which things you worry about and would like to change if it were possible, and which things you have no feelings about one way or the other.

Consider each item and encircle the number (not shown) which best represents your feelings according to the following scale:
1. Have strong feelings and wish change could somehow be made.
2. Don't like, but can put up with.
3. Have no particular feelings one way or the other.
4. Am satisfied.
5. Consider myself fortunate.

first name	sensitivity to opinions of others
morals	ability to lead
ability to express self	last name
taste in clothes	impulses
sense of duty	manners
sophistication	handwriting
self-understanding	intelligence level
life goals	athletic skills
artistic talent	fears
tolerance	happiness
moods	creativeness
general knowledge	love life
imagination	strength of conviction
popularity	conscience
self-confidence	skill with hands
ability to express sympathy	capacity for work
emotional control	conscientiousness
self-consciousness	ability to meet people
generosity	self-discipline
ability to accept criticism	suggestibility
thoughts	neatness
artistic and literary taste	vocabulary
memory	procrastination
thriftness	will power
personality	self-assertiveness
self-respect	ability to make decisions
ability to concentrate	dreams
ability to take orders	

From Secord, Jourard. J Consult Clin Psychol 1953, 17:343.

APPENDIX III. THE SECORD WORD ASSOCIATIONS TEST SHOWING NEUTRAL WORDS AND PROBE WORDS FOR SPLIT-HALF ADMINISTRATION

acid (2)[a]	function (3)	probe (3)	strip (3)
actor (1)(2)	gag (2)	pump (2)	stump (2)
acute (3)	gall (3)	quack (3)	sweet (1)(2)
arch (2)	game (1)(2)	rain (1)(3)	swell (3)
attach (3)	gas (2)	rash (2)	system (2)
back (2)	glassy (3)	rat (1)(2)	tablet (3)
bark (1)(3)	graft (2)	red (3)	tan (2)
bare (3)	index (3)	regular (2)	tape (3)
barn (1)(2)	lamp (1)(3)	run (3)	tar (1)(3)
beat (2)	layer (2)	scarlet (2)	temperature (2)
blotch (3)	light (1)(2)	scrape (3)	tender (3)
circulate (2)	limb (3)	side (2)	tent (1)(2)
colon (3)	lining (2)	sing (1)(3)	tissue (2)
collie (1)(3)	middle (3)	sling (3)	treat (3)
condition (2)	mole (2)	smart (2)	trench (2)
confine (3)	nail (3)	smear (3)	trunk (2)
contact (2)	nap (1)(3)	socket (2)	trial (1)(3)
continue (1)(2)	navel (2)	soup (1)(2)	twist (2)
contract (3)	ooze (3)	spotted (3)	vessel (3)
crisis (2)	orchard (1)(3)	spurt (2)	visit (2)
digit (3)	organ (2)	spread (3)	vote (1)(2)
enlarged (2)	pair (1)(3)	stain (2)	vogue (1)(3)
extract (3)	part (3)	stay (1)(3)	waist (3)
fiber (2)	patient (2)	still (3)	win (1)(3)
fish (1)(3)	prize (1)(2)	stitch (2)	wrench (2)

[a]Words marked (1) are neutral and are inserted for purposes of disguise. They are not scored. Words marked (2) are included in the first split-half. Words marked (3) are included in the second split-half.
From Jupp, Collins. Am J Clin Exp Hypnosis, 1983,11(2):89. Adapted from Secord. J Pers, 1953, 21:479.

APPENDIX IV. MY BODY RIGHT NOW INSTRUMENT

Fat		Thin
Beautiful		Ugly
Desirable		Undesirable
Dirty		Clean
Soft		Hard
Proportioned		Unproportioned
Light		Heavy
Powerful		Weak
Pleasant		Unpleasant
Fragile		Massive
Attractive		Repulsive
Large		Small
Inactive		Active
Firm		Flabby
Bad		Good
Uncomfortable		Comfortable

Courtesy of Gloria Leon, PhD.

APPENDIX V. MY PERSONALITY RIGHT NOW INSTRUMENT

Beautiful									Ugly
Unpleasant									Pleasant
Desirable									Undesirable
Repulsive									Attractive
Outgoing									Shy
Self-conscious									Self-assured
Preoccupied with weight									Not preoccupied with weight
Unpopular									Popular
Lovable									Hateful
Slow									Quick
Thick skinned									Sensitive
Powerful									Weak
Inactive									Active
Worthwhile									Worthless
Comfortable									Uncomfortable
Bad									Good

Courtesy of Gloria Leon, Ph.D.

REFERENCES

1. Head, H. *Asphasia and kindred disorders of speech.* London: Cambridge University Press, 1926.
2. Schilder, P. *Image and appearance of the human body.* New York: International Universities Press, 1950 (originally published in 1935).
3. Fisher, S., & Cleveland, S. *Body image and personality.* New York: Dover Publications, 1968.
4. Norris, C. The professional nurse and body image. In C. Carlson & B. Blackwell (Eds.), *Behavioral concepts and nursing intervention* (2nd ed.). Philadelphia: Lippincott, 1978, p. 5.
5. Allebeck, P., Hallberg, D., & Espmark, S. Body image—An apparatus for measuring disturbances in estimation of size and shape. *J Psychosomat Res,* 1976, *20*:583.
6. McCrea, C.W., Summerfield, A.B., & Rosen, B. Body image: A selective review of existing measurement techniques. *Br J Med Psychol,* 1982, *55*(3):225.
7. Bychowski, G. Disorders of body image in the clinical picture of psychoses. *J Nerv Ment Dis,* 1945, *97*:310.
8. Piazza, E., Rollins, N., & Lewis, F.S. Measuring severity and change in anorexia nervosa. *Adolescence,* 1983, *8*(10):293.

9. Garner, D.M., Garfinkel, P.E., Stancer, H.C., et al. Body image disturbances in anorexia nervosa and obesity. *Psychosom Med,* 1976, *38*(5):327.

10. Glucksman, M.L., & Hirsch, J. The response of obese patients to weight reduction. III. The perception of body size. *J Psychosom Med,* 1969, *31*(1):1.

11. Jupp, J.J., Collins, J.K., McCabe, M.P., et al. Change in unconscious concern with body image following treatment for obesity. *J Pers Assess,* 1983, *47*(5):483.

12. Leon, G.R. Personality, body image, and eating pattern changes in overweight persons after weight loss. *J Clin Psychol,* 1975, *31*:618.

13. Leon, G.R., Bemis, K.M., Melard, M. Aspects of body image perception in obese and normal-weight youngsters. *J Abnorm Child Psychol,* 1978, *6*(3):361.

14. Dropkin, M.J. Changes in body image associated with head and neck cancer. In L.B. Marino (Ed.), *Cancer nursing.* St. Louis: C.V. Mosby, 1981, p. 560.

15. Traub, A.C., & Orbach, J. Psychophysical studies of body image. *Arch Gen Psychiatry,* 1964, *11*:53.

16. Hall, G.S. Some aspects of the early sense of self. *Am J Psychiatry,* 1898, *9*:351.

17. Curran, F.J., & Levine, M.D. A body image study of prostitutes. *J Crim Psychopathol,* 1942, *4*:93.

18. Fisher, S. *Body experience in fantasy and behavior.* New York: Appleton-Century-Crofts, 1970.

19. Bruchon-Schweitzer, M. Body image and personality: A French adaptation of Fisher's Body Focus Questionnaire. *Percept Mot Skills,* 1978, *46*:1227.

20. Bruchon-Schweitzer, M. Dimensionality of body perception and personality. *Percept Mot Skills,* 1979, *48*:840.

21. Reihman, J., & Fisher, S. Dimensionality of body awareness. *Percept Mot Skills,* 1982, *55*:355.

22. Iagolnitzer, E.R., & Bruchon-Schweitzer, M. Dimensionality of body awareness revisited. *Percept Mot Skills,* 1984, *58*:31.

23. Reihman, J., & Seymour, F. The body focus questionnaire: Interpretive issues. *Percept Mot Skills,* 1984, *58*:356.

24. Ajzen, Y., & Iagolnitzer, E.R. Awareness in the substance of the body focus questionnaire. *Percept Mot Skills,* 1984, *59*:807.

25. Ajzen, Y., & Iagolnitzer, E.R. Dimensionality of revisited body awareness. *Percept Mot Skills,* 1985, *60*:455.

26. Gray, S. Social aspects of body image: Perception of normalcy of weight and affect of college undergraduates. *Percept Mot Skills,* 1977, *45*:1035.

27. Leon, G.R., Bemis, K.M., Melard, M. Changes in body image and other psychological factors after intestinal bypass surgery for massive obesity. *J Behav Med,* 1979, *2*(1):39.

28. Berschied, E., Waister, E., & Bohrnstedt, G. Body image: A *Psychology Today* questionnaire. *Psychology Today,* 1972, *6*(2):57.

29. Berschied, E., Waister, E., & Bohrnstedt, G. The happy American body: A survey report. *Psychology Today,* 1973, *7*(6):119.

30. Secord, P., & Jourard, S. The appraisal of body cathexis: Body cathexis and self. *J Consult Clin Psychol,* 1953, *17*:343.

31. Jourard, S.M., & Secord, P.F. Body-cathexis and the ideal female figure. *J Abnorm Soc Psychol,* 1955, *50*:243.

32. Mayer, J.D., & Eisenberg, M.G. Body concept: A conceptualization and review of paper-and-pencil measures. *Rehabil Psychol,* 1982, *27*(2):97.

33. Hammond, S.M., & O'Rourke, M.M. A psychometric investigation into the Body Cathexis Scale. *Pers Indiv Diff,* 1984, *5*(5):603.

34. Fawcett, J., & Frye, S. An exploratory study of body image dimensionality. *Nurs Res,* 1980, *29*(5):324.

35. Franzoi, S.L., & Shields, S.A. The Body Esteem Scale: Multidimensional structure and sex differences in a college population. *J Pers Assess,* 1984, *48*(2):173.

36. Rosenberg, M. *Society and the adolescent self-image.* Princeton, NJ: Princeton University Press, 1965.

37. Secord, P. Objectification of word-association procedures by the use of homonyms: A measure of body cathexis. *J Pers,* 1953, *21*:479.

38. Jupp, J.J., & Collins, J.K. Instruments for the measurement of unconscious and conscious aspects of body image. *Aust J Clin Exp Hypnosis*, 1983, *11*(2):89.
39. Leon, G.R., Lucas, A.R., Colligan, R.C., et al. Sexual, body image, and personality attitudes in anorexia nervosa. *J Abnorm Child Psychol*, 1985, *13*(2):245.
40. Osgood, C.E., Suci, G.E., & Tannenbaum, P. *The measurement of meaning.* Urbana, IL: University of Illinois Press, 1957.
41. Manchover, K. *Personality projection in the drawing of the human figure.* Springfield, IL: Chas. C Thomas, 1949.
42. Fisher, S., & Fisher, R. Style of sexual adjustment in disturbed women and its expression in figure drawings. *J Psychol*, 1952, *34:*169.
43. Berman, S., & Laffial, J. Body type and figure drawing. *J Clin Psychol*, 1953, *9:*368.
44. Silverstein, A.B., & Robinson, H.A. The representation of orthopedic disability in children's figure drawings. *J Counsel Psychol*, 1956, *20:*333.
45. Woods, W.A., & Cook, W.E. Proficiency of drawing and placement of hands in drawings of the human figure. *J Consult Psychol*, 1954, *18:*119.
46. Askevold, F. Measuring body image: Preliminary report on a new method. *Psychother Psychosom*, 1975, *25:*71.
47. Datson, P.G., & McConnell, O.L. Stability of Rorschach penetration and barrier scores over time. *J Consult Psychol*, 1962, *26:*104.
48. Hartley, R.B. The barrier variable as measured by homonyms. *J Clin Psychol*, 1967, *23:*196.
49. Dillon, D.J. Measurement of perceived body size. *Percept Mot Skills*, 1962, *14:*191.
50. Dillon, D.J. Estimation of bodily dimensions. *Percept Mot Skills*, 1962, *14:*219.
51. Slade, P.D., & Russel, G.F. Awareness of body dimension in anorexia nervosa: Cross-sectional and longitudinal studies. *Psychol Med*, 1973, *3:*188.
52. Schlachter, L. *The relation between anxiety, perceived body and personal space and actual body space among young female adults.* Unpublished doctoral dissertation, New York University, 1971.
53. Fawcett, J., & Chodil, J.J. The topographic device: Development and research. In E. Bauwens (Ed.), *Research for clinical nursing: Its strategies and findings* (Monograph Series 1979: 3). Indianapolis, IN: Sigma Theta Tau, 1980.
54. Cornelison, F.S., & Arsenian, J. A study of the response of psychotic patients to photographic self-image experience. *Psychiatr Q*, 1960, *34:*2.
55. Cornelison, F.S. Samples of psychopathology from studies of self-image experience. *Dis Nerv System* (Monograph Suppl 4), 1963, *24*(4):133.
56. Kagen, N., Kranhwehl, D., & Miller, R. Stimulated recall in therapy using videotape. A case study. *J Consul Psychol*, 1963, *10:*237.
57. Gertsma, R.H., & Reivich, R.S. Repetitive self-observation by videotape playback. *J Nerv Ment Dis*, 1965, *141*(1):29.
58. Griffiths, R.D., & Hinkson, J. The effect of videotape feedback on the self-assessments of psychiatric patients. *Br J Psychiatry*, 1973, *123:*223.
59. Griffiths, R.D., & Gillingham, P. The influence of videotape feedback on the self-assessments of psychiatric patients. *Br J Psychiatry*, 1978, *133:*156.
60. Billie, D.A. The role of body image in patient compliance and education. *Heart Lung*, 1977, *6*(1):143.
61. Padilla, G.V., & Grant M.M. Quality of life as a cancer nursing outcome variable. *Adv Nurs Sci*, 1985, *8*(1):45.
62. Champion, V.L., Austin, J.K., & Tzeng, O. Assessment of relationship between self-concept and body image using multivariate techniques. *Issues Ment Health Nurs*, 1982, *4:*299.
63. Beardslee, C., & Neff, J.A. Body-related concerns of children with cancer as compared with the concerns of other children. *Matern Child Nurs J*, 1982, *11:*121.

CHAPTER 13

Measuring Sexuality: Physiologic, Psychologic, and Relationship Dimensions

Suzanne Hearne Kaempfer, R.N., M.N. and
Susan Gross Fisher, R.N., M.S.

Human sexuality as a focus of scholarly interest has been reflected in an extensive body of literature since the first half of the twentieth century.[1–4] Psychometric instrumentation in the realm of human sexuality is relatively recent, however, with formal, serious attempts to measure sexual behavior, function, and adjustment awaiting the pioneering efforts of Masters and Johnson in the 1960s.[5–7] Since then, numerous authors have addressed a multitude of clinical and research perspectives of human sexuality.[8–25] Interest in this topic has proliferated during the past two decades to the extent that even the general notion of what defines an individual's sexual identity is undergoing radical change. Simplistically, human sexuality may be considered to reflect the degree of maleness or femaleness in a person's personality and physique. In order to operationalize the construct of sexuality for scientific investigation, however, a more refined conceptualization is needed.

Sexuality and resultant sexual behavior are a composite of physiologic, intrapsychic, and interpersonal phenomena. The physiologic dimension represents the function of the organs involved in the biology of the sexual response. The intrapsychic or psychologic dimension represents the private experience of sexual functioning, including knowledge and attitudes about sexuality, level of sexual satisfaction, sexual fantasies, gender role definition, body image, sexual experience, and basically how an individual defines himself or herself as a sexual being. The interpersonal dimension represents the nature and degree of social, interactive sexual behavior. Research on human sexuality, in order to be of clinical and scientific merit, requires the development and utilization of measurement instruments that integrate all three dimensions of sexuality.[26]

RESEARCH ON HUMAN SEXUALITY

In contrast to the energy that has been devoted to the developmental, social, and epidemiologic perspectives of sexologic research, the physiologic or somatic perspective of impairment of sexual organic function has been relatively neglected.[27–31] Research on the physiology of sexual function in men is limited, and that on the female sexual response is even more so. However, work to date suggests three avenues of inquiry: psychophysiologic, neurovascular, and gonadal. Neurovascular research pertains to mechanisms underlying autonomic innervation (glandular and smooth muscle function), regulation by central nervous system structures (e.g., the limbic system) and neurotransmitters (e.g., peptides and monoamines), and hemodynamics.

The grossly observable outcomes of neurovascular mechanisms are the subject of psychophysiologic research. Traditionally, this has entailed measurements of autonomically mediated effects on such parameters as heart rate, blood pressure, respiration, skin conduction, and pupillary response. Such indices are generally not considered to be sufficiently sensitive or discriminating. Instead, genital measures seem more reliably to distinguish sexual arousal from other emotional states. For example, in males, erectile function, including determination of penile tumescence, has been demonstrated to correlate with self-reports of sexual arousal. Pelvic vascular competency in male sexual arousal has also been investigated. In females, psychophysiologic research on sexual response has included measurement of vaginal lubrication and acidity, labia minora temperature, clitoral engorgement, and genital vasoconstriction.[27] Unlike similar studies in men, photoplethysmography of female genital vasoconstriction during sexual arousal has failed to demonstrate statistically significant correlation with self-reports of sexual arousal.

Sexuality as reflected by gonadal function has been approached through endocrine studies (e.g., circulating levels of gonadal steroids, gonadotropins, prolactin, thyroid-stimulating hormone, and thyroid hormones), fertility evaluation (e.g., menstrual history, contraceptive use, gonadal biopsy, semen evaluation), physical assessment of the genitalia and secondary sexual characteristics, and clinical manipulation of the endocrine milieu (e.g., endocrine ablation or replacement therapies).[28–31]

Psychologic research in sexuality involves psychometric documentation of affect, libido, knowledge and attitudes toward sexual function, and sexual experience. Psychosexual research not only has drawn on standard and well-established psychologic testing methods but also has begun to generate valid and reliable instruments designed specifically to measure the personal or intrapsychic dimensions of sexuality.[32]

Research on the interpersonal aspects of sexuality addresses the sexual adjustment of couples. Measurement of sexuality as it relates to dyads is less well developed than either physiologic or psychologic methodologies. Few reliable and valid instruments for the measurement of sexuality as it pertains to couples exist, whereas nonpsychometric surveys of interpersonal components of sexuality abound. In general, these have consisted of tools to be used for assessment, counseling, and discussion involving premarital, marital, and family interventions in nonresearch settings. Such tools are not and were not intended to be used for scientific investigation.[33] This lack of sophistication highlights the fact that until the organic and intrapersonal nature of human sexuality is more clearly delineated, the constructs that comprise those that are distinctively interpersonal will remain elusive both conceptually and empirically.[32]

Any illness involving distress, fatigue, pain, fear, anxiety, or depression may affect sexual function. Pathology that impairs anatomic structures alters sexual performance. Sexual drive, however, may still persist in the presence of altered sexual performance, regardless of etiology.[31]

In sexual research, it is critical to distinguish between research populations of people complaining of sexual problems and those whose sexuality is being examined in a broader context, such as physical illness.[32] Furthermore, since most psychometric instruments have been developed and used outside the context of the individual suffering from significant medical disorders, their application in these settings require concurrent reliability and validity determinations.[26]

Measures of sexuality are useful both to evaluate change resulting from therapy or dyadic experience and to conduct research on the relationship between sexual function and other variables.[34] Several reviews of research measures of human sexuality exist and provide a point of departure in organizing one's thinking on this topic.[33-40]

Schiavi et al. provide an early overview of a large number of psychometric instruments designed to measure one or more aspects of sexual activity and marital interaction with heterosexual individuals and dyads.[38] Their review provides names, authors, and descriptions of instruments, sources (some of which are outdated) of obtaining further information on instruments, and where possible, sample items and reliability and validity data.

Williams and Miller describe the criteria for evaluating the effectiveness of curricula on sexuality and summarize nine questionnaires that have been used in assessing the efficacy of educational programs on human sexuality.[39]

Sex and aging, sexual dysfunction, heterosexual relationships, rape, neurobiologic components of the sexual response, homosexuality, and psychosexual differentiation are the subject of a published collection of papers on research issues in the study of human sexuality.[40]

Conte provides a critical review of some of the self-report psychometric measures of both heterosexual and homosexual functioning, which she classifies as being either Guttman scales or inventories.[34] As conceived by Conte, Guttman-type cumulative scales assume unidimensionality of items reflecting sexual behavior, usually have few (10–20) items, and measure a narrow range of sexual function. In addition, these scales have been used in predominantly young, college-educated populations. Inventories, on the other hand, consist of questionnaires that assess a broad range of sexual behaviors and assume multidimensionality of items reflecting sexual behavior.[34]

One of the newest compilations of instrumentation for human sexuality is a publication in preparation, *Sexuality Related Measure: A Compendium*, edited by Davis and Yarber. (Charles B. White, Ph.D., Gerontology Studies Program, Trinity University, San Antonio, TX, 78284; Personal communication.)

Fundamental to psychosexual assessment, irrespective of setting, is the determination of psychologic constructs or domains that are inherent in sexual behavior, followed by the development of ways to measure them.[41] Construct validation of behaviors, characteristics, or aptitudes important to sexual functioning is in progress and is reflected in the broad range of instruments available for scrutiny. This chapter is limited to a survey of currently available methods of studying empirically the two psychosexual dimensions of human sexuality: the psychologic and the interpersonal.

Instruments are organized according to their originally intended use. An attempt has been made to contact the authors of the psychometric instruments mentioned in the literature to obtain the most current data on their reliability and validity. The results of this survey demonstrated that many instruments are either difficult to access or are no longer available or appropriate for use. Therefore, selected instruments that are of potential practical use to investigators are described in detail, with remaining tools being briefly summarized in tabular form. In view of these limitations, this chapter reflects a relatively thorough treatment of research instrumentation of human sexuality. However, in a discipline that is developing as rapidly as the study of human sexuality, new instruments or adaptations of available instruments to different subject populations are continually in progress.

COMPREHENSIVE MEASURES OF SEXUALITY

▪ SEXUAL PERFORMANCE EVALUATION QUESTIONNAIRE OF THE MARRIAGE COUNCIL OF PHILADELPHIA

Interviews are a commonly used method of obtaining information related to sexual issues. A particularly comprehensive interview guideline is that based on the Sexual Performance Evaluation Questionnaire of the Marriage Council of Philadelphia. Useful in obtaining a sexual history, the lines of inquiry addressed are under the major topic headings: childhood sexuality, onset of adolescence, orgastic experiences, feelings about self as masculine/feminine, sexual fantasies and dreams, dating, engagement, marriage, extramarital sex, sex after widowhood, separation, or divorce, sexual deviations, certain effects of sex activities, and use of erotic material. A related sexual performance evaluation outline covers investigation of specific characteristics of an individual's coital activities.[42]

Participation in an interview may be a therapeutic experience for an individual. This method of data collection, however, is very time consuming, and the resultant findings are often difficult to quantify. Research conclusions obtained in this way, therefore, become extremely tenuous.

▪ DEROGATIS SEXUAL FUNCTION INVENTORY (DSFI)

The most comprehensive and thoroughly evaluated psychometric instrument for the measurement of sexual function is the Derogatis Sexual Function Inventory (DSFI).[41,43] On the assumption that sexuality is comprised of multiple behavioral domains, ten constructs are operationalized in the subscales of the 245-item DSFI as follows:

- Information (sexual knowledge)
- Experience (sexual behavior)
- Drives (biologically determined and subject to neuroendocrine control)
- Sexual attitudes (liberal versus conservative)
- Psychologic symptoms (such as obsessive-compulsiveness or somatization)
- Affect (such as depression, anxiety, or guilt)
- Gender role definition or identity (relative masculinity or femininity is conceived along a continuum)
- Sexual fantasy (rehearsal and vicarious fulfillment/expression of sexual drives)
- Body image (self-evaluation of physical attractiveness as well as the reflected perceptions of others)
- Satisfaction (sexual frequency and novelty; achievement of orgasm; communication between partners)

These constructs are designed to permit valid clinical prediction of current sexual functional status and also provide conceptual clarity in deliberations on the nature and breadth of human sexuality as a component of personality and biologic function.

The DSFI has been well tested in a broad variety of populations, including male and female heterosexuals, homosexuals, transsexuals, and sexually dysfunctional individuals. Test–retest reliabilities for the ten subscales range from 0.42 to 0.96. Internal consistency reliability coefficients range from 0.56 to 0.97. Predictive validity of the DSFI has been demonstrated in populations of individuals suffering from sexual dysfunctions and their partners and in populations consisting of male and female transsexuals. Normed scores from 200 normal and 200 sexually dysfunctional individuals also are available. Factor analysis based on a group of 380 patient and nonpatient subjects revealed seven empirical dimensions that underlie the DSFI: body image, psychologic distress, heterosexual drive, autoeroticism, gender role, sexual satisfaction, and sexual precociousness.

The other psychometric instruments described in this chapter lack the comprehensiveness of the DSFI, being instead more focused on the dimension(s) of human sexuality they endeavor to quantify. Except where specified by a specific technique (such as factor analysis), dimensions measured reflect the conceptual framework of the researcher.

PSYCHOLOGIC DIMENSION OF SEXUALITY

Sexual Experience, Knowledge, or Attitudes

A number of instruments that assess different components of sexual experience, knowledge, or attitudes have reported reliability and validity information and are accessible to researchers.[44-59] These tools were designed for use in clinical and research settings for normal and dysfunctional individuals. Additional measures of this component of the psychologic dimension of sexuality are summarized in Table 13–1.

▪ NEGATIVE ATTITUDES TOWARD MASTURBATION SCALE

The Negative Attitudes Toward Masturbation Scale is a 30-item self-report measure that addresses three factors: (1) false beliefs about the harmful nature of masturbation, (2) positive attitude toward masturbation, and (3) personally experienced negative affects associated with masturbation.[44-46] Statements are rated on a 5-point scale (from 1, "strongly agree," to 5, "strongly disagree"). Two sample items are:

Masturbation is a normal sexual outlet.

After I masturbate, I am disgusted with myself for losing control of my body.

The Negative Attitudes Toward Masturbation Scale has been tested among psychiatric populations, normal adults, and patients with sexual dysfunctions. The split-half reliability coefficient corrected by the Spearman-Brown prophecy formula was reported to be 0.75 Point biserial correlations ranged from 0.11 to 0.57 with a median of 0.40. Evidence for instrument validity has been provided by its correlation with measures of monthly masturbation frequency for males and females, self-report of negative attitudes toward masturbation and sexual experience, and a measure of sex-related guilt.[47,48]

▪ MOSHER FORCED-CHOICE GUILT INVENTORIES (FCGI)

As originally developed, the Mosher Forced-Choice Guilt Inventories (FCGI) measured three separate aspects of guilt: hostility guilt, sex guilt, and morality (guilty) conscience using a sentence completion forced choice format.[47,48] Criticism of its format by respondents as well as multitrait method analyses has resulted in a newer version of the FCGI (which will appear in the forthcoming book, *Sexuality Related Measures: A Compendium*, edited by W.L. Yarber and C.M. Davis). The Revised Mosher Guilt Inventory, which uses a limited comparison format, consists of 114 items arranged in pairs of responses to the same sentence completion

TABLE 13–1. ADDITIONAL MEASURES OF SEXUAL ATTITUDES, EXPERIENCE, AND KNOWLEDGE OR DYSFUNCTION IN ADULTS[33,38]

Instrument Name/Author	No. of Items	Response Format	Types of Data Elicited
Sexual Pleasure Inventory/Annon	130	Rating scale	Pleasure-producing objects, behavior and people associated with sexually related activities and experiences
Sexual Fear Inventory/Annon	130	Rating scale	Fear-producing aspects of sexual experiences
Heterosexual Behavior Inventories/Robinson; Annon	77	Multiple choice	Range and frequency of heterosexual behavior, both solitary and partner-directed
Heterosexual Attitude Inventories/Robinson; Annon	77	Rating scale	Attitudes toward heterosexual activities
Sexual Response Profile/Pion	80	Rating scale; forced choice	Sexual knowledge, attitudes, and past/present practices
Sex Knowledge Inventories (SKI)/McHugh	Two versions: 80/98	Multiple choice	Sexual attitudes and knowledge
Sex Attitude Scale/Rotter	100	Likert scale	Attitudes on a variety of sexual issues
Sex Questionnaire for College Students/Shipley	156	True/False; Multiple choice; Likert scales	Knowledge and attitudes toward contraception, anatomy and physiology, sex role behaviors, child rearing and marriage
Sexual Developmental Scale for Females/ElSenoussi	177		Relation, degree, and causation of sexual frigidity among women assessed along seven factors: lack of feminine identity, free-floating anxiety, passive sex aversion, unpleasant sexual encounter, sexual insufficiency, flight into sex, and early negative conditioning
Sexuality Experience Scales (SES)/Frenken	83	Multiple formats	Four aspects of sexual behavior and experience: sex morals, psychosexual stimulation, sexual motivation, attraction to marriage
Sexual Concerns Checklist (SCC)/Kirkendall	——	Inventory	Sexual concerns, including problems of sexual function
Maferr Inventory of Masculine and Feminine Values/Steinman; Fox	34	Likert scale	Male and female sex role perceptions
Abortion Scale; Vasectomy Scale; Pill Scale; Coitometer; Gravidometer; Menometer; Sexometer/Bardis	Series of scales: 25/50	True/false; rating scales; Open-ended	Knowledge and attitudes toward abortion, vasectomy, oral contraceptives, and anatomic/physiologic aspects of coitus, pregnancy, menstruation, and human sexual function/reproduction

stem. A 7-point Likert scale [0, "Not at all true of (for) me," to 6, "Extremely true of (for) me"] is used for responses for statements, such as the following:

When I have sexual desires . . .

I enjoy it like all healthy human beings.
I fight them, for I must have complete control of my body.

Reliabilities of the Revised Mosher Guilt Inventory are not yet available. Split-half or alpha coefficients of the original FCGI averaged around 0.90. Item analysis showed item subscale total correlations ranging from 0.32 to 0.62, with a median of 0.46.

▪ SEXUAL INTEREST QUESTIONNAIRE (SIQ)

The Sexual Interest Questionnaire (SIQ) consists of 140 self-report items in semantic differential format.[49] It was designed to measure the intensity of sexual interest a male or female experiences in a given heterosexual situation. Four bipolar adjectival scales (sexy–sexless, exciting–dull, seductive–repulsive, erotic–frigid), with five scale positions each, are used to measure different aspects of sexual behavior: sexual intercourse, kissing/being kissed, and touching/being touched sexually. Examples of items and scale positions are:

Kissing my sexual partner is to me:

Quite seductive . . .
Very seductive . . .

Touching my partner sexually is to me:

Quite exciting . . .
Very exciting . . .

Test–retest reliability for the SIQ over a 3 to 5 month interval has been found to range from 0.69 to 0.92. The SIQ has discriminated between normal and sexually dysfunctional people and has been shown to be sensitive enough to document patterns of change in subjects over time.

▪ HETEROSEXUAL BEHAVIOR ASSESSMENT (HBA) SCALE

The Heterosexual Behavior Assessment (HBA) Scale is a two-version (male/female) Guttman-type scale that assesses heterosexual behaviors.[50,51] Twenty-one classes of heterosexual behavior are arranged in hierarchical manner; the total score is determined by the number of items endorsed by the subject. Behaviors sampled include:

Multual oral-genital manipulation

Sexual intercourse, ventral-dorsal

The coefficient of homogeneity of the HBA has been reported to be 0.99 with a KR reliability coefficient of 0.95. Cross-validations with different samples have been performed, and a 10-item short form is available that highly correlates (0.98) with the total scale.

SEXUAL AROUSABILITY INVENTORY (SAI)

The Sexual Arousability Inventory (female form) (SAI) is a self-report inventory of sexual arousability in women.[52,53] Descriptions of 28 sexual activities and situations are rated on a 7-point Likert scale according to degree of sexual arousal usually experienced (−1, "adversely affects arousal," "unthinkable," "repulsive," "distracting," to 5, "always causes sexual arousal," "extremely arousing"). An example of an item from the SAI is:

How you feel or think you would feel if you were actually involved in this experience:
When you hear sounds of pleasure during sex
When a loved one undresses you

The SAI has been found to discriminate between normal and sexually dysfunctional individuals when administered to women from middle and upper socioeconomic classes, including a normative sample of 370 women aged 25 or older. Criterion validity with the Bentler Heterosexual Behavior Assessment[50,51] as well as concurrent validity with measures of sexual satisfaction, frequency of intercourse, and awareness of physiologic changes of sexual arousal have been reported. Cross-validation with two different samples demonstrated alpha coefficients of 0.91 and 0.92. The test–retest reliability coefficient over an 8-week interval was 0.69.

SEX INVENTORY (SI)

The Sex Inventory (SI), developed by Thorne, is a 200-item, true/false format self-report measure of sexual attitudes and behavior in adult men.[54–56] Nine subscales have been designated: sex drive and interest, sexual maladjustment and frustration, neurotic conflict associated with sex, sexual fixation and cathexes, repression of sexuality, loss of sex controls, homosexuality, sex role confidence, and promiscuity. Sample items include:

I enjoy petting.

Seeing a person nude doesn't interest me.

It wouldn't bother me if the person I married was not a virgin.

Test–retest reliabilities for the SI have been reported to range from 0.40 to 0.50. Factorial characteristics demonstrate discrimination between normal and clinical groups and also among different clinical groups.

SEX ATTITUDE QUESTIONNAIRE

The Sex Attitude Questionnaire is a self-report measure of attitudes toward sexual behaviors and situations.[57] Using a semantic differential, 12 concepts are each evaluated on seven bipolar dimensions. An example of an item is:

An unwed mother:
good_____bad
valuable_____worthless
kind_____cruel

active_____passive

fast_____slow

understandable_____mysterious

familiar_____strange

Use of the Sex Attitude Questionnaire with a variety of populations has yielded test–retest reliability by concept that has ranged from 0.35 to 0.67 and on bipolar dimensions that has ranged from 0.52 to 0.78. Instrument validity has been demonstrated through before and after changes with participants in sex education programs.

• SEX EXPERIENCE SCALES

The Sex Experience Scales for males and females are a 12-item self-report inventory of heterosexual behaviors, for example[58]:

Feeling covered breast

Feeling nude breast

A forced choice (yes/no) Guttman scale format is utilized, and both a male and a female version are available. A coefficient of reproducibility of 0.97 has been reported.

EVALUATION OF SEXUALITY CURRICULA

Several instruments have been developed specifically to determine the effectiveness of sexual education programs as evidenced by changes in the sexual knowledge and attitudes of participants.[59–64] In these settings, success is judged by increase in sexual knowledge and/or attitudes reflecting greater permissiveness. Four instruments are described in detail. Other available measures for evaluating sexuality curricula are summarized in Table 13–2.

• SEX KNOWLEDGE AND ATTITUDE TEST (SKAT)

The Sex Knowledge and Attitude Test (SKAT), developed by Lief and Reed, is one of the most frequently used sex-related research instruments.[59] It is a 149-item self-administered measure of sexual knowledge, sexual attitudes, and level of experience in sexual activity (including biographical information). The Attitude section of the SKAT contains four subscales: sexual myths, heterosexual relations, abortion, and masturbation/autoeroticism, measured using 35 Likert format items (five alternatives ranging from "strongly agree" to "strongly disagree"). The Knowledge section of the SKAT is a single subscale that addresses psychologic, biologic, social, and psychobiologic aspects of human sexuality through the use of 71 true/false items. The sexual experience and biographical information sections are not scored. Examples of items from each section are as follows:

The spread of sex education is causing a rise in premarital intercourse. (Attitude)

Menopause in a woman is accompanied by a sharp and lasting reduction in sexual drive and interest. (Knowledge)

TABLE 13–2. ADDITIONAL INSTRUMENTS THAT HAVE BEEN USED TO EVALUATE THE SUCCESS OF SEX EDUCATION CURRICULA[39]

Instrument Name/Author	No. of Items	Response Format	Types of Data Elicited
Minnesota Sexual Attitudes Scales (MSAS)/Held et al.	35	Rating scale	Attitudes toward and feelings about designated groups of people (e.g., married adults) engaging in certain categories of sexual activities
Sexual Attitude and Behavior Survey (SABS)/Kilpatrick; Smith	40	Rating scale	Sexual attitudes and experience. Attitudinal measures elicit reported permissibility/liberality of male, female and personal behavior and fantasy
Test for Assessing Sexual Knowledge and Attitudes (TASKA)/Hawkins	122	True/false; completion; rating scale; forced choice	Biographical information, sexual attitudes, experience, changes in personal behavior, and suggestions for sexuality course development
National Sex Forum Questionnaire/ McIlvenna	26	Rating scale	Biographical information; sexual attitudes and experience
Harvard Sex Questionnaire/ Nadelson; Shaw	61	True/false; forced choice	Biographical information; sexual attitudes, experience and knowledge
Obstetrics-Gynecology Sexuality Course Evaluation Questionnaire/Montgomery; Singer	6	Likert scale	Emotional discomfort experienced in response to hypothetical clinical situations
Physicians Workshop Questionnaire/Pion	40	Essays; fill in blanks; rating scales	Sexual attitudes and knowledge; change in professional behavior; suggestions for sexuality course development

Since its publication, the SKAT has been used primarily to study a wide range of students in educational evaluation settings (including medical students, nurses, psychologists, social workers, and clergy). Fisher and Levin, for example, used the SKAT to evaluate the sexual knowledge and attitudes of nurses caring for cancer patients.[60]

Standardized scores based on results of 850 medical students from 16 U.S. medical schools tested in 1971 are available for comparison purposes. The SKAT was designed as a teaching aid and research tool for human sexuality education of health professionals. Evaluation of the sexual knowledge and attitudes of caregivers may allow the prediction of their subsequent responses to patient concerns related to sexuality.

▪ HUMAN SEXUAL KNOWLEDGE AND ATTITUDE INVENTORY (HSKAI)

The Human Sexual Knowledge and Attitude Inventory (HSKAI) was designed specifically for use with nurses.[61] It consists of 163 items (multiple choice, true/false, forced choice, and rating scales) that measure biographical information and sexual attitudes and experience. In addition, sexual knowledge of the following topics is assessed: sexual anatomy and physiology, human sexual response and inadequacy, conception, contraception, abortion, venereal disease, labor and delivery, sexual standards, sterility, sexual variations, and cultural influences. An example of an item is:

> (true or false) Orgasm during intercourse greatly increases a woman's ability to become pregnant.

Test–retest reliability for the HSKAI has been reported to be 0.84, and construct validity for its sexual knowledge content was established by jury rating.

Recently Taylor measured before and after sexual attitudes among 115 students in a human sexuality course.[62] Her 18-item instrument consists of ratings scales, open-ended questions, and personal interviews.

• SEX QUESTIONNAIRE

The Sex Questionnaire is a multidimensional self-report measure of sexual attitudes and behaviors comprised of eight subscales: Heterosexual Experience, Attitudes Toward Heterosexual Behavior, Parental Attitudes, Orgasmic Experience, Homosexual Experience, Masturbatory Experience, Number of Heterosexual Partners, and Desire to View Erotic Movies.[63] Responses are rated on a 5-point scale. A sample of 555 male and female college students was used to determine test–retest reliabilities for each subscale. For example, the 14-item Heterosexual subscale demonstrated values ranging from 0.80 to 0.95, and those for the 4-item Homosexual subscale ranged from 0.49 to 0.84. Coefficients of reproducibility and coefficients of scalability have been reported for four of the subscales.

SEXUAL ORIENTATION AND ROLES

Sexual orientation and sexual roles are viewed here from three perspectives: gender role definition, gender identity, and sexual deviancy. Gender role definitions and attitudes are the focus of several instruments.[65–68]

• ATTITUDE TOWARD WOMEN SCALE (AWS)

The Attitude Toward Women Scale (AWS) is a 55-item self-report measure of attitudes pertaining to female roles, including vocational, educational, social, and intellectual dimensions of freedom, interpersonal relationships, and sexual behaviors.[65] Subjects indicate the degree of agreement/disagreement with declarative statements, such as the following, on a 4-point scale:

> It is all right for wives to have an occasional, casual, extramarital affair.

> Husbands and wives should be equal partners in planning the family budget.

The AWS has been administered to both males and females, and normative data from samples of psychology students and their parents are available.

• BEM SEX ROLE INVENTORY (BSRI)

The Bem Sex Role Inventory (BSRI) is a 60-item self-report measure of gender role definition through categorizing personality characteristics on independent dimensions of masculinity and femininity.[66] Responses are rated on a 7-point Likert scales and produce masculinity, femininity, and androgeny subscale scores. A social desirability scale is also included. Two items on the BSR are:

Defend my own beliefs

Sensitive to needs of others*

Test–retest reliability of the BSRI has been reported to range from 0.89 to 0.93 over a 4-week interval. Coefficient alpha for three of the BSRI scales in two separate samples ranged from 0.70 to 0.86. The BSRI has demonstrated concurrent validity with other measures of masculinity and femininity, and normative data are available.

• SEX ROLE SURVEY (SRS)

The Sex Role Survey (SRS) is a 53-item self-report measure of attitudes toward sex roles, including four dimensions: power in the home, sex role-appropriate behavior, equality in business and the professions, and equal involvement in social and domestic work.[67] Declarative statements are rated on a 9-point scale from "I agree very much" through "I disagree very much." A sample item is:

As head of the household, the father should have final authority over children.

The SRS has been used in populations of various ages and educational and social class backgrounds. Alpha coefficients for the four factors and total score have been reported to range from 0.85 to 0.96. In addition, cross-validation studies have been performed, and normative data are available. Construct validity of the SRS has been evaluated using measures of values and characteristics, such as cognitive rigidity, support for premarital sex, authoritarianism, and values orientation.

• ATTITUDES TOWARD HOMOSEXUALITY SCALE (ATHS)

Attitudes toward homosexuality along three dimensions (general, lesbian, and male) are addressed by the Attitudes Toward Homosexuality Scale (ATHS).[68] This 28-item self-report measure contains such statements as:

Homosexuals should not be permitted to raise children.

Respondents rate along a 9-point scale (from "strongly agree" to "strongly disagree"). The ATHS has been tested using college students and faculty. Split-half reliability has been reported to be 0.93, with alpha coefficients ranging from 0.93 to 0.94.

---

*Reproduced by special permission of the Publisher, Consulting Psychologists Press, Inc., Palo Alto, CA, from *Bem Sex Role Inventory* by Sandra L. Bem, 1981 Manual.

• SEXUAL ORIENTATION METHOD

Gender identity, in terms of both a continuum of masculine/feminine personality qualities and relative homo-eroticism or hetero-eroticism, may be addressed psychometrically.[69,70] The Sexual Orientation Method, is a self-report test of the relative hetero-erotic and homo-erotic orientation of homosexual men.[69] In it, 120 paired questions, half concerning attitudes toward men and half concerning attitudes toward women, are rated using a 5-point scale of degree of sex attributes: attractive, interesting, hot, handsome, exciting, and pleasurable. Test–retest reliability for the Sexual Orientation Method was reported to range from 0.80 to 0.94 in samples of control subjects consisting of adult males. The authors have found the scores of homosexual patients to be significantly different from those of control subjects.

• FEMININE GENDER IDENTITY SCALE (FGI)

The Feminine Gender Identity Scale (FGI) is a 19-item, multiple choice measure of feminine qualities in homosexual males.[70] An example of an item from the FGI is:

Do you think your appearance is:

very masculine
masculine
a little feminine
quite feminine

The alpha reliability coefficient for the complete FGI has been found to be 0.93. Part-whole correlations of individual items with the full scale have ranged from 0.29 to 0.84. Work to date indicates that the FGI is able to discriminate between transsexual and heterosexual males with no overlap.

Extremes in sexual behavior, or sexual deviation, may be conceived as distortions of gender role definitions and identity. Interest in ascertaining the efficacy of clinical interventions with people exhibiting such behaviors has begun to generate tools to accomplish this.[71,72]

• SEMANTIC DIFFERENTIAL AS A MEASURE OF SEXUAL ATTITUDES

The Semantic Differential as a Measure of Sexual Attitudes is a self-report measure of attitudinal change during treatment for sexual deviation.[71] Twenty sexual or nonsexual concepts (such as "call girl") are rated on 13 bipolar semantic differential scales consisting of three dimensions: anxiety ("placid–jittery"), general evaluation ("bad–good"), and sex evaluation ("seductive–repulsive"). A short form is available; however, correlation with the longer version has not been reported.

The Semantic Differential, which has been used with patients exhibiting sexual deviations, has demonstrated test–retest reliability of 0.60 over a 24-hour interval, and component factor analysis has yielded factor scores that all exceed 0.70. The Semantic Differential has been validated clinically by observations of clinical improvement varying in relation to the attitudinal scores. Similarly, it has been used both for assessment of progress during treatment and for 2-year posttreatment follow-up of patients with sexual deviancy or dysfunction.

▪ CLARKE SEX HISTORY QUESTIONNAIRE (SHQ)

The Clarke Sex History Questionnaire (SHQ) was developed and tested over a 10-year period of clinical practice involving a wide variety of sexually anomalous people and sex offenders.[72] It is a 225-item self-administered questionnaire that elicits information on a broad range of normal and anomalous sexual behavior, including frequency, desire for, and aversion to the behavior. Behaviors addressed are extreme and relatively uncommon, as illustrated by a sample item:

> How often have you . . . exposed yourself in a more or less public place?

Discriminant and criterion-related validity of SHQ items has been reported for clinically discrete subject groups versus controls. Item factor analysis and discriminant and convergent validity data for the SHQ subscales are also available.

SEXUAL DYSFUNCTION

Sexual dysfunction is a broad concept that can encompass both physiologic and psychologic components. Approaches to the medical evaluation of infertility or sterility, as well as problems with sexual performance or response, have been described.[32] This discussion is limited to psychometric determination of the nature and extent of an individual's sexual health.

▪ MULTIAXIAL PROBLEM-ORIENTED SYSTEM FOR SEXUAL DYSFUNCTION

The Multiaxial Problem-Oriented System for Sexual Dysfunction is a comprehensive measure, using a history format, of specific behavioral sexual problems associated with the different phases of the sexual cycle.[73] It was designed to produce a normed computerized profile of sexual function. Examples of items that elicit information according to phase of the sexual cycle are:

> Desire: "Aversion to sex"
>
> Arousal: "Difficulty maintaining erections"
>
> Orgasm: "Inorgasmic"
>
> Coital pain: "Dyspareunia"
>
> Frequency dissatisfaction: "Desired frequency much higher than current activity level"

▪ SEX HISTORY FORM

The Sex History Form is an instrument derived from the Multiaxial Problem-Oriented System. A questionnaire consisting of 28 multiple-choice items has been developed to permit a more psychometric evaluation of sexual dysfunction, and norms are available for sexually well-functioning people. An example of one of the items is:

> If you try, is it possible for you to reach orgasm through having your genitals caressed by your mate?

1. Nearly always, over 90 percent of the time
2. Usually, about 75 percent of the time
3. Sometimes, about 50 percent of the time
4. Seldom, about 25 percent of the time
5. Never
6. Have never tried to

Both the Multiaxial Problem-Oriented System and the Sex History Form may be used to classify sexual dysfunctions in clinical situations and research.

• MALE IMPOTENCE TEST (MIT)

The Male Impotence Test (MIT), is a self-report questionnaire of male potency intended to discriminate among psychogenic impotency, organic impotency, and nonimpotency.[74] Several areas are assessed: reaction to female rejection, flight from male role, reaction to male inadequacy, and an organic dimension. Sleep laboratory measures of nocturnal penile tumescence in conjunction with administration of the MIT were performed with 32 males complaining of impotence. Questions about the validity of the MIT resulting from lack of correlation between these independent determinations of male impotence have yet to be resolved.

• SEXUAL ANXIETY SCALE (SAS)

The Sexual Anxiety Scale (SAS) is a 22-item self-report measure of cognitively experienced sexual and social anxieties, with separate versions for males and females.[75] Reported reliability of the SAS is 0.92, with a 0.62 validity coefficient with a measure of intensity of sexual dysfunction.

BODY PERCEPTION

Body perception or image is an integral component of an individual's sexuality and can make a significant contribution to sexual health or dysfunction. Because of the growing recognition of and interest in body image disturbance among people suffering from physical illness and disability, it is given separate consideration here.

• BODY CONTACT QUESTIONNAIRE (BCQ)

The Body Contact Questionnaire (BCQ) measures desire for body contact using 12 self-report items rated on a 5-point Likert scale (1, "never," to 5, "always").[76] A sample item is:

If you have trouble falling asleep, it is helpful to:

a. Sleep with your husband (wife)
b. Be held by your husband (wife)
c. Hold your husband (wife)
d. Hold a pillow or some other object
e. Drink alcohol

The BCQ was tested in samples of psychiatric patients in whom responses correlated with open-ended interview responses. Test–retest reliability was reported to be 0.94 for a 1-day to 2-week interval, with an internal consistency reliability coefficient of 0.82.

▪ BODY ATTITUDE SCALE (BAS)

The Body Attitude Scale (BAS) is a self-report semantic differential rating scale of attitude toward outward body form.[77–80] Thirty different body concepts or parts are rated on a 7-point (from "most negative" to "most positive") bipolar adjective scale, containing constructs that comprise three primary attitude dimensions (evaluative, such as "good–bad," potency, such as "weak–strong," and activity, such as "fast–slow"). Examples of body concepts that are evaluated are:

Color of my hair

Size of my arms

Size of my bust

The BAS was developed in populations of adults for whom generalizability coefficients for both sexes were reported to range from 0.93 to 0.98. Individual differences in body attitude scores were found to relate to gross variations in physique. Furthermore, the BAS distinguishes between normal and chronically ill subjects on evaluation of body appearance.

AGING AND DEVELOPMENTAL ADAPTATIONS

The elderly and the developmentally disabled are two special nonpatient populations that have been the focus of psychosexual inquiry.[81–83]

▪ AGING SEXUALITY KNOWLEDGE AND ATTITUDES SCALE (ASKAS)

The Aging Sexuality Knowledge and Attitudes Scale (ASKAS) measures sexual attitudes and knowledge in the context of age-related changes and sexuality for the elderly.[81] The 61 items can be either self-administered or administered in interview format. The Knowledge section consists of 35 true/false questions. The Attitude section uses a 7-point Likert scale response format in which extent of agreement or disagreement with the item statement is determined. Sample items from the ASKAS are:

Males over the age of 65 usually experience a reduction in intensity of orgasm relative to younger males. (Knowledge)

If family members object to a widowed relative engaging in sexual relations with another resident of a nursing home, it is the obligation of the management and staff to make certain that such sexual activity is prevented. (Attitude)

The ASKAS has been used extensively with staff and residents of nursing homes and with aged people in the community and their families. Reported split-half reliabilities for both sections of the ASKAS range from 0.83 to 0.91. Test–retest reliabilities range from 0.72 to 0.97. Alpha reliabilities range from 0.76 to 0.93. Factor analysis and change scores before and after a sexual education program among aged subjects, people who work with the aged, and family members of elderly persons have demonstrated validity of the ASKAS. Furthermore, in contrast to control groups, experimental groups showed significant changes in the direction of greater knowledge and more permissive attitudes.

▪ SOCIO-SEXUAL KNOWLEDGE AND ATTITUDES TEST (SSKAT)

The Socio-Sexual Knowledge and Attitudes Test (SSKAT) was originally developed to measure sexual knowledge and attitudes of developmentally disabled adults who are not verbally proficient or whose speech is unintelligible.[82,83] However, the SSKAT is also applicable for use with nonretarded persons provided they have visual and verbal comprehension. A 227-page *Stimulus Picture Book* presents realistic pictures requiring "yes/no" and "point to" responses to questions on 14 socio-sexual topic areas, including anatomy, terminology, menstruation, intimacy, intercourse, pregnancy and childbirth, birth control, masturbation, homosexuality, and venereal disease. Sample items from one section of the SSKAT are:

I. Anatomy terminology:
"What is this called?" point to vulva (naked female, front view)

"What is this for?" point to vulva (naked female, front view) . . . probe once and ask, *"Is there anything else this is for?"**

Although content and predictive validity for the SSKAT remain to be established, test–retest reliability for a 7- to 10-day interval in a sample of 100 retarded men and women for both knowledge and attitude subscales ranged from 0.76 to 0.91. In addition, KR reliability coefficients for SSKAT subscale items have ranged from 0.53 to 0.83.

INTERPERSONAL DIMENSIONS OF SEXUALITY

Measures of the interpersonal dimension of sexuality address marital/dyadic characteristics, including a range of parameters and indicators of adjustment and satisfaction. Instruments with reported reliability and validity are described.[3,84-99] Additional measures of this dimension of sexuality are summarized in Table 13–3.

▪ LOCKE-WALLACE MARRIAGE INVENTORY

One of the earliest self-report measures of marital adjustment and satisfaction is the Locke-Wallace Marriage Inventory.[3] This instrument consists of 15 items using several formats: multiple choice, a 6-point rating scale (from "always agree" to "always disagree"), selection of applicable items from a checklist, and a 7-point rating scale (from "very unhappy" to "perfectly happy"). Sample items include:

Have you ever wished you had not married?
- a. Frequently
- b. Occasionally
- c. Rarely

---

*Courtesy of Stoelting Co., 1350 S Kostner Ave., Chicago, IL 60623.

TABLE 13–3. ADDITIONAL MEASURES OF INTERPERSONAL DIMENSIONS OF HUMAN SEXUALITY IN ADULTS[33,36,38,98]

Instrument Name/Author	No. of Items	Response Format	Types of Data Elicited
Background Schedule/Marriage Council of Philadelphia	39	Demo-graphic; opinions	Religion, activities shared with partner, occupation, siblings, parental data, and interaction between self and parents at various phases of life
Marital Satisfaction Inventory/ Snyder	280	True/false	Dimensions of potential marital distress: affective and problem-solving communication, time together, finances, role orientation, sexual satisfaction, family history of problems, childrearing problems
Self-Disclosure Questionnaire/ Bodin	52	Rating scale	Degree to which subject has revealed self to partner about the topic of each item, and then the expected spouse response to the same item. Topics of disclosure include aspects of personality, childhood and family, body and health, and marital relationship
Index of Marital Satisfaction/ Hudson	25	Rating scale	Interpersonal aspects of a marital relationship
Index of Sexual Satisfaction/ Hudson	25	Rating scale	Sexual aspects of a marital relationship
Four Relationship Factor Questionnaire/Lawlis	44	Rating scale	Perceptions of a specific relationship with another individual along four dimensions, such as sexual/affectional
California Marriage Readiness Evaluation/Manson	115	True/false	Eight areas of potential marital maladjustment and conflict: character structure, emotional maturity, marriage readiness, family experiences, planning ability, dealing with money, compatibility and marriage motivation
Caring Relationship Inventory/ Shostrom	83	True/false	Elements of caring and love in a relationship, including affection, eros, friendship, empathy, self-love, being love, and deficiency love
Couple's Pre-Counseling Inventory/ Stewart	133	Inventory	Areas of marital life, including behaviors pleasing to each partner, happiness with relationship, level of communication, ways of handling conflict, moods, sexual

TABLE 13–3. *(Continued)*

Instrument Name/Author	No. of Items	Response Format	Types of Data Elicited
			satisfaction, commitment to relationship, willingness to change, effectiveness in daily life
Courtship Analysis (CA) and Dating Problems Checklist (DPCL)/ McHugh	150	Inventory	Dynamics of partners in courtship, specifically, character traits and behaviors of partners; perceived problem areas in the relationship
Engagement Schedule/Marriage Council of Philadelphia	41	Demo-graphic; opinions	Facts about own engagement; feelings about parents, in-laws, confiding, affection, sharing interests and activities, need for information on sex, family planning
Dating Scale/Bardis	25	Likert scale	Attitudes toward various aspects of dating
Erotometer (for measuring heterosexual love)/Bardis	50	Likert scale	Intensity of love for a member of the opposite sex as reflected by desires, attitudes, feelings, wishes
Love Attitudes Inventory (LAI)/Knox	30	Inventory; long answer	Aspects of romantic and realistic love
Marital Check-up Kit/Bienvenu	6	Exercises adminis-tered by a counselor	Personality traits, communication strengths and weaknesses, understanding of feelings and attitudes, such as related to spouse and marriage; self-evaluation of strengths
Marriage Adjustment Form (MAF)/ Burgess	93	Multiple choice	Areas of marital adjustment
Marriage Adjustment Inventory/ Manson; Lerner	157	Multiple choice	Common problems in marriage: dominance, family relations, immaturity, neurotic traits, sociopathic traits, children, money management, interests, sexual compatibility
Marriage Adjustment Schedule/ Marriage Council of Philadelphia	Two versions: 34/36	Inventory	Feelings, attitudes, behavior regarding shared activities, sex, problems, shared responsibility
Marriage Analysis (BGMA)/Blazier; Goosmans	113	Multiple choice	Areas of marriage: self-image, role concepts, feelings toward partner, emotional openness, sexual adjustment
Marriage Evaluation (ME)/Blount	60	Multiple choice	Perceptions of marriage in such areas as values, decision making, personal growth,

(continued)

TABLE 13–3. (*Continued*)

Instrument Name/Author	No. of Items	Response Format	Types of Data Elicited
			communication, commitment, expectation
Marriage Expectation Inventory/ McDonald	58	Inventory	Marital expectations in such areas as love, communication, sex, money, freedom, religion
A Marriage Prediction Schedule (AMPS)/Burgess	74	Multiple choice	Areas of premarital expectations regarding marriage
Marriage Role Expectation/Dunn; DeBonis	71	Multiple choice	Areas of marital expectation: authority, personal characteristics, homemaking, social participation, employment/support, child care
Marriage Scale/White	21	Likert scale	Factors related to compatibility and marital life: mutual understanding, communication, love, habits, sex, occupation, interests, finances, plans
Mirror-Couple Relationship Inventory/J.A. Hunt; R.A. Hunt	336	Inventory	Attitudes toward self and partner
Pair Attraction Inventory (PAI)/ Shostrom	224	Inventory	Attitudes about the nature of a heterosexual relationship
Premarital Communication Inventory/Bienvenu	40	Inventory	Areas of communication, such as differences, anger, feelings, sex, beliefs, problem-solving, future expectations
Premarital Counseling Inventory/ R.B. Stuart; F. Stuart	94	Inventory	Attitudes and expectations toward and understanding of one's partner
Premarital Counseling Kit (PCK)/ Bienvenu, Sr.	6	Counseling guidelines	Areas of marriage, such as communication, compatibility, strengths, problem areas
Relationship Satisfaction Survey/ Lucas	120	Inventory	Marital conflicts and issues, such as values, communication, affection
Sex Attitudes Survey/McHugh	107	Rating scale	Sexual attitudes on intercourse, sex roles, sexual orientation
Sexual Communication Inventory (SCI)/Bienvenu	30+	Open ended; inventory	Frequency and pattern of sexual communication
Biographical Marital Questionnaire/Greene	22	Open ended	Affectional aspects of marriage, division of responsibility in the home, feelings about kinship networks, views on source of marital problems

On the scale line below, check the mark which best describes the degree of happiness, everything considered, of your marriage.

The Locke-Wallace Marriage Inventory demonstrates discrimination between adjusted and maladjusted couples. Split-half reliability has been reported to be 0.90.

• SEXUAL COMPATIBILITY TEST

The Sexual Compatibility Test is a 101-item self-administered measure of sexual activity, attitudes, satisfaction, and responsiveness in couples.[84] Specific sexual activity involving the couple is rated along six dimensions, and normative data are available. In a study of 100 couples, reported alpha coefficients ranged from 0.90 to 0.96, and product moment correlations ranged from 0.79 to 0.97. A concurrent validity study reported an omega-squared ranging from 0.08 to 0.48.

• DYADIC ADJUSTMENT SCALE

The Dyadic Adjustment Scale is a 32-item self-report measure of marital or similar dyads according to dimensions of dyadic satisfaction, dyadic consensus, dyadic cohesion, and affectional expression.[85] Items are rated on a 6-point scale. A sample item is:

Most persons have disagreements in their relationships. Please indicate below the approximate extent of agreement or disagreement between you and your partner for each item on the following list:
Demonstrations of affection
Making major decisions

Cronbach coefficient alpha for the total Dyadic Adjustment Scale and its component subscales ranges from 0.73 to 0.96. Criterion-related and construct validity have been demonstrated by the scale's ability to differentiate between married and divorced people. Correlation coefficients of 0.86 and 0.88 with scores on the Locke-Wallace Marriage Inventory[3] have been reported for married and divorced individuals, respectively.

• REISS PREMARITAL SEXUAL PERMISSIVENESS SCALES (PSP)

The Reiss Premarital Sexual Permissiveness Scales (PSP) is a 12-item self-report attitudinal scale assessing three categories of premarital physical acts: kissing, petting, and coitus, each considered under four conditions of affection: engagement, no affection, strong affection, and love.[86] Subjects indicate the degree of agreement or disagreement with statements, such as the following, on a rating scale:

I believe that full sexual relations are acceptable for the (fe)male before marriage when (s)he feels strong affection for his (her) partner.

I believe that full sexual relations are acceptable for the (fe)male before marriage even if (s)he does not feel particularly affectionate toward his (her) partner.

Reliability and validity of the PSP have been evaluated by Guttman scale analysis, factor analysis, and construct validity procedures. The PSP meets Guttman Scale reliability criteria, with a coefficient of reproducibility above 0.90, coefficient of scalability above 0.65, and pure scale types between 50 and 60 percent of the samples studied.

• INVENTORY OF MARITAL CONFLICTS (IMC)

The Inventory of Marital Conflicts (IMC) is a measure of conflict resolution and decision-making process in couples.[87] Eighteen vignettes (12 conflict and 6 nonconflict) describe marital conflicts. For each vignette, subjects answer questions pertaining to person responsible for the problem, way of resolving the problem, personal experience with the problem, and knowledge of other couples who have experienced the problem. Members of a couple complete the scale individually, then discuss their responses in order to decide jointly responsibility for and resolution of the conflicts in each vignette. The discussions are tape-recorded, then coded in 29 categories to measure the interaction process objectively. Using the Spearman-Brown correction, split-half reliabilities based on win scores for outcomes of the 18 items on the IMC have been reported to average 0.41.

• BARRETT-LENNARD RELATIONSHIP INVENTORY (RI)

The Barrett-Lennard Relationship Inventory (RI) measures four dimensions of interpersonal relationships from the perspective of either an observer or the members of the relationship: congruence, level of regard, empathic understanding, and unconditionality.[88,89] Sixty-four items (8 positively worded, i.e., "yes" weighs positively, and 8 negatively worded, i.e., "no" weighs positively, for each of the four dimensions of interpersonal relationships) are rated from +3, strongly true, to −3, strongly not true. A scale score is computed for each dimension. Several versions of the scale are available depending on the measurement setting and intent. Examples of items include:

He/she respects me as a person. (Level of Regard scale)

He/she usually senses or realizes what I am feeling. (Empathy scale)

The RI has been used in more than 100 studies of relationships between parents and children, partners, supervisors and advisees, and marital clients and counselors. Split-half and test–retest reliabilities of component scales of the RI have been found to average 0.85, and the RI has been found to correlate with other measures of marital relationship adequacy.

• STRUCTURED AND SCALED INTERVIEW TO ASSESS MALADJUSTMENT (SSIAM)

The Structured and Scaled Interview to Assess Maladjustment (SSIAM) is a 60-item structured interview format measure of maladjustment in five areas: work, family, marriage, sex, and social.[90,91] Also included are assessments of friction with others, deviant behavior, environmental stress, and aspects of positive mental health. Eleven dimensions for each area addressed are rated on a 10-point scale. A sample item is:

Is there any tension, coolness, or outright quarreling in your (marital) family?

Interrater reliability of the SSIAM has been reported for three interviewers with a sample of 15 patients. Using a population of 164 adults receiving outpatient psychotherapy, correlation coefficients of reliability for the SSIAM subscales were found to range from 0.78 to 0.97. Patient self-ratings of maladjustment yielded correlation coefficients ranging from 0.20 to 0.70 with ratings of close informants.

▪ SEXUAL INTERACTION INVENTORY (SII)

The Sexual Interaction Inventory (SII), developed by LoPiccolo and Steger, is a self-report inventory of sexual adjustment and satisfaction of heterosexual couples to determine the outcome of treatment for sexual dysfunction.[92,93] Six questions on each of 17 items that cover a range of heterosexual behaviors are rated on a 6-point scale. Issues include degree of satisfaction with frequency and range of sexual behaviors, sexual pleasure, self-acceptance, partner acceptance, and knowledge of partner's sexual preferences. Scores provide ratings of real–ideal sexual frequency and satisfaction for both members of a couple. An example of an item on the SII is:

The male and female having intercourse.
When you and your mate engage in sexual behavior, does this particular activity usually occur? Currently occurs:

1. Never
2. Rarely (10 percent of the time)
3. Occasionally (25 percent of the time)
4. Fairly often (50 percent of the time)
5. Usually (75 percent of the time)
6. Always

The SII has been used with normal and sexually dysfunctional couples. The authors report test–retest reliabilities of 0.53 to 0.90 over a 2-week period and a Cronbach coefficient alpha of 0.85 to 0.93. The validity of the SII has been demonstrated by its ability to reflect changes produced by therapy in patients with sexual dysfunctions. The SII also discriminates between sexually satisfied couples and sexually dysfunctional couples, and its scales correlate with global ratings of sexual satisfaction.

▪ MARITAL COMMUNICATION SCALE (MCS)

The Marital Communication Scale (MCS) is a measure of nonverbal communication accuracy in which couples participate in a dyadic, face-to-face testing situation.[94] Sixteen hypothetical situations are presented, 8 in which one member of the couple is the expresser and the other the receiver, 8 in which the roles are reversed. The score is the total number of items accurately identified by the receiver as being the intent of the sender. One hypothetical situation in the MCS is the following:

You and your husband are sitting alone in your living room on a winter evening. You feel cold.
a. You wonder if he is also cold or is it only you who are cold.
b. You want him to warm you with physical affection.
c. You want him to turn up the heat.

"I'm cold. Aren't you?"

The MCS has discriminated between satisfied and dissatisfied couples. Split-half reliability using the Spearman-Brown correction had demonstrated coefficients of 0.87 for two groups of 10 college couples and 0.70 for an odd–even split of items on a sample of 97 college couples. Test–retest reliability for a 7-week interval was reported to be 0.92.

▪ MARITAL COMMUNICATION INVENTORY (MCI)

The Marital Communication Inventory (MCI) is a self-report measure of success or failure in marital communication with respect to emotions, feelings, economics, behaviors, and communication patterns.[95] Forty-six items are rated "usually," "sometimes," "seldom," or "never." Separate male and female versions exist. Examples of items from the MCI are:

Does your spouse have a tendency to say things which would be better left unsaid?

Do you and your spouse engage in outside interests and activities together?

The MCI has been evaluated in samples of married couples with a reported corrected odd–even split-half correlation coefficient of 0.93 using the Spearman-Brown correction formula. Using the Mann-Whitney U test, the MCI has demonstrated a significant difference between two matched groups, one receiving marital counseling and one without apparent marital problems.

▪ PERSONAL ASSESSMENT OF INTIMACY IN RELATIONSHIPS (PAIR)

The Personal Assessment of Intimacy in Relationships (PAIR) Inventory is a 75-item measure that elicits information on five types of intimacy: social, emotional, intellectual, sexual, and recreational.[96] Subjects respond to statements using a 5-point Likert scale in two steps: perceived ("as it is now") and expected ("how he or she would like it to be"). Sample statements are:

Sexual expression is an essential part of our relationship.

I am satisfied with our sex life.

Factor analysis and split-half reliabilities of the PAIR have been evaluated, and validity has been demonstrated by its correlation with measures of marital adjustment, self-disclosure, and family environment. Cronbach alpha reliability coefficients for each of the six subscales of the PAIR have been reported to be 0.70 or greater.

▪ WARING INTIMACY QUESTIONNAIRE (WIQ)

The Waring Intimacy Questionnaire (WIQ) is a 160-item true/false format instrument that assesses eight components of marital intimacy: sexuality, cohesion, affection, conflict resolution, identity, expressiveness, autonomy, and compatibility.[97] A social desirability section is included to assess independence of subscales and response bias. Evaluation of the WIQ using several large samples of married people has yielded test–retest reliabilities that range from 0.70 to 0.90. KR 20 reliabilities have ranged from 0.52 to 0.87. The WIQ demonstrates a highly significant correlation with the PAIR Inventory.[96]

▪ SEX-LOVE-MARRIAGE SCALE (SLM)

The Sex-Love-Marriage Scale (SLM) consists of eight 5-point Likert-type items for which subjects provide responses ranging from "strongly disagree" to "strongly agree." The scale, which measures the degree to which sex, love, and marriage are cognitively associated was developed using samples composed of students from universities.[99] Examples of items include:

> Sexual intercourse is better—more enjoyable, intense, and satisfying—if the sex partners are married to each other.

> Sex thoughts about someone other than the sex partner during intercourse with the partner are a form of unfaithfulness.

The eight items yielded a Cronbach alpha reliability coefficient of 0.80. In addition, a reliability of 0.75 or greater was obtained with separate samples drawn from four universities. Concurrent validity of the SLM scale was evaluated using the Reiss Premarital Sexual Permissiveness Scale.[86] A principal components factor analysis with oblique rotation has indicated that a single variable accounts for 75 percent of the SLM scale variance.

APPLICATIONS IN SPECIFIC CLINICAL POPULATIONS

All of the instruments described in this chapter were developed for use with people of varying age, developmental level, and sexual health but who were not suffering from a concurrent physical illness or disability. The use of these instruments in special populations requires adaptation of items and evaluation of their reliability and validity. Research into the demands imposed on one's sexuality by the presence of physical illness is being conducted by researchers in a wide variety of disciplines. To illustrate the form this has taken in different realms of clinical expertise, efforts to assess psychosexual impacts in the presence of several types of chronic illness are briefly presented.[100-111]

▪ BULLARD ET AL. QUESTIONNAIRE

Bullard et al. developed a 67-item questionnaire and interview schedule designed to help ascertain the need for sexual health services as perceived by cancer patients.[100] Likert-type and open-ended questions address content related to perceived importance, satisfaction, and frequency of a variety of behaviors, ranging from verbal communication, kissing, touching, and hugging to more explicit sexual activity, such as intercourse.

▪ HARRIS ET AL. QUESTIONNAIRE

Harris et al. used a 63-item sexual behavior questionnaire to study 96 gynecologic cancer patients hospitalized and diagnosed within the previous 6 weeks.[101] The concerns and perceptions of both the patients and their partners were elicited on a broad range of topics, including satisfaction and frequency of coitus, masturbation, and orgasm. Also of interest were the changes in sexual function brought about by the symptoms, diagnosis, and treatment of the malignancy.

• FISHER INTERVIEW GUIDE

Fisher used a flexible open-ended interview guide to study patients, aged 36 to 60, who had undergone total pelvic exenteration 3 to 10 years before the interview.[102] Subjects were allowed maximum opportunity to delve into specific areas such as:

Feelings concerning surgery and changes in body function in the early postoperative phase of recuperation

Postoperative feelings concerning femininity

Recently, Fisher suggested some further possible research applications of available psychosexual measurement instruments with oncology populations.[103]

• SEXUAL ADJUSTMENT QUESTIONNAIRE (SAQ)

Waterhouse and Metcalfe developed a three-part questionnaire, the Sexual Adjustment Questionnaire (SAQ), that measures changes in the cancer patient's sexual expression from before to after cancer diagnosis.[104] Subsections consist of activity level, desire, relationship, arousal, orgasm, and techniques. Additional items inquire about willingness to discuss sexual concerns with others, feelings about the effects of cancer and surgery on sexual relationships, and whether health caregivers do or should discuss sexual concerns with patients. An example of an item on the SAQ is:

How soon after surgery did you resume sexual activity (alone or with another person)?
In hospital
Less than 1 month
1–2 months
2–4 months
4–6 months
More than 6 months
Have not yet

Test–retest reliabilities for a combined sample of 92 head and neck cancer patients and nonpatients ranged from 0.5389 to 0.9374, with a mean of 0.6721. Construct validity was demonstrated by the finding that the scores of subjects with head and neck cancer were significantly lower on the activity level, techniques, and relationships subsections of the SAQ.

• SEXUAL BEHAVIOR ASSESSMENT SCHEDULE: ADULT (SEBA)

Greenberg has suggested the possible use of the Sexual Behavior Assessment Schedule: Adult (SEBA) in oncology settings.[32,105] The SEBA is an interview schedule that assesses sexual orientation, sexual dysfunction, libido, and psychosexual development and was developed originally for studies of potential long-term effects on sexuality of concurrent medical conditions.

• ALTHOF ET AL. SEMISTRUCTURED INTERVIEW

Althof et al. developed a semistructured interview schedule to evaluate both preoperative and longitudinal postoperative effects of coronary bypass surgery on the sexual adaptation of female patients.[106]

• SEXUAL FUNCTIONING QUESTIONNAIRE

The Sexual Functioning Questionnaire is a 17-item instrument designed for use with people involved in an antihypertensive medication program.[107] Items are rated on a 5-point Likert-type scale, with a high score indicating positive sexual functioning. The major elements of sexual experience (such as perceptions of arousal, desire, satisfaction, and orgasm) are assessed through such items as the following:

> During the past 2 months, have you been too tired to have sex?

> When sexually excited were you able to get an erection?

Test–retest reliability for 72 hours was 0.83 for a sample of healthy people. Cronbach alpha ranged from 0.55 to 0.65 among different samples.

• HANSEN ASSESSMENT OF SEXUAL HEALTH (HASH)

The Hansen Assessment of Sexual Health (HASH) was developed to assess the impact on sexuality of nine functional impairments associated with chronic illness: pain, fatigue, appetite change, sleep problems, breathing problems, bowel and bladder problems, mobility problems, hand problems, and mood changes.[108] Sixty subjects suffering from a wide range of medical problems were used to develop the scale. Sampling problems, however, prevented adequate reliability and validity testing, and the instrument awaits further development.

• PERCEPTION OF DIABETES MELLITUS QUESTIONNAIRE (PDM)

Methods to evaluate sexuality in relation to diabetes mellitus have been addressed.[109–111] The Perception of Diabetes Mellitus Questionnaire (PDM) assesses the perceived impact of diabetes on sexual functioning and relationships with a spouse or partner.[109] The PDM consists of a seven-item Relationship Score (RS) section and a six-item Sexual Function (SF) score. Items are rated on a 7-point scale ranging from 1 ("minimal effect") to 7 ("great effect"). The PDM was initially evaluated in Caucasian diabetic women. Coefficient alphas of 0.79 and 0.83 for the RS and SF scores, respectively, have been obtained.

• JENSEN SEXUAL HISTORY FORM

Jensen has studied sexual dysfunction in male and female insulin-treated diabetics.[110,111] His instrument is an adaptation of the Sexual History Form (from the Multiaxial Problem-Oriented System for Sexual Dysfunction).[73]

SUMMARY

Research in the field of human sexuality must acknowledge several special limitations. First, due to the sensitive nature of sexuality, it is often quite difficult to obtain objective data from the subject and/or partner. Some people are unwilling to participate in research related to sexual matters because of embarrassment, denial, fear, and desire for privacy. Similarly, people who have sexual problems and are seeking help may self-select themselves to partici- pate in such studies, thus creating a biased sample. Some subjects may respond to inquiries based on what they suppose to be the desirable or socially acceptable response because of reluctance to reveal unusual or nonconventional sexual values and practices. Psychometric instrumentation in the field of sexuality is a relatively recent phenomenon. The growing recognition of sexuality as an issue of overall health and well-being has permitted the evolution of a growing number of instruments to measure human sexuality in both research and clinical practice. Many of these instruments, however, need more complete testing, particularly when applied to medically ill or physically handicapped populations.

The explicit nature of instruments that measure dimensions of an individual's sexuality need not negate their use. For patient populations in particular, introduction of sexual assess- ment early in the diagnostic and therapeutic plan may enable the establishment of an environ- ment of openness and comfort in what has been regarded traditionally as a highly personal and sensitive topic.

ACKNOWLEDGMENT

This work was supported in part by National Cancer Institute predoctoral training grant 1F31 CA08000.

REFERENCES

1. Kinsey, A.C., Pomeray, W.B., & Martin, C.E. *Sexual behavior in the human male.* Philadelphia: Saunders, 1948.
2. Kinsey, A.C., et al. *Sexual behavior in the human female.* Philadelphia: Saunders, 1953.
3. Locke, H., & Willimson, R.C. Marital adjustment: A factor analysis study. *Am Soc Rev,* 1958, *23*(5):562.
4. Thompson, A.P., & Cranwell, F.R. Frequently cited sources in human sexology. *J Sex Marital Ther,* 1984, *10*(1):63.
5. Masters, W.H., & Johnson, V.E. *Human sexual response.* Boston: Little, Brown, 1966.
6. Masters, W.H., & Johnson, V.E. *Human sexual inadequacy.* Boston: Little, Brown, 1970.
7. Masters, W.H., Johnson, V.E., & Kolodny, R.C., *Human sexuality.* Boston: Little, Brown, 1982.
8. Bancroft, J.H.J. *Human sexuality and its problems.* New York: Churchill-Livingstone, 1983.
9. Beyer, C. (Ed.). *Endocrine control of sexual behavior.* New York: Raven Press, 1979.
10. Cook, M. (Ed.). *The bases of human sexual attraction.* New York: Academic, 1981.
11. Feldman, P., & MacCulloch, M. *Human sexual behavior.* New York: Wiley, 1980.
12. Fromer, M.J. *Ethical issues in sexuality and reproduction.* St. Louis: Mosby, 1983.
13. Gagnon, J.H. *Human sexualities.* Glenview, IL: Scott, Foresman, 1977.
14. Hogan, R.M. *Human sexuality: A nursing perspective.* New York: Appleton-Century-Crofts, 1980.
15. Katchadourian, H.A., & Lunde, D.T. *Biological aspects of human sexuality* (2nd ed.). New York: Holt, Rinehart and Winston, 1980.
16. Katchadourian, H.A., & Lunde, D.T. *Fundamentals of Human Sexuality.* 3rd ed. New York: Holt, Rinehart, and Winston, 1980.

17. Kolodny, R.C. et al. *Textbook of human sexuality for nurses.* Boston: Little, Brown, 1979.
18. Kolodny, R.C., Masters, W.H., & Johnson, V.E. *Textbook of sexual medicine.* Boston: Little, Brown, 1979.
19. Lion, E.M. (Ed.), *Human sexuality in nursing process.* New York: Wiley, 1982.
20. Mims, F.H., & Swenson, M. *Sexuality: A nursing perspective.* New York: McGraw-Hill, 1979.
21. Money, J., & Musaph, H. (Eds.). *Handbook of sexology.* New York: Elsevier, 1978.
22. Siemen, S., & Brandzel, R.C. *Sexuality: Nursing assessment and intervention.* Philadelphia: Lippincott, 1982.
23. Victor, J.S. *Human sexuality: A social psychological approach.* Englewood-Cliffs, NJ: Prentice-Hall, 1980.
24. Weinberg, J.S. *Sexuality, human needs and nursing practice.* Philadelphia: Saunders, 1982.
25. Woods, N.F. *Human sexuality in health and illness* (3rd ed.). St. Louis: Mosby, 1984.
26. Derogatis, L.R. Response: The measurement of sexual dysfunction in cancer patients. *Cancer* [Suppl], 1984, *53*(10):2285.
27. Abramson, P.R., Perry, L.B., Rothblatt, A., et al. Negative attitudes toward masturbation and pelvic vasocongestion: A thermographic analysis. *J Res Pers,* 1981, *15*:497.
28. Schiavi, R.C. Psychophysiological research and human sexuality (Editorial). *J Sex Marital Ther,* 1976, *2*(3):163.
29. Schiavi, R.C. Sex therapy and psychophysiological research. *Am J Psychiatry,* 1976, *133*(5):562.
30. Schiavi, R.C., & White, D. Androgens and male sexual function: A review of human studies. *J Sex Marital Ther,* 1976, *2*(3):214.
31. Schiavi, R.C., & Schreiner-Engel, P. Physiologic aspects of sexual function and dysfunction. *Psychiatr Clin North Am,* 1980, *3*(1):81.
32. Greenberg, D.B. The measurement of sexual dysfunction in cancer patients. *Cancer* [Suppl], 1984, *53*(10):2281.
33. Sweetland, R.C., & Keyser, D.J. (Eds.). *Tests: A comprehensive reference for assessments in psychology, education and business.* Kansas City: Test Corporation of America, 1983.
34. Conte, H.R. Development and use of self-report techniques for assessing sexual functioning: A review and critique. *Arch Sex Behav,* 1983, *12*(6):555.
35. Buros, O.K. (Ed.). *The seventh mental measurement yearbook.* Highland Park, NJ: Gryphon Press, 1972.
36. Comrey, A.L., et al. (Eds.). *A source book for mental health measures.* Los Angeles: Human Interaction Research Institute, 1973, p. 187.
37. Schiavi, R.C. The assessment of sexual and marital function (Editorial). *J Sex Marital Ther,* 1979, *5*(3):167.
38. Schiavi, R.C., et al. The assessment of sexual function and marital interaction. *J Sex Marital Ther,* 1979, *5*(3):169.
39. Williams, A.M., & Miller, W.R. The design and use of assessment instruments and procedures for sexuality curricula. In N. Rosenzweig and F.P. Pearsall (Eds.), *Sex education for the health professional: A curriculum guide.* New York: Grune & Stratton, 1978, p. 137.
40. Green, R., & Wiener, J. (Eds.). *Methodology in sex research.* Rockville, MD: DHHS: National Institute of Mental Health, 1981.
41. Derogatis, L.R. Psychological assessment of psychosexual function. *Psychiat Clin North Am,* 1980, *3*(1):113.
42. Group for the Advancement of Psychiatry. *Assessment of sexual function: A guide to interviewing.* New York: Jason Aronson, 1974.
43. Derogatis, L.R., & Melisaratos, N. The DSFI: A multi-dimensional measure of sexual functioning. *J Sex Marital Ther,* 1979, *5*(3):244.
44. Abramson, P.R., & Mosher, D.L. Development of a measure of negative attitudes toward masturbation. *J Consult Clin Psychol,* 1975, *43*(4):485.
45. Mosher, D.L., & Abramson, P.R. Subjective sexual arousal to films of masturbation. *J Consult Clin Psychol,* 1977, *45*(5):796.
46. Abramson, P.R., & Mosher, D.L. An empirical investigation of experimentally induced masturbatory fantasies. *Arch Sex Behav,* 1979, *8*(1):27.

47. Mosher, D.L. The development and multitrait-multimethod matrix analysis of three measures of three aspects of guilt. *J Consult Psychol*, 1966, *30*:35.
48. O'Grady, K.E., & Janda, L.H. Factor analysis of the Mosher Forced-Choice Guilt Inventory. *J Consult Clin Psychol*, 1979, *47*:1131.
49. Harbison, J.J.M., Graham, P.J., Quinn, J.T., et al. A questionnaire measure of sexual interest. *Arch Sex Behav*, 1974, *3*(4):357.
50. Bentler, P.M. Heterosexual behavior assessment. I. Males. *Behav Res Ther*, 1968, *6*(1):21.
51. Bentler, P.M. Heterosexual behavior assessment. II. Females. *Behav Res Ther*, 1968, *6*(1):27.
52. Hoon, E.F., Hoon, P.W., Wincze, J.P. An inventory for the measurement of female sexual arousability: The SAI. *Arch Sex Behav*, 1976, *5*(4):291.
53. Chambless, D.L., & Lifshitz, J.L. Self-reported sexual and anxiety arousal: The Expanded Sexual Arousability Inventory. *J Sex Res*, 1984, *20*(3):241.
54. Allen, R.M., & Haupt, T.D. The Sex Inventory: Test–retest reliabilities of scale scores and items. *J Clin Psychol*, 1966, *22*(4):375.
55. Thorne, F.C. The Sex Inventory. *J Clin Psychol*, 1966, *22*(4):367.
56. Thorne, F.C., & Haupt, T.D. The objective measurement of sex attitude and behavior in adult males. *J Clin Psychol*, 1966, *22*(4):395.
57. Fretz, B.R. An attitude measure of sexual behaviors. Paper presented at American Psychological Association Convention, 1974.
58. Zuckerman, M. Scales of sex experience for males and females. *J Consult Clin Psychol*, 1973, *41*(1):27.
59. Miller, W.R., & Lief, H.I. The sex knowledge and attitude test (SKAT). *J Sex Marital Ther*, 1979, *5*(3):282.
60. Fisher, S.G., & Levin, D. The sexual knowledge and attitudes of professional nurses caring for oncology patients. *Cancer Nurs*, 1983, *6*(1):55.
61. Woods, N.F., & Mandetta, A. Changes in students' knowledge and attitudes following a course in human sexuality: Report of a pilot study. *Nurs Res*, 1975, *24*(1):10.
62. Taylor, M.E. A discriminant analysis approach to exploring changes in human sexuality attitudes among university students. *J Am Coll Health*, 1982, *31*(3):124.
63. Zuckerman, M., Tushup, R., & Finner, S. Sexual attitudes and experience: Attitude and personality correlates and changes produced by a course in sexuality. *J Consult Clin Psychol*, 1976, *44*(1):7.
64. Williams, H.A., Wilson, M.E., Hongladorum, G., et al. Nurses' attitudes toward sexuality in cancer patients. *Oncol Nurs Forum*, 1986, *13*(2):39.
65. Spence, J.T., & Helmrich, R. Who likes competent women? Competence, sex role, congruence of interests, and subjects attitudes toward women as determinants of interpersonal attraction. *J Appl Soc Psychol*, 1972, *2*(3):197.
66. Bem, S. The measurement of psychological androgyny. *J Consult Clin Psychol*, 1974, *42*(2):155.
67. MacDonald, A.P., Jr. Identification and measurement of multidimensional attitudes toward equality between the sexes. *J Homosex*, 1974, *1*(2):165.
68. MacDonald, A.P., Jr., Huggins, J., Young, S., et al. Attitudes toward homosexuality: Preservation of sex morality of the double standard? *J Consult Clin Psychol*, 1973, *40*:161.
69. Sambrooks, J.E., & MacCullock, M.J. A modification of the sexual orientation method and an automated technique for presentation and scoring. *Br J Soc Clin Psychol*, 1973, *12*(2):163.
70. Freund, K., Nagler, E., Langevin, R., et al. Measuring feminine gender identity in homosexual males. *Arch Sex Behav*, 1974, *3*(3):249.
71. Marks, I.M., & Sartorius, N.H. A contribution to the measurement of sexual attitude. The semantic differential as a measure of sexual attitude in sexual deviations. *J Nerv Ment Dis*, 1967, *145*(6):441.
72. Paitich, D., Langevin, R., Freeman, R., et al. The Clarke SHQ: A clinical sex history questionnaire for males. *Arch Sex Behav*, 1977, *6*(5):421.
73. Schover, L.R., Friedman, J.M., Weiler, S.J., et al. Multiaxial problem-oriented system for sexual dysfunction. *Arch Gen Psychiatry*, 1982, *39*(5):614.

74. Beutler, L.E., Karacan, I., Anch, A.M., et al. MMPI and MIT discriminators of biogenic and psychogenic impotence. *J Consult Clin Psychol*, 1975, *43*(6):899.
75. Obler, M. Systematic desensitization in sexual disorders. *J Behav Ther Exp Psychiatry*, 1973, *4*(2):93.
76. Hollender, M.H., Luborsky, L., Scaramella, T.J. Body contact and sexual enticement. *Arch Gen Psychiatry*, 1969, *20*(2):188.
77. Kurtz, R., & Hurt, M. Body attitude and physical health. *J Clin Psychol*, 1970, *26*(2):149.
78. Kurtz, R.M., Sex differences and variations in body attitudes. *J Consult Clin Psychol*, 1969, *33*(5):625.
79. Kurtz, R. The relationship of body attitude to sex, body size, and body build in a college population. Doctoral dissertation, University of Cincinnati, 1966. *Dissertation Abstracts International*, 1966, *27*(6):1928A.
80. Kurtz, R. Body attitude and self-esteem (Summary). *Proceedings of the 79th Annual Convention of the American Psychological Association*, 1971, *6*:467.
81. White, C.B. A scale for the assessment of attitudes and knowledge regarding sexuality in the aged. *Arch Sex Behav*, 1982, *11*(6):491.
82. Edmonson, B., & Wish, J. Sex knowledge and attitudes of moderately retarded males. *Am J Ment Defic*, 1975, *80*(2):172.
83. Wish, J.R., et al. *The Socio-Sexual Knowledge and Attitude Test: Instruction manual.* Chicago: Stoelting Co., 1980.
84. Foster, A.L. The sexual compatibility test. *J Consult Clin Psychol*, 1977, *45*(2):332.
85. Spanier, G.B. Measuring dyadic adjustment: New scales for assessing the quality of marriage and similar dyads. *J Marr Fam*, 1976, *38*(1):15.
86. Reiss, I.L. *The social context of premarital sexual permissiveness.* New York: Holt, Rinehart and Winston, 1967, p. 211.
87. Olson, D.H., & Ryder, R.G. Inventory of Marital Conflicts (IMC): An experimental interaction procedure. *J Marr Fam*, 1970, *32*(3):443.
88. Barrett-Lennard, G.T. The Relationship Inventory: Later developments and adaptations. *JSAS Catalog of Selected Documents in Psychology*, 1978, *8*:68 (MS. No. 1732).
89. Barrett-Lennard, G.T. The Relationship Inventory now: Issues and advances in theory, method and application. In L. Greenberg & W.M. Pinsof (Eds.), *The psychotherapeutic process: A research handbook.* New York: Guilford Press (In Press).
90. Gurland, B.J., Yorkston, N.J., Stone, A.R., et al. The Structured and Scaled Interview to Assess Maladjustment (SSIAM). I. Description, rationale and development. *Arch Gen Psychiatry*, 1972, *27*(2):259.
91. Gurland, B.J., Yorkston, N.J., Goldberg, K., et al. The Structured and Scaled Interview to Assess Maladjustment (SSIAM). II. Factor analysis, reliability and validity. *Arch Gen Psychiatry*, 1972, *27*(2):264.
92. LoPiccolo, J., & Steger, J. The Sexual Interaction Inventory: A new instrument for assessment of sexual dysfunction. *Arch Sex Behav*, 1974, *3*(6):585.
93. McCoy, N.N., & D'Agostino, P.A. Factor analysis of the Sexual Interaction Inventory. *Arch Sex Behav*, 1977, *6*(1):25.
94. Noller, P. *Nonverbal communication in marital interactions.* Elmsford, NY: Pergamon, 1984.
95. Bienvenue, M.J., Sr. Measurement of marital communication. *Fam Coordinator*, 1970, *19*(1):26.
96. Schaefer, M.T., & Olson, D.H. Assessing intimacy: The PAIR Inventory. *J Marital Fam Ther*, 1981, *7*(1):47.
97. Waring, E.M., & Reddon, J.R. The measurement of intimacy in marriage: The Waring Intimacy Questionnaire. *J Clin Psychol*, 1983, *39*(1):53.
98. Greene, B.L. *A clinical approach to marital problems* (2nd ed.). Springfield, IL: Chas. C Thomas, 1981.
99. Weis, D.L., Slosnevick, M., Cate, R., et al. A survey instrument for assessing the cognitive association of sex, love, and marriage. *J Sex Res*, 1986, *22*(2):206.
100. Bullard, D.G., Causey, G.C., Newman, A.B., et al. Sexual health care and cancer: A needs assessment. *Front Radiat Ther Oncol*, 1980, *14*:55.

101. Harris, R., Good, R.S., Pollack, L. Sexual behavior of gynecologic cancer patients. *Arch Sex Behav,* 1982, *11*(6):503.
102. Fisher, S.G. Psychosexual adjustment following total pelvic exenteration. *Cancer Nurs,* 1979, *2*(3):219.
103. Fisher, S.G. Sexuality as a variable in oncology nursing research. *Oncol Nurs Forum,* 1985, *12*(1):87.
104. Waterhouse, J., & Metcalfe, M. Development of the sexual adjustment questionnaire. *Oncol Nurs Forum,* 1986, *13*(3):53.
105. Meyer-Bahlburg, H.F.L., & Ehrhardt, A.A. Sexual Behavior Assessment Schedule: Adult (SEBA-A), 1983.
106. Althof, S.E., Coffman, C.B., & Levine, S.B. The effects of coronary bypass surgery on female sexual, psychological and vocational adaptation. *J Sex Marital Ther,* 1984, *10*(3):176.
107. Watts, R.J. Sexual functioning, health beliefs and compliance with high blood pressure medications. *Nurs Res,* 1982, *31*(5):278.
108. Hansen, E.I., & Brouse, S.H. Assessing sexual implication of functional impairments associated with chronic illness. *J Sex Educ Ther,* 1983, *9*(2):39.
109. Pieper, B.A., et al. Perceived effect of diabetes on relationship to spouse and sexual function. *J Sex Educ Ther,* 1983, *9*(2):46.
110. Jensen, S.B. Diabetic sexual dysfunction. A comparative study of 160 insulin-treated diabetic men and women—An age-matched control group. *Arch Sex Behav,* 1981, *10:*493.
111. Jensen, S.B. Sexual dysfunction in insulin-treated diabetics: A six year follow-up study of 101 patients. *Arch Sex Behav,* 1986, *15*(4):271.

CHAPTER 14

Measuring Dietary Intake and Nutritional Outcomes

Nancy Bergstrom, R.N., Ph.D.

The role of nutrition in the etiology and treatment of cancer and other diseases is a topic of a great deal of current research. Dietary habits have been related to the development of certain diseases, including cancer and heart disease (e.g., dietary fat has been related to higher incidences of colon cancer, with correlation coefficients as high as 0.85[1]). Nutritional status has been related to favorable outcomes after surgery[2-4] or after such therapies as radiation[5] and chemotherapy.[6,7] Morbidity and mortality rates of special groups of subjects have been shown to increase when the subjects were diagnosed as having protein or protein/calorie malnutrition or anergy.[2-4,8,9]

A multitude of techniques is available to study both the dietary intake of subjects and the clinical outcomes. Two major factors are important when selecting a method to measure either dietary intake or nutritional outcomes. The first is the reliability of the data, that is, the degree to which the data are accurate when collected. The second is the validity of the data— the degree to which the recorded data are representative of the true or actual dietary intake or the nutritional outcomes. Each of these factors is addressed in connection with the related methods.

COLLECTING DIETARY INTAKE DATA

Methods used to collect dietary intake data include diet recall, dietary records or histories, dietary observation, food frequency recordings, and dietary score methods. Each of the methods has advantages and disadvantages, which are usually related to the reliability or validity of the collected data, the resources required to collect the data, and the expertise of the investigators.

▪ DIET RECALL

Diet recall (most often 24-hour recall) is one type of diet interview modified from the work of Burke.[10] Data are obtained by interviewing a subject and asking the subject to recall all food and drinks ingested from rising through the last snack of the evening of the previous day.[11-14] The interviewer generally guides the subject through the day, asking:

What time did you get up yesterday?

Did you eat anything on arising?

What did you have for lunch?

Did you eat anything during the afternoon?

Food items usually are not suggested by the interviewer to avoid leading the subject to report items that were not eaten, but the interviewer may jog the memory of the subject by asking questions, such as:

Did you eat your toast dry?

Did you eat your baked potato plain?

Did you have anything to drink during the afternoon?

The quantity of food eaten is determined by asking the subject to describe the amount. Plastic food models and measuring cups and spoons are used to assist the subject in recalling the serving size.

The advantages of the 24-hour diet recall method that have been recognized by nutritionists include[12,15,16] (1) data are collected rather quickly, (2) the interview can be conducted by health care professionals without a great deal of training, and (3) data may be obtained by telephone interview. Major disadvantages of the method are[12,13,15-20] (1) memory or ability to recall may be incomplete, (2) subjects may have a tendency to report what they believe the data collector wants to hear, (3) many people have difficulty estimating serving size, (4) one 24-hour period may not be representative of the subject's usual dietary intake (women, in particular, have been noted to have day-to-day variations in intake), and (5) analysis of the data is time consuming and costly.

Interrater reliability has been and should continue to be established for any investigation where two or more interviewers collect dietary intake data. The use of manuals, such as the staff procedure manual for the Hanes II study, helps investigators to obtain reliable data from subjects.[14]

Twenty-four-hour recall data have been validated on one level by observing actual intake of measured foods surreptitiously and later obtaining recall data from the subject. A high correlation between data obtained by both methods has been taken as a measure of validity. This approach to establishing validity has been used with elderly people participating in a congregate meal program,[21,22] with children in lunch programs,[23,24] with morbidly obese subjects,[25] with obese and nonobese boys,[26,27] and with hospitalized lactating women.[28]

Many of the studies performed to establish the reliability or validity data fell short of the objective. The majority only calculated total caloric intake or the intake of calories, protein, and fat.[12,27] Work remains to be done in this area, and these weaknesses must be considered when selecting this method of data collection.

▪ DIETARY RECORDS

Dietary records or diaries (1-, 3-, 7-day) have been used to collect what investigators hope will be more precise data. Subjects are interviewed about the purpose of the study and instructed in the keeping of records. Each food or fluid item ingested is recorded as close to the time of eating as possible to reduce memory-related inaccuracies. Subjects may or may not be asked to weigh or measure the food.[12,13]

The advantages of the dietary record or diary are[12,13] (1) memory or ability to recall is not relied on to as great an extent, (2) serving size data may be more accurate if subjects measure or weigh food, (3) data may be obtained for a longer period of time than when using recall methods, hence increasing the representativeness of the dietary intake data, and (4) personnel are not required to be present to collect data and costs of data gathering are thus minimized.

Major disadvantages of dietary record or history methods include[12,13] (1) subjects must be highly motivated to remember to record data and to be willing to weigh or measure food, (2) memory-related errors may be replaced by recording errors, (3) the consciousness-raising experience of writing down what one has eaten may result in a Hawthorne effect, thus reducing the representativeness of the data, and (4) more data are generated and more time may be required to analyze the data.

Attempts to establish the validity or representativeness of data collected by this method have been made by asking subjects to keep dietary records for 2 consecutive weeks[29] or at 1- to 9-month intervals.[30,31] Correlations have been fairly adequate ($r = 0.70$ to 0.85) for the 1- to 9-month interval. There were no significant differences between dietary intakes of individuals on two consecutive 1-week records.[29] Most studies made at two different time periods have fairly good agreement.[29-32] Hence, many investigators believe that this method, with the identified limitations, does produce useful data.

▪ DIETARY OBSERVATIONS

Direct observations of dietary intake by trained observers may increase the reliability and validity of dietary intake data. Direct observations can be very precise when subjects are eating and are being observed in an institutional setting. Daily menus from the dietary department, including the food items to be served, variations in food items based on special diets, and serving size, are known. When casseroles, soups, or other mixed dishes are created, recipes are obtained to assist in computer estimation of nutrient intake.[32] The investigator observes the tray just before delivery to the patient to verify that all food items are present. Observations during the meal ensures that the patient, rather than someone else, is eating the food. As trays are collected, the amount actually eaten is recorded by the observer after determining that food was not saved or discarded.

Advantages of dietary observations include (1) a trained observer, working with known serving sizes and recipes, records all food, and (2) subject memory or motivation is not crucial to the study. Disadvantages may include (1) a potential Hawthorne effect if patients feel they are being watched, (2) a potential Hawthorne effect if staff put more effort into assisting patients with eating, (3) subjects must be in an institution or at a meal site to be observed cost effectively, hence independently living subjects could not be studied as easily, and (4) a great deal of observer time is spend recording data.[31]

The reliability of this method of recording data can be assured by having pairs of observers record intake independently. A high correlation between pairs of observers has been obtained and supports the belief that data can be reliable.[33]

The validity of the data, when viewed from the perspective of how representative it is of the true or real intake of the subject, can be questioned on the basis of potential Hawthorne effects. This potential may decrease as the number of days of observation increase and may have no effect on anorexic, elderly, or other patients with eating disorders.

• FOOD FREQUENCY RECORDINGS

Questionnaires or interviews that ask only how often one eats specific foods over a given timeframe are useful in large epidemiologic studies. The subject is given a list of foods and asked to indicate the number of times per specified interval he or she has eaten each item. Items on the checklist are selected because they have properties of interest to the problem to be studied (e.g., foods high in calcium would be listed for studies of osteoporosis). The data are generally used to divide subjects into broad categories of intake adequacy, such as quartiles or quintiles for the purpose of assessing risk factors in relation to levels of intake[34–40] —that is, four or five categories of subjects may be established based on 1 = the lowest 20 percent, 2 = 21 to 40 percent, 3 = 41 to 60 percent, 4 = 61 to 80 percent, 5 = 81 to 100 percent.

Advantages of this method are that (1) data can be collected in brief interviews (as short as 15 minutes), by telephone, or as part of a mailed questionnaire, and (2) little personnel time is necessary to collect and interpret the data.

Disadvantages of the method are numerous:

1. Data about the intake of specific nutrients is not obtained.
2. The list presented to the subject may not be extensive enough to include all foods containing properties of interest.
3. Only general food intake data are obtained.

The reliability of this method has been demonstrated in a number of investigations.[35–40] Correlations have been established between dietary records of food eaten over a 7-day period and recall of frequency data on the eighth day. Subjects have been asked to recall the immediate 24-hour period and the 7-day period, with agreements between recall and records ranging from 78 to 100 percent.[36] Validity has been reported in two studies that assumed that if spouses reported the same food frequency as the subject, validity was established. A high level of agreement was established between spouses.[41,42]

• DIETARY SCORE

The dietary score method for obtaining and analyzing dietary intake is based on the Basic Four Food Guide[43] and, more recently, on the Daily Food Guide.[44] The premise of this method is that each food group contributes unique nutrients to the diet. In this method, points are assigned for food items eaten from a specific food group. A serving from the milk or meat group would be assigned 2 points, whereas the fruit–vegetable and bread–cereal groups are assigned 1 point for each serving. A maximum of 4 points is allotted per food group, giving each food group equal weight. A total of 16 points is possible for the normal diet.[45]

Guthrie and Scheer[45] did not record the actual serving size of foods eaten when assigning a dietary score. It may be especially important to consider serving size when assessing cancer patients, elderly patients, or anyone with anorexia. *The Hassel Free Guide to a Better Diet* was used to add this dimension in one study.[33]

The reliability of the scoring has been evaluated by graduate nursing students who observed the dietary intake of oncology patients in a demonstration project. Pairs of student observers, student and staff members, or student and patient or family members scored dietary intake. Correlations between pairs of observers were high ($r = 0.80$ or better).[46]

The validity of this method was evaluated by Guthrie and Scheer,[45] who assigned dietary scores to the 24-hour dietary records obtained from 212 university students. In this instance, the instrument would be judged valid to the degree that the adequacy of intake between 24-hour records and dietary scores were similar. A nutrient adequacy ratio was calculated using the RDA for age and sex as the standard by which to judge the reported intake from the 24-hour recall. The method was demonstrated to be valid, since a score of 16 (the total possible points) met the RDA for 7 of 12 nutrients as calculated from the 24-hour intake, and the remaining 5 nutrients met 80 percent of the RDA.

Major advantages of the method are:

1. With little training, it can be easily administered and analyzed by most staff nurses, many clients, and families.
2. The method is flexible and can be easily modified to assess needs of specific groups.
3. Data analysis takes only moments.

Disadvantages of the dietary score method are:

1. Mixed types of food (e.g., casseroles) require judgment in rating.
2. It is difficult to rate fast foods.
3. A wide range of caloric and nutrient levels may be ingested, especially if subject eats more or less than the minimum serving size.

Computer Programs for Analyzing Dietary Intake Data

Once data regarding dietary intake have been collected, the nutritive value of foods must be calculated using established tables. The USDA's Bulletin 72, *Nutritive Value of Food,*[47] and Handbook 8, *Composition of Foods,*[48] list food items, quantities, and the nutrient content of many food items. These source books are updated frequently and represent a reliable source of information for estimating nutritive contents of food. In fact, the only more reliable source of information about nutritive content would be laboratory analysis of a portion of the food actually eaten by the subject. This is usually only done in metabolic studies where exact intake and output data are required.

The process of using the USDA references to calculate nutrient intake by hand is laborious and time-consuming. Approximately 100 computer programs are available currently to facilitate these analyses. Each program is designed to meet specific needs. Programs vary from highly sophisticated (generally expensive) mainframe systems to very simple (often inexpensive) microcomputer programs designed for home meal planning.

According to Wilson[49] and Wheeler and Wheeler,[50] the user should give highest priority to selecting a program with a current, well-documented database. The USDA's Handbook 8 is generally considered the preferred and most reliable database. A second highly important selection criterion is whether or not the program analyzes the specific nutrients of concern to the research project. Some programs have a limited database and calculate a limited number of nutrients.

The database for fast foods, convenience foods, and special dietary formulations is contained in some programs. A number of the programs permit the user to update values in the database, add recipes, or add data about additional nutrients.

Wilson[49] suggested that results be reported both in absolute values and as a percentage of the most recent RDA for age–sex categories. An additional capacity to store data and calculate mean intake values over specified periods may be useful for some investigators.

Several computer programs with which the author is familiar or that have been reviewed in computer journals are listed below.

Inexpensive Programs. These programs cost less than $100.

▪ DINE

DINE has a database of about 3500 foods and 10 nutrients. It has been rated as being only "fair" by Wheeler and Wheeler.[50]

▪ NUTRI-PACK

Nutri-pack is a very simple program that analyzes 600 foods for 12 nutrients. Wilson[49] stated it had few other features.

▪ HEALTH-AIDE

Health-Aide has had several updates and, according to Wilson,[49] has an excellent program for analyzing energy expenditure, but it has been faulted as using some questionable references for the database.

Moderately Priced Programs. The costs of these programs range between $100 and $1000.

▪ NUTRITIONIST III

Nutritionist III has an 1800-food database that includes brand names, vitamins, and formulas. Sixty-one nutrients are analyzed by the program. The program uses USDA databases 8.1– 8.10 and has received high marks from both Wilson[49] and Wheeler and Wheeler.[50] It is my experience that the program is user friendly and efficient and has impressive graphics and knowledgeable support people to answer questions by phone.

▪ NUTRI-CALC

Nutri-Calc is similar to Nutritionist III in both intent and usefulness, according to Wilson[49] and Wheeler and Wheeler.[50] The program feature that analyzes recipes is reputed to be easier to use than the Nutritionist III.

Any computer program should be updated periodically. For this reason, it is insufficient to rely on a list of available programs when selecting a program to purchase. The user is well advised to seek current specifications from the developer and to determine if the program of interest meets all the user's needs.

Summary

A number of methods for quantifying nutrient intake data have been briefly described. Reliability and validity have been established at some level for all of these methods, but reliability and validity continue to be ongoing issues in the selection of any method.

The precision of the data being sought, the advantages and disadvantages of the major methods, and the skill and resources of the investigator all must be considered when selecting methods for collecting dietary intake data. A well-documented database is essential for estimating the nutrient intake of several of the methods presented. Computer programs can greatly assist in calculating nutrient intake data.

METHODS TO ASSESS NUTRITIONAL OUTCOMES

The outcomes of dietary intake, digestion, absorption, and utilization are reflected in the health of the individual and by a number of subjective and objective measurements. The history and physical examination, anthropometric measurements, clinical evaluation of blood and serum, and skin testing are all components of nutritional assessment. Singly, none of these methods provides definitive data about the nature of nutritional alterations in patients due to reliability, validity, sensitivity, and pathophysiologic factors. More commonly, multiple indicators are selected to add credibility to conclusions. However, each method is discussed here singly, followed by examples of multiple indicators used by clinicians to diagnose protein/calorie malnutrition or to predict surgical or other treatment outcomes.

• HISTORY AND PHYSICAL EXAMINATION

The oldest and no doubt the most widely used method of nutritional evaluation is the history and physical examination. There are numerous textbooks and journal articles designed to teach health care providers the "how to" of systematic history and head to toe physical examinations. [51,52]

The history seeks to identify factors that may reflect changes in health and/or nutrient intake or digestion that provide clues to potential changes in nutritional status. The history seeks to elicit information about usual weight, current weight, weight changes, changes in the pattern or variety of food intake, changes in appetite, and signs and symptoms of related problems, for example, anorexia, nausea, vomiting, and diarrhea. [52,53] Positive findings from the history can provide a focal point for further evaluation.

The systematic physical examination seeks to document physical signs and symptoms of nutritional deficiencies, adequacy, and excesses. Tables listing descriptions of normal and abnormal findings for each system are often found in textbooks and may include descriptors of potential deficiencies causing specific symptoms, or they may list the major nutrients and give examples of signs and symptoms of deficiencies and excesses. [52,54-56] For example, the Michigan Department of Health in a booklet, *Basic Nutrition Facts,* provides such a table [56]; one subsection of the nutrient list is given as Table 14–1.

Such tables are useful resources, but additional training is necessary to learn to identify signs and symptoms clinically. Medical specialty textbooks often have pictorials depicting different degrees of malnutrition on specific body systems. For example, the effect of hypovitaminosis A on the eye has been shown pictorially. [57]

Additional factors that deserve consideration when conducting a history and physical examination are (1) what disease process, medication side effect, or metabolic abnormality can account for the signs and symptoms, (2) what effect does age have on expected findings (e.g., calcium deficiency may result in rickets in children and osteoporosis in elderly women), (3) what are the normal changes related to aging, and (4) what are the half-lives of nutrients suspected to be deficient (evidence of depletion or repletion is difficult to document due to the long half-lives of many nutrients).

The advantages of the physical examination as a source of nutritional status data is that thousands of examinations are performed in the U.S. annually. The clinician who is aware of the signs and symptoms of nutritional deficits is in a position to evaluate further and treat the clients with potential problems.

The disadvantages of physical examinations as a routine method of detecting abnormalities are (1) physical examinations are time consuming and costly, (2) data obtained cannot stand alone, and further investigation is required, (3) examiners vary in ability to observe,

TABLE 14—1. NUTRIENTS FOR HEALTH

Nutrient	1980 RDA Level	Dietary Sources	Major Body Functions	Effects of Inadequacy	Effects of Excess
Vitamin A (retinol equivalents, mcg)	M[a] F C 1000 800 700	liver, carrots sweet potato, dark green leafy vegetables, broccoli, winter squash, apricots, cantaloupe, peaches, milk, fish liver oil	important component in visual process of the eye including adaptation to dark; assists in formation and maintenance of skin, mucous membranes, bones, teeth	xerophthalmia (an eye condition leading to blindness), night blindness, permanent blindness, poor growth	yellow pigmentation of skin, loss of appetite, vomiting

[a]C, child; F, female; M, male.
From Basic nutrition facts, 1980, p. 15. Courtesy of Michigan Department of Public Health.

correctly interpret, and differentially diagnose problems, and (4) deficiencies must be severe and/or persistent enough to produce visible symptoms.

The reliability of physical examination data has been evaluated in many nutritional studies. Interrater reliability, as indicated by the percentage agreement between two examiners in a developing country, ranged from 33 to 75 percent for selected physical signs.[58] Three examiners working in a given area during the Ten State Nutrition Survey also had highly variable instances of given signs and symptoms.[58] These investigators had received similar training and would have been expected to have greater reliability.

Two clinical examiners reported agreement on the classification of patients as having or not having protein/calorie malnutrition in 81 percent of the cases.[59] Results of a study in New Zealand in which two surgeons classified subjects as obese, normal, mildly depleted, moderately depleted, and severely depleted based on history and physical examination, however, demonstrated only a 51 percent agreement.[60] Thus, there may be a great deal of variability in findings by different observers. This variability requires that training and ongoing evaluation of observations be a part of any study.

The validity of the physical examination has been studied by documenting agreement between objective findings, such as laboratory values, and subjective findings, such as clinical impression. In the previously mentioned study by Pettigrew et al.,[60] clinical judgment by two surgeons was correct when verified by laboratory data in only 60 percent and 65 percent of the cases. Perhaps this is best explained by the lack of correlations between laboratory findings and clinical examination, factors that can be influenced by nutrient stores in the body and prolonged half-lives of some blood components.

▪ ANTHROPOMETRY

Anthropometry, the measurement of the human body, is an additional method of clinical assessment. Anthropometric measurements, such as height, wrist circumference, elbow breadth, weight, triceps skinfold thickness, upper arm circumference, and in infants head circumference, are nonspecific indicators of growth and development and nutritional status. Each of these measurements contributes to the clinician's ability to evaluate nutritional status and growth and development.

Weight. Weight is interpreted in relation to height with or without consideration of frame size determined by wrist circumference or elbow breadth. It is a composite measure of leanness or obesity. A loss of 5 percent of the usual body weight, weight less than 90 percent of the ideal body weight, or a loss of 10 pounds in a brief period of time all may reflect nutritional risk.

Weight and height are interpreted in relation to age in children. Visits to pediatricians and school health evaluations almost always include evaluation of growth. Chronic nutritional deficiencies and other physical and psychosocial factors are potential causes for failure to grow.

Midupper Arm Circumference. The midupper arm circumference is a composite view of both protein (muscle mass) and energy (skinfolds) stores. Norms have been established for midupper arm circumference, but the data are rarely interpreted without considering the triceps skinfold.

Triceps Skinfold. The triceps skinfold thickness reflects body fat stores. Fat stores are indicative of chronic undernutrition or overnutrition and do not change rapidly on a day-to-day basis. Caution must be exerted when interpreting these results, since an obese person may have excessively thick fat folds, yet be malnourished and losing weight.

Arm Muscle Area. The arm muscle area reflects lean body mass and is derived by the following formula[61]:

$$\text{Arm muscle mass (cm)} = \frac{\text{midupper arm circumference (cm)} -}{[0.314 \times \text{triceps skinfold (mm)}]}$$

Decreases in muscle area can be the result of muscle wasting due to nutritional deficiencies and muscle disease. Severe depletion is defined as an arm muscle area in the lowest 5th percentile on established tables. People in the 5th to 25th percentiles are considered moderately depleted.

Reliability and Validity. The reliability of anthropometric measurements is a matter of concern, especially when multiple investigators or clinicians are performing the measurements over a timespan. Three major considerations are (1) instrument selection, quality, design, and standardization, (2) training and supervision of personnel, and (3) periodic replication.

Instrument selection can be facilitated by data from a variety of sources. Manufacturer's design and operating specifications, reports of previous studies in which like instruments were compared, the experience of other investigators, and personal experience are all useful when evaluating instruments. Instruments should have clearly identified standards against which values can be verified. For instance, the Lange calipers[62] to measure skinfold thickness apply 10 g/mm^2 of pressure on the contact surface of the skin. Accuracy can be determined by using a standard calibration block available from the manufacturer. Each step on the calibration block is 10 mm. If the caliper registers 10 mm while resting on the first step and 10 ($\pm$ 0.5) additional mm on each of the four subsequent steps, it is assumed to be precise. When the instrument is not in calibration, it is returned to the manufacturer for servicing. The manufacturer addresses quality and design issues in the specifications and provides a case for storage and suggestions for maintenance.

The training and supervision of personnel have been facilitated by the use of established measurement protocols. Detailed descriptions of each measurement protocol have been published to reduce measurement error.[61,63–65] Recently published tests have devoted many pages to protocols for anthropometric measurements of adults, including photographs and diagrams.[66,67]

Protocols provide step-by-step directions for performing anthropometric measurement, but training and skill acquisition are necessary. For instance, in a protocol to measure triceps skinfold, the patient is asked to stand erect. The tip of the olecranon process of the ulna and the acromial process of the scapula are palpated and marked. The midpoint between these points is identified and marked. Skinfold thickness is measured by picking up a double fold of fat and skin and applying the calipers.[67]

Sources of error in the measurement of skinfold thickness can include the selection of different skin sites, variations in body and hand positions, which influence the amount of tissue in the skinfold, and the length of time the caliper is applied before taking the reading.[63,68] Adequate training sessions and supervision reduce the amount of variability of measurement. Periodic planned interrater reliability testing is necessary at intervals to maintain the stability of measurement techniques over time. This author conducts reliability evaluations once a month during long term studies.

Interpretation of Data. Once data have been precisely and accurately collected, equal care must be given to evaluating the results. Table 14–2 presents several anthropometric measurements and sources of standards for interpretation. When interpreting data, the investigator should evaluate the methods by which the standards were developed. The characteristics of the study subjects on which the standard was developed will more likely be representative and, hence, valid if the characteristics of the study subjects are similar. Race, sex, and age are important characteristics.

▪ LABORATORY STUDIES

Laboratory studies can be performed on blood, serum, plasma, tissues, hair, nails, urine, sweat, and stools. Laboratory studies are believed to offer an objective assessment of nutritional status and to provide evidence of preclinical deficiencies. There are multiple factors to be considered when using laboratory studies as part of a nutritional evaluation. Special considerations include selecting the study, sample collection details, sample handling, sample analysis, and interpretation of findings.

Selecting the Study. Laboratory studies are performed to determine nutrient concentrations, balance status, nutrient needs, changes in blood components related to intake, and responses to tests, doses, or loads. The investigator must be familiar with all of the alternative laboratory tests and determine which tests provide the most direct, reliable, and valid data. Direct tests of water-soluble vitamins, for instance, include studies of plasma, serum, or red blood cell concentrations. Such direct tests would be preferable to indirect tests, such as

TABLE 14–2. INTERPRETING RESULTS OF ANTHROPOMETRIC MEASUREMENTS

Measurement	Sources of Standards
Weight/height	HANES[69]
Adults	Metropolitan Life[70]
	Jensen et al.[67]
	National Center for Health Statistics[76]
	Blackburn et al.[61]
	Simko et al.[66]
Children	Waterlow et al.[69]
	Hamill & Moore[72]
	Hamill et al.[75]
	Roche[73]
	DHEW[77]
Midupper arm circumference	Friscancho[71]
	Simko et al.[66]
	Jensen et al.[67]
Triceps skinfold	Frisancho[71]
	Jelliffe[74]
	Simko et al.[66]
	Jensen et al.[67]
Arm muscle area	CDC, 1975
	Friscancho[71]
	Simko et al.[66]
	Jensen et al.[67]

urine concentrations of excreted metabolites, since these metabolites could be influenced by many intervening variables (e.g., renal function, intermediary metabolism).

Many clinical researchers possess a degree of expertise in the selection and interpretation of laboratory studies. Texts and journal articles provide useful background information about selection among available studies, but consideration also must be given to many minute details during the planning stages. Hence, many investigators consult a nutritional biochemist or a biochemist at a reputable clinical laboratory. Christakas[64] suggested that the best single source for advice is the Nutritional Biochemistry Section, Center for Disease Control (CDC) in Atlanta. Other potential consultants are those people most frequently referred to in journal articles in relation to specific nutrients.

Sample Collection and Handling. Optimal attention must be given to specimen collection, preservation, and transportation. The timing of sample collection is an important initial detail. Food and fluid intake influences the results of some tests. It generally is most appropriate to obtain fasting blood samples and urine samples on arising in the morning, but when this is not possible or not absolutely essential to the study, data should be collected in as similar a fashion as possible. Subjects require adequate instruction about necessary test preparations or expectations.

Special equipment may be needed to collect the sample. For example, vacuum tubes may need preservatives, and glass tubes must either be treated or avoided when collecting samples for zinc analysis.[78] As much preparation of the sample as possible should be done immediately at the site of sample collection. Some samples require immediate chilling on ice and/or freezing, whereas others require immediate centrifuging and pipetting. When transporting the samples, care must be taken to assure that warming or defrosting does not occur.

Selecting a Clinical Laboratory. Few clinical investigators have the expertise and equipment to perform all assays required. A certified clinical laboratory must maintain high standards in order to maintain certification, since patient care decisions are based on these results. In most instances, these laboratories are more than adequate for performing assays.

Because of the infrequency with which some assays are performed, a laboratory may not analyze certain factors of interest to the investigator. In this case, contracts may be made with specialty laboratories. The investigator should elicit information about the sensitivity, precision, and accuracy of the desired assay. The sensitivity is important when perhaps thousandths of a milliliter may be crucial to the interpretation of data. If only the nearest hundredth is determined, the assay may not be adequately sensitive for the study.

The reliability or precision of the analysis can be demonstrated by analyzing samples in duplicate or triplicate. In this instance, the investigator decides what value to use when interpreting the data and what margin of variability is acceptable. Reliability is worthless, however, if the assay is not valid or accurate. The validity or accuracy of the assay itself can be assured by calibrating equipment appropriately and by using known standards. Results that agree with known standards across a range of values (highest to lowest expected) provide evidence on one level to support the validity of the assay. The investigator can expect to receive from the laboratory on request data for both reliability and validity.

Interpretation of Laboratory Data. Interpretation of laboratory results requires careful judgments. Clinical laboratories generally provide information about acceptable normal values for the laboratory. Christakas[64] cautions investigators to consider the variations due to diet and intercurrent disease. Certainly, age and gender must be considered as a source of variation.

When using published norms, the investigator needs to determine if the norms were

TABLE 14–3. INTERPRETING LABORATORY STUDIES USING PUBLISHED NORMS

Laboratory Study	Published Norm
Hemoglobin and hematocrit	King & Fauker[79]
	Christakas[64]
Serum retinol (vitamin A)	Smith & Goodman[80]
25-Hydroxy vitamin D (25-OHD)	Mawer[81]
Zinc	Solomons[82]
Zinc	Iyengar et al.[83]
Plasma	Iyengar et al.[83]
Urinary	Fredricks et al.[84]
Erythrocyte	Auerbach[85]
	Rosner & Gorfien[86]

established on a sample similar to the study sample. The rationale for the cutoff points created by the authors of tables may be controversial. The rationale for the cutoff should be clear and acceptable to the investigator interpreting the data.

Tables of normal values can be found in journal articles that provide original data to support the tables. Several references giving examples of tables of normal values and cutoff points are shown in Table 14–3.

• SKIN TESTING

Skin testing as an indicator of cell-mediated immunity and visceral protein stores is often a part of nutritional assessment. A reactive response is one in which an area of induration equal to or greater than 5 mm occurs in 24 to 48 hours after intradermal injection of an antigen. When there is a lesser response or no response, the patient is judged to be anergic and at increased risk for infection, sepsis, and mortality.[87–94] Nutritional supplementation has been shown to reverse anergy and increase immune competence.[95–98]

The procedure for measuring and interpreting skin tests has been carefully outlined and clearly described.[67] The selection of antigens for skin tests varies according to the investigators who select them. The list of potential antigens includes stretokinase-streptodornase (SK-SD), mumps, *Candida,* tuberculin purified protein derivative (PPD), trichophyton, histoplasmin, and coccidioidin. A number of investigators have reported the percentage of subjects reactive to each antigen and to combinations of antigens.[99–104] There appears to be some consensus that multiple antigens should be used.[101]

The skin tests are read at both 24 and 48 hours, since at least one study found that some antigens cause an early reaction that subsides and others respond later. The author concluded that measurement at exclusively one of these times would have missed some positive reactions.[99]

• NUTRITIONAL ASSESSMENT

A number of nutritional assessment techniques have been discussed in the preceding paragraphs. These techniques are often combined to obtain data for specific purposes. Investigators and clinicians have attempted (1) to study the nutritional status of the community,[74] (2) to evaluate the health benefits of specific government programs,[105] (3) to define a program of assessment to identify children at risk due to nutritional deficits,[64] (4) to direct a complete assessment of hospitalized patients,[61,67] (5) to perform an instant nutritional assessment based on readily available patient data (e.g., serum albumin and total lymphocyte count),[2,49] and (6) to create a prognostic index for specific groups based on nutritional status.[6,88] Each of these references provides insight into the fine art of matching the purposes of a study with appropriately selected outcome variables.

SUMMARY

The primary starting point when selecting measures to study the nutritional status of patients is to have clearly stated purposes or specific aims. Knowledge of the purpose of the study will aid in selecting appropriate methods. A thorough understanding of the methods of interest and all the related alternative methods is essential to the selection of the most appropriate instruments. Although there are many issues involved in the selection of the most sensitive, reliable, and valid instruments in any study, studies of nutritional status require meticulous attention to numerous details. Since no one method for measuring dietary intake or nutritional status is perfect in relation to reliability, validity, and sensitivity, the author recommends that investigators consider using multiple indicators of dietary intake and nutritional status. For instance, generalizations about the dietary intake of a subject are limited to those days for which records or observations are available. The data can be strengthened by obtaining anthropometric measurements that may support the conclusion that the dietary intake of a subject reflects a usual pattern.

REFERENCES

1. Armstrong, B., & Doll, R. Environmental factors and cancer incidence and mortality in different countries with special reference to dietary practices. *Int J Cancer,* 1975, *15*(5):617.
2. Seltzer, M.H., Fletcher, H.S., Slocum, B.A., et al. Instant nutritional assessment in the intensive care unit. *JPEN* 1981, *5*(1):70–72.
3. Klidjian, A.M., Archer, T.J., Foster, K.J., et al. Detection of dangerous malnutrition. *J Parenter Enter Nutr,* 1982, *6*(2):119.
4. Hickman, D.M., Miller, R.A., Rombeau, J.L. Serum albumin and body weight as predictors of postoperative course in colorectal cancer. *J Parenter Enter Nutr,* 1980, *4*(3):314.
5. Harvey, K.B., Bothe, A., & Blackburn, G.L. Nutritional assessment and patients outcome during oncological therapy. *Cancer,* 1979, *43*(5):2065.
6. Freeman, M., Frankmann, C., Beck, J., et al. Prognostic nutrition factors in lung cancer patients. *J Parenter Enter Nutr,* 1982, *6*(2):122.
7. Issell, B.F., Valdivieso, M., & Zaren, H.A. Protection against chemotherapy toxicity by intravenous hyperalimentation. *Cancer Treat Resp,* 1978, *62*(8):1139.
8. Mullen, J.L., Gertner, M.H., Buzby, G.P., et al. Implications of malnutrition in the surgical patient. *Arch Surg,* 1979, *114*(2):121.
9. Seltzer, M.H., Bastidas, J.A., Cooper, D.M., et al. Instant nutritional assessment. *J Parenter Enter Nutr,* 1979, *3*(3):157.
10. Burke, B.S. The dietary history as a tool in research. *J Am Diet Assoc,* 1947, *23*(12):1041.
11. Karvetti, R.-L., & Knuts, L.-R. Agreement between dietary interviews: Nutrient intake measured by dietary history and 24-hour and seven-day recalls. *J Am Diet Assoc,* 1981, *79*(12):654.
12. Block, G. A review of validations of dietary assessment methods. *Am J Epidemiol,* 1982, *115*(4):492.

13. Young, C.M., Chalmers, F.W., Church, H.N., et al. A comparison of dietary study methods. II. Diet history vs. seven-day record and 24-hour recall. *J Am Diet Assoc,* 1952, *28*(3):218.
14. United States Department of Health, Education and Welfare. Hanes II—Examination staff procedures manual for the health and nutrition examination survey 1976–1979. (Instructions manual, part 15a.) Rockville, MD: National Center for Health Statistics, 1976.
15. Beaton, G.H., Milner, B.A., Corey, P., et al. Sources of variance in 24-hour dietary recall data: Implications for nutrition study design and interpretation. *Am J Clin Nutr,* 1979, *32*(12):2546.
16. Posner, B.M., Borman, C.L., Morgan, L., et al. The validity of a telephone-administered 24-hour dietary recall methodology. *Am J Clin Nutr,* 1982, *36*(3):546.
17. Fidanza, F. Sources of error in dietary surveys. *Bibl Nutr Dieta,* 1974, *20:*105.
18. Balogh, M., Kahn, H., & Medalie, J.H. Random repeat 24-hour dietary recalls. *Am J Clin Nutr,* 1971, *24*(3):304.
19. White, E.C., McNamara, D.J., & Abrens, E.H. Jr. Validation of a dietary record system for the estimation of daily cholesterol intake in individual outpatients. *Am J Clin Nutr,* 1981, *34*(2):199.
20. Garn, S.M., Larkin, F.A., & Cole, P.E. Commentary: The problem with one-day dietary intakes. *Ecol Food Nutr,* 1976, *5*(4):245.
21. Gersovitz, M., Madden, J.P., & Smiciklas-Wright, H. Validity of the 24-hour recall and seven-day record for group comparisons. *J Am Diet Assoc,* 1978, *73*(1):48.
22. Madden, J.P., Goodman, S.J., & Guthrie, H.A. Validity of the 24-hour recall. Analysis of data obtained from elderly subjects. *J Am Diet Assoc,* 1976, *68*(2):143.
23. Meredith, A., Matthews, A., Zickefoose, M., et al. How well do school children recall what they have eaten? *J Am Diet Assoc,* 1951, *27*(9):749.
24. Emmons, L., & Hayes, M. Accuracy of 24-hour recalls of young children. *J Am Diet Assoc,* 1973, *62*(4):409.
25. Bray, G.A., Zachary, B., Dahms, W.T. et al. Eating patterns of massively obese individuals: Direct vs. indirect measurements. *J Am Diet Assoc,* 1978, *72*(1):24.
26. Waxman, M., & Stunkard, A.J. Caloric intake and expenditure of obese boys. *J Pediatr,* 1980, *96*(2):187.
27. Stunkard, A.J., & Waxman, M. Accuracy of self-reports of food intake. *J Am Diet Assoc,* 1981, *79*(11):547.
28. Linusson, E.F.I., Sanjur, D., & Erikson, E.C. Validating the 24-hour recall method as a dietary survey tool. *Arch Latinoam Nutr,* 1975, *24:*277.
29. Adelson, S. Some problems in collecting dietary data from individuals. *J Am Diet Assoc,* 1960, *36*(5):453.
30. Heady, J.A. Diets of bank clerks. Development of a method of classifying the diets of individuals for use in epidemiological studies. *J R Stat Soc [A],* 1961, *124:*336.
31. Morris, J.N., Marr, J.W., & Heady, J.A. Diet and plasma cholesterol in 99 bankmen. *Br Med J,* 1963, *1:*571.
32. Bergstrom, N., & Wiese, R.A. Feeding institutionalized elderly: 3-versus 5-meals a day. (Manuscript unpublished.)
33. Bergstrom, N. The consistency of diet intake observed weekly among elderly residents in a nursing home. (Manuscript unpublished.)
34. Willett, W.C., & MacMahon, B. Diet and Cancer—An overview. *N Engl J Med,* 1984, *310*(10):633.
35. Morgan, R.W., Jain, M., & Miller, A.B. A comparison of dietary methods in epidemiologic studies. *Am J Epidemiol,* 1978, *107*(6):488.
36. Hankin, J.H., Rawlings, V., & Nomura, A. Assessment of a short dietary method for prospective study on cancer. *Am J Clin Nutr,* 1978, *31*(2):355.
37. Abramson, J.H., Slome, C., & Kosovsky, C. Food frequency interviews as an epidemiologic tool. *Am J Public Health,* 1963, *53*(7):1093.
38. Balogh, M., Kahn, H., Medalie, J., et al. The development of a dietary questionnaire for an ischaemic heart disease survey. *Israel J Med Sci,* 1968, *4*(2):195.
39. Browe, J.H., Gofstein, R.M., Morley, D.M., & McCarty, M.C. Diet and heart disease study in the cardiovascular health center. *J Am Diet Assoc,* 1966, *48*(2):95.
40. Hankin, J.H., Rhoads, G.G., & Glober, G.A. A dietary method for an epidemiological study of gastrointestinal cancer. *Am J Clin Nutr,* 1975, *28*(9):1055.

41. Marshall, J., Priore, R., Haughey, B., et al. Spouse-subject interviews and the reliability of diet studies. *Am J Epidemiol,* 1980, *112*(5):675.
42. Kolonel, L.N., Hirohata, T., & Nomura, A.M.Y. Adequacy of survey data collected from substitute respondents. *Am J Epidemiol,* 1977, *106*(6):476.
43. U.S. Department of Agriculture, Agricultural Research Service. *Essentials of an adequate diet.* Home Economics Research Report No. 3, Washington, DC: Government Printing Office, 1957.
44. U.S. Department of Agriculture. Agricultural Research Service. *Food for fitness—A daily food guide.* Leaflet No. 424, Washington, DC: Government Printing Office, 1977.
45. Guthrie, H.A., & Scheer, J.C. Validity of a dietary score for assessing nutrient adequacy. *J Am Diet Assoc,* 1981, *78*(3):240.
46. Bergstrom, N. Quantifying dietary intake of cancer patients: A quick and reliable method. *Proceedings of the Ninth Annual Congress of the Oncology Nursing Society,* 1984.
47. U.S. Department of Agriculture. Science and Education Administration. *Nutritive value of foods.* Home and Gardens Bulletin. No. 72, Washington, DC, 1981.
48. Watt, B.K., & Merrill, A.L. *Composition of foods.* Agriculture Handbook No. 8, Washington, DC: U.S. Department of Agriculture, 1983.
49. Wilson, A.K. Nutrition analysis programs. *Med Electronics, 24*(5), Sept. 1984.
50. Wheeler, L.A., & Wheeler, M.L. Review of microcomputers nutrient analysis and menu planning programs. *MD Computing,* 1984, *1*(2):42.
51. Malasano, L. *Health assessment* (2nd ed.). St. Louis: Mosby, 1981.
52. The Nurses' Reference Library. *Assessment.* Springhouse, PA: International Communications, Inc., 1982.
53. Keithley, J.K. Proper nutritional assessment can prevent hospital malnutrition. *Nursing 79,* 1979, *9*(2):68.
54. Centers for Disease Control and Health Services Administration. *A guide in pediatric weighing and measuring.* Atlanta: CDC, 1981.
55. Reed, P.B. *Nutrition: An applied science.* New York: West Publishing Co., 1980, p. 421.
56. Michigan Department of Public Health. *Basic nutrition facts.* Lansing, MI: Michigan Department of Public Health, 1980.
57. Spalton, D.J., Hitchings, R.A., & Hunter, P.A. *Atlas of clinical ophthalmology.* Philadelphia: Lippincott, 1984.
58. Hansen, R.G., & Monroe, H.N. (Eds.). *Problems of assessment and alleviation of malnutrition in the Unites States.* Proceedings of a workshop sponsored by Vanderbilt University, January 1970.
59. Baker, J.P., Detsky, A.S., Wesson, D.E., et al. Nutrition assessment: A comparison of clinical judgement and objective measurements. *N Engl J Med,* 1982, *306*(16):969.
60. Pettigrew, R.A., Charlesworth, P.M., Farmilo, R.W., & Hill, G.L. Assessment of nutritional depletion and immune competence: A comparison of clinical examination and objective measurements. *J Parenter Enter Nutr,* 1984, *8*(1):21.
61. Blackburn, G.L., Bistrian, B.R., Maini, B.S., et al. Nutritional and metabolic assessment of the hospitalized patient. *J Parenter Enter Nutr,* 1977, *1*(1):11.
62. Lange, Skinfold caliper. Cambridge Scientific Industries. Cambridge, MD.
63. Werner, J.S., & Lourie, J.A. *Human biology: A guide to field methods.* Oxford: Blackwell Scientific Publications, 1969.
64. Christakis, G. (Ed.). *Nutritional assessment in health programs.* Proceedings of the Conference on Nutritional Assessment, American Public Health Association, Inc., Washington, DC, 1972.
65. Johnson, C.L., Fulwood, R., Abraham, S., & Bryner, J.D. Basic data on anthropometric measurements and angular measurements of hip and knee joints for selected age groups 1–74 years of age. United States, 1971–1974. Vital Health Statistics, Series II, No. 219. Hyattsville, MD: DHHS Publication No (PHS 81-1669), 1983.
66. Simko, M.D., Cowell, C., & Gilbride, J.A. *Nutrition assessment: A comprehensive guide to planning intervention.* Rockville, MD: Aspen, 1984, p. 60.
67. Jensen, T.G., Englert, D.M., & Dudrick, S.J. *Nutritional assessment: A manual for practitioners.* E. Norwalk, CT: Appleton-Century-Crofts, 1983.

68. Burkinshaw, L., James, P.R.M., & Krupowiczy, D.W. Observer error in skinfold thickness measurements. *Hum Biol,* 1973, *45*(2):273.
69. Waterlow, J.C., et al. The presentation and use of height and weight data for comparisons of nutritional status of groups of children under the age of 10 years. *Bull WHO,* 1977, *55:*489.
70. Society of Actuaries and Association of Life Insurance Medical Directors of America. Metropolitan Height and Weight Tables, Metropolitan Life Insurance Company, 1983.
71. Frisancho, A.R. New Norms of upper limb fat and muscle areas for assessment of nutritional status. *Am J Clin Nutr,* 1981, *34*(11):2540.
72. Hamill, P.V.V., & Moore, W.M. Contemporary growth charts: Needs, construction and application. *Pediatr Nurs Curr,* 1976, *23*(5):17.
73. Roche, A.F. Growth assessment of handicapped children. *Diet Curr,* 1979, *6*:25.
74. Jelliffee, D.B. *The assessment of the nutritional status of the community.* Geneva: World Health Organization, 1977, p. 63.
75. Hamill, P.V.V., et al. NCHS Growth curves for children, birth–18 years, United States. *Vital Health Stat,* Series 11, No. 165, DHEW Publ. No. (PHS) 78-1650, 1977.
76. National Center for Health Statistics. Weight by height and age of adults 18–74 years: United States, 1971–1974. Rockville, MD. National Center for Health Statistics, DHEW publication No. (PHS) 79-1656, 1979.
77. Department of Health, Education and Welfare—Region V. *Proceedings of the nutrition assessment of children and youth workshop.* Columbus, OH: Ross Laboratories, 1977.
78. Prasad, A.S. (Ed.). *Clinical biochemical and nutritional aspects of trace elements.* New York: Alan R. Liss, 1982.
79. King, J.W., & Fauker, W.R. (Eds.). *Critical resources in clinical laboratory sciences.* Cleveland, OH: CRC Press, 1963.
80. Smith, F.R., & Goodman, D.S. Vitamin transport in human vitamin A toxicity. *N Engl J Med,* 1974, *194*(7):805.
81. Mawer, E.B. Critical implication of measurements of circulating vitamin D metabolities. *Clin Endocrinol Metab,* 1980, *9*(1):63.
82. Solomons, N.W. On the assessment of zinc and copper nutriture in man. *Am J Clin Nutr,* 1979, *32*(4):856.
83. Iyengar, C.V., Kollmer, W.E., & Bowen, H.J.M. *The elemental composition of human tissues and body fluids.* New York: Verlag Chemic, Weinhern, 1978.
84. Fredericks, R.E., Tanak, K.R., & Valentine, W.N. Variations of human blood cell zinc in disease. *J Clin Invest,* 1964, *43*(2):304.
85. Auerbach, S. Zinc content of plasma, blood and erythrocytes in normal subjects and in patients with Hodgkin's disease and various hematologic disorders. *J Lab Clin Med,* 1965, *65*(4):628.
86. Rosner, R., & Gorfien, P.C. Erythrocyte and plasma zinc and magnesium levels in health and disease. *J Lab Clin Med,* 1968, *72*(2):213.
87. Biena, R., Ratcliff, S., Barbour, G.L., et al. Malnutrition and hospital prognosis in the alcoholic patient. *J Parenter Enter Nutr,* 1982, *6*(4):301.
88. Buzby, G.P., Muller, J.L., Mathews, D.C., et al. Prognostic nutritional index in gastrointestinal surgery. *Am J Surg,* 1980, *139*(1):160.
89. Dionigi, P., Nazari, S., Bonoldi, A.P., et al. Nutritional assessment and surgical infections in patients with gastric cancer or peptic ulcer. *J Parenter Enter Nutr,* 1982, *6*(2):128.
90. MacLean, L.D., Meakins, J.L., Taguchi, K., et al. Host resistance in sepsis and trauma. *Ann Surg,* 1975, *182*(3):207.
91. Morath, M.A., Miller, S.F., & Finley, R.K. Nutritional indicators in post-burn bacteremic sepsis. *J Parenter Enter Nutr,* 1981, *5*(6):488.
92. Meakins, J.L., Pietsch, J.B., Bubenick, O., et al. Delayed hypersensitivity: Indicator of acquired failure of host defense in sepsis and trauma. *Ann Surg,* 1977, *186*(3):241.
93. Kaminski, M.V., Fitzgerald, M.T., Murphy, R.J., et al. Correlation of mortality with serum transferrin and anergy. *J Parenter Enter Nutr,* 1977, *1*:27.
94. Willcutts, H.D., Linderme, D., Chlastawa, D., et al. Anergy: Is nutritional reversal possible outcome significant? *J Parenter Enter Nutr,* 1979, *3*(2):292A.

95. Law, D.K., Dudrick, S.J., & Abdouw, N.I. Immounocompetence of patients with protein-caloric malnutrition. The effects of nutritional repletion. *Ann Intern Med,* 1973, *79*(4):545.
96. Bistrian, B.R., Blackburn, G.L., Scrimshaw, N.S., et al. Cellular immunity in semistarved states in hospitalized adults. *Am J Clin Nutr,* 1975, *28*(10):1148.
97. Bistrian, B.R., Sherman, M., Blackburn, G.L., et al. Cellular immunity in adult marasmus. *Arch Intern Med,* 1977, *137*(11):1408.
98. Blackburn, G.L., Gibbons, G.W., Bothe, A., et al. Nutritional support in cardiac cachexia. *J Thorac Cardiovasc Surg,* 1977, *73*(4):489.
99. Jensen, T.G., Englert, D.M., Durdrick, S.J., et al. Delayed hypersensitivity in skin testing. Response rates in surgical population. *J Am Diet Assoc,* 1983, *82:*17.
100. Blackburn, G.L., Bistrian, B.R., Mani, B.S., et al. Nutritional and metabolic assessment of the hospitalized patient. *J Parenter Enter Nutr,* 1977, *1*(11):11.
101. Winborn, A.L., Banazek, N.K., & Freed, B.A. A protocol for nutritional assessment in a community hospital. *J Am Diet Assoc,* 1981, *78*(2):129.
102. Israel, L., Mugica, J., & Chahinian, P. Prognosis of early bronchogenic carcinoma. Survival curves of 451 patients after rejection of lung cancer in relation to results of preoperative tuberculin skin test. *Biomed,* 1973, *19*(1):68.
103. Daly, J.M., Dudrick, S.J., & Copeland, E.M. Evaluation of nutritional indices as prognostic indicators in the cancer patient. *Cancer, 1979, 43*(3):925.
104. Palmer, D.L., & Reed, W.P. Delayed hypersensitivity skin testing. Response rates in a hospital population. *J Infect Dis,* 1974, *130*(2):132.
105. United States Department of Agriculture. Food and Nutrition Service. *Evaluating the nutrition and health benefits of the special supplemental food program for women, infants and children.* Washington, DC: United States Printing Office, FNS-165, 1977.

CHAPTER *15*

Measuring Sleep

Susan Larsen Beck, R.N., M.N.

Sleep is defined as the natural suspension of consciousness during which the processes of the body are restored.[1] According to Guyton, sleep is a state of unconsciousness from which a person can be aroused by appropriate sensory and other stimuli.[2] Although sleep previously was considered to be a completely passive phenomenon, it is now known to be a rich and active process. Sleep functions both physiologically and psychologically to restore and replenish the body's resources.

Disturbances of sleep due to various causes are among the most common disorders of the central nervous system.[3] Several surveys have suggested that the number of people in the United States who complain of insomnia, disorders of initiating and maintaining sleep, may well be in the millions. It is estimated that between 8 and 15 percent of the U.S. adult population have frequent and chronic complaints about the quality and quantity of their sleep. This prevalence is supported by the extensive use of hypnotic drugs in this country. A 1977 survey by the National Institute on Drug Abuse estimated that 9 percent of the U.S. adult population used a hypnotic sedative in the preceding year.[4] There has been some evidence to support the idea that insomnia may be a risk factor for certain chronic diseases.[5]

In primary health care, sleep pattern disturbance is more prevalent as normal sleep/wakefulness patterns are disrupted by the physical and emotional response to illness, drugs and treatments, and changes in environment due to hospitalization. As a nursing diagnosis, sleep pattern disturbance has been defined as a disruption of sleep time causing discomfort or interference with desired life activities.[6] Sleep deprivation has been of particular concern in critically ill patients and has been associated with intensive care unit syndrome, mental status alterations occurring in people subjected to the intensive care unit environment. Sustained lack of sleep can affect both psychologic and physical well-being. Initially, it can cause mood changes, irritability, and aggressiveness.[7] Prolonged sleep deprivation results in psychologic dysfunctions, such as forgetfulness, disorientation, and confusion. Neurologic changes also have been observed in those who are sleep deprived. These include mild nystagmus, hand tremor, ptosis of the eyelids, change in speech quality, and decreased pain tolerance.[8,9]

In order to obtain a greater understanding of the problem and to test interventions to manage sleep pattern dysfunction, it is necessary to have available reliable, valid, and clinically appropriate instruments to measure sleep. The purpose of this chapter is to describe the current state of the science of sleep measurement.

BACKGROUND

The modern conceptualization of sleep as an active and functional process began in 1937, when Loomis, Harvey, and Hobart discovered different stages of sleep based on the amplitude and activity of the brain during sleep.[10] These findings were the result of electroencephalographic (EEG) monitoring during sleep. In 1953, periods of rapid eye movements (REM) were observed during sleep by Aserinsky and Kleitman.[11] Further studies built on these findings and led to the now accepted classification of REM sleep and four stages of non-REM sleep. Human beings thus alternate between three states: wakefulness, non-REM sleep, and REM sleep.

Wakefulness
Wakefulness is characterized by a state of alertness and appropriate response to stimuli. An EEG in an awake individual reflects spontaneous, low-voltage, random, and fast electrical activity.[12] There are usually alpha wave patterns of 8 to 12 cycles per second. Muscular activity is high, and only rapid eye movements are recorded on electrooculogram.

Non-REM sleep begins as a person falls asleep and brain activity slows. The moment that a person disengages from the outside world can be measured precisely within several seconds. Following the onset of sleep, the brain activity gradually decreases. Four stages of non-REM sleep have been identified on the basis of EEG activity. Progression from stage 1 to stage 4 is characterized by progressively slower brain wave activity.[13]

Stage 1. EEG activity slows from alpha waves to beta and theta waves (1 to 6 cycles per second). There are primarily irregular, low-amplitude, mixed-frequency signals. Brain activity slows with the onset of stage 2 sleep, which usually occurs within a few minutes after falling asleep.

Stage 2. EEG activity consists primarily of theta waves. Two electrical phenomena, spindles and K-complexes, are also present.

Stage 3. Slow, high-amplitude delta waves characterize this stage of sleep. These waves average 1 to 4 cycles per second and may comprise 20 to 50 percent of the sleep record.

Stage 4. This stage is characterized by more than 50 percent slow, delta waves. It represents the lowest level of physiologic and possibly psychologic activity. It may be the most essential part of the sleep cycle.

REM Sleep
REM sleep has also been termed "activated sleep." The brain is intensely active, and this stage of sleep is thought to correspond to dreaming. REM sleep is characterized by profound motor inhibition, central nervous system stimulation, penile erection, short-acting physiologic events, such as rapid eye movements, and the ability to recall dreams on awakening.

Little is known about the exact functions of these two different sleep states. Some evidence suggests that non-REM sleep helps to restore the brain's biochemical balance. REM sleep may be the time during which the brain sorts, files, and stores information. It is believed to be associated with memory and learning.

Just as wakefulness and sleep alternate rhythmically, non-REM and REM sleep also form a rhythmic cycle. The progression through the stages of non-REM sleep is also systematic. A normal single night of sleep usually consists of four to six 90-minute cycles of non-REM/REM sleep.

MEASUREMENT OF SLEEP

There are three approaches to sleep measurement: polysomnography, self-reports, and observations. Although polysomnography is considered the most accurate, self-reports and observations have been used more often by nurse investigators.

Polysomnography

Polysomnography or all-night sleep recordings are considered the most accurate measure of sleep.[14,15] They are the standard to which all other measures are compared. This phenomenon flows logically from the fact that the stages of sleep were initially characterized on the basis of EEG activity. A standardized technique for using and scoring polysomnography was published by Rechtschaffen and Kales in 1968.[15]

The standard involves the use of readings from eight electrodes that are fed into eight channels on a polygraph machine. A variety of equipment has been used in various sleep investigations, including phone-transmitted systems.[14] The bipolar EEG is recorded from two midline frontoparietal electrodes and measures fluctuations in brain wave activity. The electrooculogram (EOG), which measures eye movements, is recorded from four electrodes secured to the outer canthi of the eyes. The electromyogram (EMG), read from two electrodes placed on the diagastric chin muscles, records absence of muscle activity, an indicator of REM sleep.

The polysomnographic technique involves a thorough cleansing of the face and scalp at the various attachment points. The scalp electrodes are attached by means of a specially prepared gauze pad; the facial electrodes are secured with tape. The wires are then gathered in a ponytail, and each is connected to the appropriate channel of the polygraph machine.

According to the standard, two experienced scorers rate the sleep on the basis of epochs. An epoch is a 30-second sample of the EEG that falls on one page of a continuous polygraph record when chart speed is 10 mm/second. Automatic analysis of sleep records via an analog spectrum analyzer has been described. However, the reliability of such analysis decreases in subjects with disturbed sleep.[16]

Multiple sleep parameters or variables have been used to estimate sleep based on the results of polysomnography. These parameters are included in Table 15–1, which compares the variables used in the three types of sleep measurement.

Polysomnography has been used in a variety of sleep investigations. Such sleep recordings have been used in descriptive studies of sleep patterns in acute schizophrenics,[17] psychotic and nonpsychotic depressives,[18,19] and alcoholics.[20,21] Carskadon et al. located 20 reports of polysomnographic sleep studies in clinically defined insomniacs.[22] Broughton and Baron used polysomnography to describe sleep patterns after acute myocardial infarctions,[23] and Calvery et al. used this measurement technique to evaluate the effect of oxygenation on sleep quality in chronic obstructive pulmonary disease.[24] Porter and Horne measured the effect of different carbohydrate levels on sleep via polysomnography.[25]

TABLE 15–1. VARIABLES USED TO ESTIMATE SLEEP

Variable	Polysomnography	Self-report	Observation
Total sleep time	X	X	X
The time of onset of the end of stage 1 sleep until morning awakening	X		
Sleep latency (time to sleep onset)	X	X	X
Elapsed time from turning out the lights to three consecutive 30-second epochs of stage 1 or first epoch of stage 2	X		
Percentage of sleep time	X	X	X
Wake time after sleep onset	X	X	X
Number of arousals lasting 15 seconds or longer	X	X	X
Minutes and/or percentage of time for stages 1,2,3,4, and REM sleep	X		
REM density (percentage of 2-second mini-epochs containing one or more REMS)	X		
Number of sleep stage shifts/night	X		
Sleep efficiency (percentage of time in bed spent asleep)	X	X	X
Soundness of sleep		X	
Movement during sleep	X	X	X
Difficulty in falling asleep	X	X	X
Difficulty in falling back to sleep	X	X	X
Sleep interruption (number of nights/week and number of times/night awakened spontaneously)	X	X	X

Self-Reports

Nonphysiologic measures of sleep are of two types: self-reports and observations. Self-reporting measures vary widely and have been used to gather both qualitative and quantitative data.

▪ GENERAL SLEEP HABITS (GSH) QUESTIONNAIRE

In the classic study of psychologic and physiologic differences between good and poor sleepers, Monroe developed the General Sleep Habits (GSH) Questionnaire.[26] Content validity of this ten-item questionnaire was based on the results of three preliminary investigations that showed that people have definite impressions about whether they are good or poor sleepers. Good sleepers usually fall asleep in less than 10 but never more than 15 minutes, as a rule never wake up during the night, and as a rule have no difficulty in falling or remaining asleep. Poor sleepers usually take 60 minutes or longer (and always more than 30 minutes) to fall asleep, usually wake up at least once during the night, and report subjective difficulty in falling asleep.

Although no reliability data are provided, the predictive validity of the GSH Questionnaire was supported by the results of this study of 16 good and 16 poor sleepers. Subjects were classified as "good" or "poor" based on the results of the questionnaire. EEG sleep recordings revealed that poor sleepers had significantly less sleep time, a higher proportion of stage 2 sleep, markedly less REM sleep, more awakenings, and more required time to fall asleep than good sleepers.

The GSH Questionnaire elicits quantitative data through questions, such as:

How many nights per week do you awaken during the night?

Answers to such questions produce score data for each question. No composite scoring mechanism is described. Qualitative data are obtained through questions, such as:

How much do you enjoy sleep?

much enjoyment
moderate enjoyment
little enjoyment
no enjoyment

Responses to this type of question are presented by Monroe as frequency data, specifically as a percent of subjects who selected each category.[26]

• PARSONS AND VERBEEK ADAPTATION

In a nursing investigation of sleep–awake patterns in 15 patients following cerebral concussion, Parsons and VerBeek adapted this tool.[27] However, their instrument is reported to contain 50 items, and its validity and reliability are not addressed. Their questionnaire included collection of retrospective baseline data. Because their study involved head-injured patients, the researchers often had to help the subject read or complete the questions. They thought that injury-associated impairment of memory and comprehension may have influenced the results obtained with this tool. Such factors are of concern when using any questionnaire.

• SLEEP PATTERN QUESTIONNAIRE (SPQ)

Baekeland et al. developed a Sleep Pattern Questionnaire (SPQ) that they "used to advantage in a number of studies."[28,29] This instrument consists of 11 items that measure both qualitative and quantitative characteristics of sleep. Three items are filled out just before retiring, and 8 items are completed immediately after arising. This instrument is somewhat unique in that it includes such variables as subject's ratings of state of fatigue, soundness of sleep, and state of rest on awakening. An example from the SPQ is as follows:

State of rest on awakening
  A. Refreshed
  B. Still tired
  C. More tired than when you went to bed

Eight of the items are treated categorically, and three items are scored on a scale. The scored items include soundness of sleep (3 = deep, 2 = moderately deep, 1 = light), movement during sleep (3 = hardly moved, 2 = moved a little, 1 = tossed all night), and state of rest on awakening (3 = refreshed, 2 = still tired, 1 = more tired than when you went to bed). No composite scoring is described.

In comparing the SPQ to sleep recordings in 21 subjects, Baekeland and Hoy found that the subjects could accurately estimate sleep latency, number of awakenings longer than 4 minutes, and frequency of body movements.[29]

The SPQ was adapted for use in an experimental study by Browman and Tepas.[30] In a sample of nine subjects, they found that although there was a tendency to underestimate total sleep time and to overestimate sleep latency and awakenings, these subjective estimates did not differ statistically from EEG estimates, thus supporting the validity of this tool. Reliability was not addressed. Pacini and Fitzpatrick, two nurse investigators, used this instrument to examine sleep patterns of 38 hospitalized and nonhospitalized elderly patients.[31]

▪ DAILY SLEEP DIARY

Numerous other approaches to obtain subjective estimates of sleep have been used. Coates et al. used a Daily Sleep Diary in which subjects reported minutes to onset of sleep, minutes awake after sleep onset, number of awakenings, bedtime, and time awakened.[14]

▪ CARSKADON ET AL. SLEEP QUESTIONNAIRE

Carskadon et al. used a sleep questionnaire, which was given to 122 subjects before access to clocks in the morning.[22] Little information is provided about this questionnaire. The subjects were asked to estimate total sleep time, sleep latency, and number of arousals. They found that subjects consistently underestimated the amount of time they slept and the number of arousals and overestimated the amount of time it took them to fall asleep. Weiss et al. asked patients how many hours (to the nearest half-hour) they had slept. In addition, each patient was asked to rate the quality of his sleep on a scale of 1 to 5 (1 = very poor, 2 = poor, 3 = fair, 4 = good, 5 = very good).[32]

▪ SLEEP DYSFUNCTION SCALE

The Sleep Dysfunction Scale[33] is an easily administered questionnaire of four questions that measure number of days in which there were problems in falling asleep, staying asleep, early awakening, and awakening tired. The exact response categories are not described, but scores range from 4 (no sleep disturbance) to 20 (high sleep disturbance). The index of reliability is reported as 0.79 (Cronbach coefficient alpha). This scale has been used as part of a quality of life index in two studies, one on the impact of coronary artery bypass surgery[34] and the other on the effect of antihypertensive therapy.[33]

▪ LAMB SELF-REPORT QUESTIONNAIRE

Lamb developed a Self-Report Questionnaire in her study of newly diagnosed oncology patients.[35] Her instrument contained 34 questions about the participant's normal sleeping habits over the past year. This pretest questionnaire was adapted to a posttest form to assess sleep habits during hospitalization. This instrument is reported to include many items from questionnaires found in the literature plus categories, such as bedtime rituals, effects of menstruation on sleep, and aids used to enhance sleep. A sample question is as follows.

Do you ever have trouble falling asleep at home (or on the posttest in the hospital)?

always
sometimes
never

Although numerical scores are reported, the scoring of the questionnaire is not described. The questionnaire was pilot-tested in interview format on approximately ten oncology patients; however, the results of Lamb's study indicated that the sleep patterns of both samples of 30 hospitalized patients remained fairly equal in spite of significantly higher levels of depression in the oncology patients. This result led her to question the sensitivity of her instrument.

▪ SLEEP CARD

Another approach to obtaining self-reported sleep estimates is the use of a graph. In their study of sleep and wakefulness in the Arctic, Lewis and Masterton developed a Sleep Card that depicted a sleep pattern over a month.[36] Pacini and Fitzpatrick used the Sleep Card in addition to the SPQ in their study of geriatric patients in order to estimate total sleep time, a variable that is not included in the SPQ.[31]

▪ MODIFIED SLEEP CHART (MSC)

This original sleep card was modified by Floyd. The Modified Sleep Chart (MSC) (Fig. 15–1) consists of a graph with boxes representing 20-minute segments of a 24-hour period. The instructions are for the subject to place an S in the box if they judged that they had been sleeping for more than 10 minutes or an A if they were awake the whole time or slept less than 10 minutes.[37]

The validity and reliability of the original Sleep Card have not been established. Floyd checked the validity of the MSC by comparing it to nursing observations. For the 97 percent of the time when nurses were certain about the subject's sleeping or waking state, there were no discrepancies between staff and patient estimates of sleeping and waking. To date, no correlations between estimates obtained from Sleep Charts and polysomnography have been published.

Another point to consider is the time interval used on the chart. On the basis of her investigation of 70 psychiatric patients, Floyd believed that the use of a 20-minute interval was somewhat problematic, since patients are more accustomed to 15 or 30 minute time-frames.

Observations
Observations have been used to measure sleep. In Hagemann's study of hospitalized children, observations were made every 5 minutes, and the behavior was categorized as sleep, wakefulness, or arousal.[38] These variables were operationalized based on specific criteria. For example, "sleep was present when the child was lying motionless in bed, eyes were closed, respirations were slow and regular, body tone was relaxed, and the child was unresponsive to environmental stimuli, such as noise or light" (p. 5).[38] Sleep onset was determined by the time of the initial observation of sleep. Total sleep duration was the amount of time from sleep onset until termination, minus the total time lost by sleep disruptions. In this study, only one researcher observed the children. Using more than one observer would improve the reliability of the data.

INSTRUCTIONS

1. This chart will be used to record those times when you are sleeping or awake.
2. Each row of three boxes represents one hour; each box stands for one-third of an hour, i.e., 20 minutes.
3. For each 20-minute block of time, put an "S" in the box if you judge yourself to have *slept* 10 or more minutes.
4. If you slept less than 10 minutes or were *awake* the whole 20 minutes, put an "A" in the box.
5. Put an "S" only for the times actually spent sleeping; put an "A" for time spent awake in bed.
6. Please record the sleep times as honestly and accurately as possible.

		0–20 min. after	20–40 min. after	40–60 min. after
AFTERNOON	12 noon to 1 p.m.			
	1 to 2			
	2 to 3			
	3 to 4			
	4 to 5			
	5 to 6			
EVENING	6 to 7			
	7 to 8			
	8 to 9			
	9 to 10			
	10 to 11			
	11 to 12			
NIGHT	12 to 1 a.m.			
	1 to 2			
	2 to 3			
	3 to 4			
	4 to 5			
	5 to 6			
MORNING	6 to 7			
	7 to 8			
	8 to 9			
	9 to 10			
	10 to 11			
	11 to 12			

Figure 15–1. Modified Sleep Chart (MSC). (*Courtesy of Judith A. Floyd, R.N., Ph.D.*)

▪ FALLING ASLEEP BEHAVIORAL INVENTORY

In a study of falling asleep behavior of hospitalized children, White et al. developed a computer-compatible method for recording behavior data using the Senders Signals and Receivers System.[39] Such electronic keyboard systems have been shown to yield more accurate data on the order and timing of behavior.[40] These investigators developed a Falling Asleep Behavioral Inventory composed of 54 behaviors observed in children falling asleep. The behaviors were coded and grouped into mutually exclusive categories. An example set of codes with their corresponding behaviors is:

PO   Pouting
X   Crying
WH   Whimpering

Content validity was established through review of the instrument by experienced pediatric nurses. During the training period, an interrater reliability of 86 percent was obtained. The investigators then used this method to observe 18 hospitalized children for three consecutive nights.

▪ BAHR AND GRESS HOURLY OBSERVATIONS

In two descriptive pilot studies of sleep patterns in the institutionalized elderly, Bahr and Gress used hourly observations made independently by two observers.[41,42] Major categories that were coded included "sleeping," "restless," "awake," and "up out of bed." Awake activities were both physiologic (i.e., elimination, drinking, eating, and complaining of pain) and psychosocial (i.e., expression of feelings, activities, and talking). Of a total of 297 observations on 11 subjects, there was 93.9 percent agreement between observers.[41]

▪ OTHER STUDIES

Helton et al. measured sleep deprivation in 62 ICU patients by recording, via a flow sheet at the bedside, all interruptions per 15 minute blocks over a 24-hour period for 5 days.[43] An interruption was defined as any stimulus that decreased the time available for sleep. The total number of sleep cycles the subject experienced while in ICU was compared to the total ordinarily experienced in order to determine the cumulative degree of sleep deprivation. Subjects were then categorized on the basis of their cumulative deprivation (no sleep deprivation, moderately deprived—less than 50 percent loss of sleep, or severely deprived—more than 50 percent loss).

Weiss et al. had nurses observe if a patient was asleep or awake on the basis of regular respiration, closed eyes, relaxation and immobility, and relative lack of response to minor environmental stimuli.[32] In the previously cited study by Coates et al.,[14] spouses were used as observers and completed the same sleep diary as the subject.

VALIDITY, RELIABILITY, AND FEASIBILITY

Because EEG equipment is expensive and not widely available and because sleep recordings may be inappropriate in many clinical settings in which the measurement technique could in fact confound the results, there is a real need for a more practical yet valid measure of sleep. Although there have been numerous studies in which subjective and observational measurement were used, some serious concerns about the validity of such measures exist. In addition to the previously cited findings of Carskadon et al.,[22] a study comparing nurses' estimates, patients' self-reports, and polysomnograms found that nurses correctly estimated the amount of sleep of only 2 of the 14 subjects.[31] Only 4 of the 14 subjects correctly estimated the duration of their own sleep.

In a step beyond these simple correlational studies, Coates et al. applied the more powerful approach of the Multitrait Multimethod (MTMM) analysis.[14] By this method, two or more traits are measured by two or more methods in order to assess convergent validity, discriminant validity, and reliability. The matrix produced by this method presents intercorrelations resulting when each of several traits is measured by each of several methods.[44]

Rather than using various constructs, the traits in this study are variables that can be considered to estimate sleep. The variables included were minutes to sleep onset, number of awakenings, and minutes awake. These three parameters were then measured by three methods: self-report, spouse report, and sleep recordings. Reliability was established by using three recording nights. The investigation was conducted with two groups: one of 12 good sleepers and one of 12 insomniacs.

Convergent validity is found by the correlations for the same trait measured by different methods. For good sleepers, the correlations for minutes to sleep onset (0.99, 0.78, and 0.84) were significantly large. For insomniacs, both minutes to sleep onset (0.98) and minutes awake (0.88) were significant.

The study results support the use of self-reports of minutes to sleep onset as a reliable and valid measure for good sleepers and minutes awake and minutes to sleep onset as valid and reliable for insomniacs. Spouse reports were not found to be reliable or valid for either group. In fact for the insomniacs, data were unobtainable, since the spouses slept all night.

The use of the MTMM analysis in this study provided some important initial information on alternative measures of sleep. The use of this psychometric technique can make a significant contribution to future investigation in this area.

FUTURE PROJECTIONS

The MTMM analysis could be used to test reliability and validity of various instruments to measure sleep across various methods, across sleep parameters, and across groups or samples. In projecting a series of investigations, one could consider the following variants.

Methods
In comparison with the standard of sleep recordings, various forms of self-reporting (diaries, questionnaires, and interviews) could be evaluated. Observations of nurses, parents, or others could also be considered. It would be important to standardize the use of polysomnographic equipment across investigations.

Sleep Parameters
Multiple variables to measure sleep have been identified. Not all of these could be measured across methods, however (i.e., stages of non-REM sleep). Priority might rest on total sleep time, sleep efficiency, and percentage of sleep time. Phases of REM/non-REM sleep also could be considered via observations. The variables of onset of sleep and time awake should

be further studied in larger and different groups. Additionally, the whole concept of perceived quality of sleep could be investigated.

Samples

The study by Coates et al.[14] was with small samples (12 each) of good and poor sleepers. In addition to further investigation with larger samples in these groups, study in various clinical populations would be important. For example, it would be fruitful to use samples of depressed patients, psychotics, and alcoholics—all who have a tendency toward sleep dysfunction. It would be important to test in hospitals and in homes, in ICUs and on general floors, and in individuals with specific diseases, such as cancer, coronary disease, or diabetes.

By systematically altering these variables and using the MTMM analysis, it is hoped that an adequate self-report or observation instrument could be developed and tested in order to provide a practical, reliable and valid measure of sleep.

SUMMARY

The past 50 years have been marked by tremendous advances in the knowledge of sleep and its measurement.[45] The stages of REM/non-REM sleep have been identified on the basis of polysomnography. This method serves as a standard for quantitative measurement of sleep. However, the use of polysomnography is expensive and not always clinically feasible in nursing research. Instruments based on self-reports and observations also have been developed and used to some extent in nursing research. Additionally, instruments have been developed to qualitatively measure sleep. Further work to establish the validity and reliability of these instruments is needed.

REFERENCES

1. *Websters Third International Dictionary.* Springfield, MA: G & C Merriam, 1968.
2. Guyton, A.C., *Structure and function of the nervous system.* Philadelphia: Saunders, 1976.
3. Pletscher, A. Opening remarks. In R.G. Priest, A. Pletscher, & J. Ward (Eds.), *Sleep research.* Baltimore: University Park Press, 1979.
4. Weitzman, E.D. Sleep and its disorders. *Annu Rev Neurosci,* 1981, *4*:381.
5. Hammond, E.C., & Garfinkel, L. Coronary heart disease, stroke and aortic aneurysm: Factors in the etiology. *Arch Environ Health,* 1969, *19*(8):167.
6. Gordon, M. *Manual of nursing diagnosis.* New York: McGraw-Hill, 1982.
7. Gerner, R.H., Post, R.M., Gillen, J.C., & Bunney, W.E. Biological and behavioral effects of one night's sleep deprivation in depressed patients and normals. *J Psychiatr Res,* 1979, *15*(1):21.
8. Ross, J.J. Neurological findings after prolonged sleep deprivation. *Arch Neurol,* 1965, *12*(4):399.
9. Kollar, E., Namerow, N., Pasnaw, R., Naitoh, P. Neurological findings during sleep deprivation. *Neurology,* 1968, *18*(9):836.
10. Loomis, A.L., Harvey, E.N., & Hobart, G.A. Cerebral states during sleep, as studied by human brain potentials. *J Exp Psychol,* 1937, *21*:127.
11. Aserinsky, E., & Kleitman, N. Regularly occurring periods of eye motility, and concomitant phenomena during sleep. *Science,* 1953, *118*:273.
12. Chuman, M.A. The neurological basis of sleep. *Heart Lung,* 1983, *12*(2):177.
13. Usden, G., & Hawkins, D. *The office guide to sleep disorders.* New York: KPR Infor/Media, 1980.
14. Coates, T., George, J., Killen. J., et al. Estimating sleep parameters: A multitrait multimethod analysis. *J Consult Clin Psychol,* 1982, *50*(3):345.

15. Rechtschaffen, A., & Kales, A. (Eds.). *A manual of standardized terminology, techniques, and scoring system for sleep stages of human subjects.* Los Angeles: UCLA Brain Information Service/Brain Research Institute, 1968.

16. Hasan, J. Automatic analysis of sleep recordings: A critical review. *Ann Clin Res,* 1985, *17*(5):220.

17. Kupfer, D., Wyatt, R., Scott, J., et al. Sleep disturbance in acute schizophrenic patients. *Am J Psychiatry,* 1970, *126*(9):1213.

18. Hawkins, D., Mendels, J., Scott, J., et al. The psychophysiology of sleep in psychotic depression: A longitudinal study. *Psychosom Med,* 1967, *29*(4):329.

19. Snyder, F. Dynamic aspects of sleep disturbance in relation to mental illness. *Biol Psychiatry,* 1969, *1*(2):119.

20. Gross, M., Goodenough, D., Tobin, M., et al. Sleep disturbance and hallucinations in acute alcoholic psychoses. *J Nerv Ment Dis,* 1966, *142*(6):493.

21. Williams, H.L., & Rundell, O.H. Altered sleep physiology in chronic alcoholics. *Alcohol Clin Exp Res,* 1980, *5*(2):318.

22. Carskadon, M., Dement, W., Mitler, M., et al. Self-report versus sleep laboratory findings in 122 drug-free subjects with complaints of chronic insomnia. *Am J Psychiatry,* 1976, *133*(12):1382.

23. Broughton, R., & Baron, R. Sleep patterns in the intensive care unit and on the ward after acute myocardial infarction. *Electroencephalogr Clin Neurophysiol,* 1978, *45*:348.

24. Calvery, P., Brezenova, V., Douglas, N., et al. The effect of oxygenation on sleep quality in chronic bronchitis and emphysema. *Am Rev Respir Dis,* 1982, *126*(2):206.

25. Porter, J.M., & Horne, J.A. Bedtime food supplements and sleep: Effects of different carbohydrate levels. *Electroencephalogr Clin Neurophysiol,* 1981, *51*(4):426.

26. Monroe, L. Psychological and physiological differences between good and poor sleepers. *Abnorm Psychol,* 1967, *72*(3):255.

27. Parsons, L.C., & VerBeek, D. Sleep–awake patterns following cerebral concussion. *Nurs Res,* 1982, *31*(5):260.

28. Baekeland, F. Correlates of home dream recall: Reported home sleep characteristics and home dream recall. *Compr Psychiatry,* 1969, *10*(6):482.

29. Baekeland, F., & Hoy, P. Reported vs. recorded sleep characteristics. *Arch Gen Psychiatr,* 1971, *24*(6):548.

30. Browman, C., & Tepas, D.I. The effect of presleep activity on all-night sleep. *Psychophysiology,* 1976, *13*(6):536.

31. Pacini, C., & Fitzpatrick, J. Sleep patterns of hospitalized and nonhospitalized aged individuals. *J Gerontol Nurs,* 1982, *8*(6):327.

32. Weiss, B., McPartland, R., & Kupfer, D. Once more: The inaccuracy of non-EEG estimations of sleep. *Am J Psychiatry,* 1973, *130*:1282.

33. Croog, S.H., Levine, S., Testa, M.A., et al. The effects of antihypertensive therapy on the quality of life. *N Engl J Med,* 1986, *314*(26):1657.

34. Jenkins, C.D., Stanton, B.A., Savageau, J., et al. Coronary artery bypass surgery: Physical, psychological, social, and economic outcomes six months later. *JAMA,* 1983, *250*(6):782.

35. Lamb, M.A. The sleeping patterns of patients with malignant and nonmalignant diseases. *Cancer Nurs,* 1982, *5*(5):389.

36. Lewis, H.E., & Masterton, J.P. Sleep and wakefulness in the Arctic. *Lancet,* 1957, *1*:1262.

37. Floyd, J. Interaction between personal sleep-wake rhythms and psychiatric hospital rest-activity schedule. *Nurs Res,* 1984, *33*(5):255.

38. Hagemann, V. Night sleep of children in a hospital. Part 1: Sleep duration. *Matern Child Nurs,* 1981, *10*(2):1.

39. White, M., Wear, E., & Stephenson, G. A computer-compatible method for observing falling asleep behavior of hospitalized children. *Res Nurs Health,* 1983, *6*(3):191.

40. Simpson, M. Problems of recording behavioral data by keyboard. In M.E. Lamb, S.J. Suomi, & G.R. Stephenson (Eds.), *Social interaction analysis: Methodological issues.* Madison, WI: University of Wisconsin Press, 1979.

41. Gress, L., Bahr, R.T., & Hassanein, R. Nocturnal behavior of selected institutionalized adults. *J Gerontol Nurs,* 1981, *7*(2):86.

42. Bahr, R.T. Sleep-awake patterns in the aged. *J Gerontol Nurs,* 1983, *9*(10):534.
43. Helton, M., Gordon, S., & Nunnery, S. The correlation between sleep deprivation and the intensive care unit syndrome. *Heart Lung,* 1980, *9*(3):464.
44. Campbell, D.T., & Fiske, D.W. Convergent and discriminant validation by the Multitrait Multimethod Matrix. *Psychol Bull,* 1959, *56*(2):81.
45. Karnovsky, M. Progress in sleep. *N Engl J Med,* 1986, *315*(16):1026.

CHAPTER 16

Measuring Attitudes Toward Chronic Illness

Rebecca F. Cohen, R.N., Ed.D.

Chronic diseases constitute a major health threat to modern populations. Such diseases tend to be progressive, and as they progress, they affect adversely ever more aspects of daily life. The following four instruments were included not only because of their usefulness in measuring the impact of chronic illness on the patient's ability to function but also because of their unique, broad approach to the concept of human health. The Rapid Disability Rating Scale-2 (RDRS-2) and Simplified Disability Assessment Scales are geared toward what the patient actually does, not what he or she is able to do, as well as certain psychologic functioning. The Sickness Impact Profile (SIP) measures the impact of illness in terms of dysfunction, not levels of positive functioning, and evaluates psychosocial as well as physical health. The Arthritis Impact Measurement Scale (AIMS) measures physical health and emotional and social well-being.

MEASURES OF ABILITY TO FUNCTION

With the increasing numbers of elderly in our society and a similar increase in need for long-term care, there have been many instruments developed to measure physical functioning in order to determine the patient's needs so that they can be assigned to the appropriate level of care. These instruments are used also to assess the adequacy and composition of staff and to determine how patients respond to various modes of treatment. Some scales, such as the Sickness Impact Profile (SIP)[1] and Rand Measures of Health Status,[2] measure health status, that is, the patient's overall health described by diagnoses, doctor visits, days in bed, number of therapeutic drugs, self-assessed health, pain, and other variables, including the ability to perform everyday activities. Other measures, such as the Cumulative Illness Rating Scale (CIRS),[3] measure impairment, that is, the extent of organic pathologic change determined by a physician. Disability, or how impairment affects the person in regard to limitations of activities and functioning, is often measured by using the Barthel Index[4,5] and the Evaluation of Levels of Subsistence.[6]

Parts of scales that measure disability can be divided further into items that specifically measure either activities of daily living (ADL) or the instrumental activities of daily living (IADL). Examples of ADL scales are the Index of ADL[7] and the Physical Self-Maintenance Scale.[8] Examples of IADL scales are the Instrumental Activities of Daily Living Scale[8] and a subsection of the Multidimensional Functional Assessment (OARS) Scale. Some scales combine ADL and IADL items or may also include other health status variables.[9]

Chronic illness is the Number one health problem in the United States. Between 1900 and 1970, a shift was seen in mortality patterns from death from acute infections to the chronic illnesses, along with an increase in mortality rates from major chronic diseases of more than 250 percent. These changes have brought about the need for a new arrangement of values, priorities in policy, financing, and management of health care.[10,11]

Traditionally, professionals approached chronic symptom management in terms of compliance and service utilization and attempted to engineer the patient to the health team's treatment goals. However, it has been noted that this approach fails to incorporate an appreciation of the role played by personality variables in the development and outcome of chronic illness as well as how the chronic illness affects the individual emotionally and psychologically.

If health care providers are to influence the patient's adaptation to chronic illness, they must recognize the lay perception of illness and understand what the patient, as an individual, sees as relevant. A strong relationship has been shown between coping styles and attitudes and treatment results. This is important to remember because ineffective coping styles and damaging attitudes can affect treatment outcomes adversely and, therefore, need to be identified early in the course of diagnosis. By studying coping styles, perceptions, attitudes, beliefs, and illness behavior, we may be able to affect not only treatment outcomes (including mortality rates) and adaptation to chronic illness but also the initial development of the illness process itself.[10,11]

There has been a proliferation of investigations to study chronic illness from a wide variety of perspectives designed to evaluate the outcome of physical illness and its treatments, as well as the patient's response to physical disease.[12] Some of the instruments used to measure a patient's attitudes toward chronic disease discussed in this chapter also appear in other chapters. This overlapping of instruments, in terms of function, should be considered when determining which tool to use for a research project. There are many ways that chronic illness effects an individual: physically, psychologically, spiritually, emotionally. Often what appears simple on the surface is really quite complicated; for example, when measuring disability, it is important to consider not only what the patient cannot do but also what he or she will not do, for each may result in the same degree of confinement. As we learn more about the human mind and body, the measurement tools utilized grow more comprehensive in terms of approaching the patient as a whole rather than as separate entities. This chapter points out and emphasizes the growth that has occurred in the development of tools to measure patient attitudes.

Linn and Linn[9] point out that in institutions most of these functional status tests are completed by nurses or nursing attendants according to their observations of the patients. When used in the community, rating systems are often self-report inventories. Scales vary regarding the numbers of response choices, ranging from simple dichotomous (yes–no) scales to the 11-point SIP scale. Although the purpose of the yes–no response is to allow untrained people to rate reliably the answers, one disadvantage is that less variance in behavior can be described, and, thus, the scale may not be sensitive to treatment changes or to discrimination between levels of functioning. On the other hand, even trained raters find it difficult to distinguish between 11 different levels of an item, such as bathing. Generally, scales that maintain the best discrimination while still being easy to administer involve only four to seven responses.

Another problem with most of the instruments available to measure physical functioning is that they lack specificity for item definitions and can lead to unreliability. For example, does one measure whether an activity "is" or "can be" performed? A person may be physically able to dress unassisted but does not do so because of severe depression. One observer could rate the subject as able to dress without assistance, and another could rate the subject as requiring full assistance. Another source of discrepancy arises from lack of specificity about conditions for making assessments. The scale may not indicate whether the person is to be evaluated with or without glasses, a hearing aid, or other types of protheses.[9]

· RAPID DISABILITY RATING SCALE-2 (RDRS-2)

In response to the limitations of currently available instruments, Linn and Linn[9] revised Linn's Rapid Disability Rating Scale[13] into the Rapid Disability Rating Scale-2 (RDRS-2). Ratings in the RDRS-2 are made on the basis of what the person does and not on what he or she is able to do. There are 18 items, with 4-point scales ranging from "no assistance or disability" to "severe." The first group of items measures the ADL, and later items assess related disabilities and special problems of confusion, depression, and uncooperativeness in order to provide clues concerning the reasons for disability. Sample questions include:

1. **Assistance with activities of daily living**   **Degree of Disability**

   a. Eating   None   a little   a lot   spoon-fed   IV tube

   b. Walking (with cane or walker, if used)   None   a little   a lot   doesn't walk

   c. Dressing (include help in selecting clothes)   None   a little   a lot   must be bathed

2. **Degree of disability**

   a. Communication (expressing self)   None   a little   a lot   does not communicate

   b. Sight (with glasses, if used)   None   a little   a lot   does not see

   c. In bed during day (ordered or self-initiated)   None   a little (<3 hrs)   a lot   most/all of time

3. **Degree of special problems**

   a. Mental confusion   None   a little   a lot   extreme

   b. Depression   None   a little   a lot   extreme (p. 380)[9]

Items on the RDRS-2 are scored from 1 = none to 4 = severe. Therefore, total scores can range from 18 (no disability) to 72 (if the responses indicating the most severe disabilities are chosen for all items). Since the scale is short, it is sometimes useful to examine item scores between groups when more detailed information is needed about types of disabilities. Item definitions and instructions for ratings appear on the scale, so that little training is needed in making assessments. The scale can be used by any person who knows the subject to be rated and who has observed him or her in the activities of daily living.[9]

Intraclass correlations between the findings of two nurses who independently rated the same 100 patients were found to range from $r = 0.62$ to a high of $r = 0.98$; all were statistically significant. Reliability was also shown by testing the same 50 patients twice within a 3-day period. Test–retest values ranged from $r = 0.58$ to $r = 0.96$ between the first and second ratings by Pearson product moment correlations.[9]

Rating scale measurements using both the RDRS-2 and the Maryland-Barthel Disability Index[5] found that the test of functional status is useful in predicting outcome. Items on the RDRS-2 were used to predict mortality in a stepwise multiple regression as well as by discriminant function analysis. All items together reached an r of 0.20, with the best predictors of mortality being the need for assistance with eating, incontinence, time in bed, diet, and depression. For accuracy of classification, the scale correctly identified patients who would die 72 percent of the time.[9]

In another study to validate the RDRS-2, ratings on the RDRS-2 were correlated significantly with ratings of impairment on a 13-item scale made independently by physicians ($r = 0.27$) and with the patient's self-reports of health on a 6-point scale ($r = 0.43$). Thus, the RDRS-2 appears to be an easy to use, reliable, and valid measure of physical functioning that may provide a more comprehensive look at disability than other instruments. However, it must be remembered that subjects used in the development of this instrument were all elderly, and their degree and type of physical problem were not stated.[9]

▪ SIMPLIFIED DISABILITY ASSESSMENT SCALE

A test for the evaluation of patients with chronic illness developed by Sett[14] is also important because it, too, was an attempt to simplify the measurement of disability in hospitalized patients. Although developed some time ago, it can still serve as a useful tool in caring for patients with chronic illnesses and should be expanded beyond its experimentation with patients with cerebrovascular accident.

Sett[14] studied other disability instruments and chose from the ADL three areas that he considered the most essential factors for the independence of the patient in caring for himself or herself at home: ambulation, self-care, and communication. Four examiners performed the testing procedures separately on 20 patients who had had a cerebrovascular accident. They were instructed not to communicate their findings until each had tested the patient in the designated ADL areas. The Chi-square test was applied to the data to determine the statistical significance. The p value was less than 0.01 in all three areas. The simplified disability test was conducted as follows:

Ambulation
The examiners were told to have the patient demonstrate his ability to walk or perform a transfer to or from a wheel chair. A scale of 0 = patient is confined to bed to 5 = patient walks without assistance was utilized.

Self-care
This was a test of the patient's ability to carry out such activities of daily living as eating, dressing, bathing, and toilet-care. A scale of 0 = patient is unable to perform any of the activities of daily living (ADL) without assistance to 5 = patient performs ADL using both upper extremities was developed. In arriving at scores for self-care; seven questions were used in addition to observing the movements of the patient.

Communication
Communication scores ranged from 0 = patient has severe expressive-receptive (global) aphasia to 5 = patient has neither aphasia nor dysarthria. The test used was a modification of the Schuell technique. The score was based on the patient's responses to approximately 9 commands and questions (p. 1096).[14]

The Sett[14] test for evaluating disability levels in patients with chronic illness was used initially by medical students to measure a patient's improvement or regression relative to his environment or continued therapy. The elaborate tests employed by physical therapists and occupational therapists were considered complex and time-consuming, and, therefore, the simplified tests were needed to provide quick, yet comprehensive, data-gathering techniques.

• SICKNESS IMPACT PROFILE (SIP)

The Sickness Impact Profile (SIP) was developed to provide a measure of perceived health status that is sensitive enough to detect changes or differences in health status that occur over time or between groups. It is useful for a variety of types and severity of illness and across demographic and cultural subgroups. Also, the SIP, which measures the behavioral impacts of illness in terms of dysfunction, not levels of positive functioning, is intended to provide a measure of the efforts or outcomes of health care that can be used for evaluation, program planning, and policy formulation.[1]

The SIP, which was discussed at length in Chapter 2, contains 136 statements about health-related dysfunction in 12 areas of activity. It includes not only measures of physical functioning but also four psychosocial categories: social interaction, alertness behavior, emotional behavior, and communication. It can be administered by an interviewer in 20 to 30 minutes or can be self-administered. In completing the SIP, the subject is asked to endorse or check only those statements that he or she is sure describe him or her on a given day and are related to his or her health.[15]

The test–retest reliability ($r = 0.92$) and internal consistency ($r = 0.94$) of the SIP were investigated using different interviewers, different forms, different administration procedures, and a variety of subjects who differed in type and severity of dysfunction. Overall, the reliability of the SIP in terms of score was high ($r = 0.75$ to 0.92), and reliability in terms of items checked was moderate ($r = 0.45$ to 0.60). Reliability did not appear to be affected significantly by the variables examined, which suggests that the SIP is useful potentially for measuring dysfunction under a variety of administrative conditions and with a variety of subjects.[16] Convergent and discriminant validity of the SIP was assessed using the Multitrait Multimethod technique and deemed appropriate for an instrument that attempts to measure a characteristic for which there is no criterion.[17]

An interesting question that must be addressed in relation to the results of the SIP Scale, as useful and beneficial as it may be, is that of the reliability of self-ratings versus service provider ratings when analyzing disability and dysfunction. This question was undertaken by a team of researchers in Finland, and their results provide some interesting information about the ability of patients to self-assess their own functional levels.

Kivela[18] points out that there are three main methods by which disability can be measured: clinical assessment of the individual's performance, questioning the individual about his current level of daily performance, and standard tests of individual performance conducted by a trained observer. The purpose of this study was to compare the questionnaire-based disability with the evaluation made by health care professionals. In all, 205 chronic patients and elderly people who were receiving home nursing or home help services or both were included in the study. A questionnaire was developed using activities listed in standardized measurements of ADL and IADL. Comparisons between the questionnaire-based and rater assessments of performance were then made for individual activities of self-care and domestic duties, including the following six activities: dressing, eating, daily washing, bathing or sauna, cooking, and cleaning.[18]

For rating the activities of dressing, eating, and daily washing, the patients were asked to perform the activity. When rating the activities of bathing or sauna, cooking, and cleaning, the home nursing personnel relied on their previous knowledge of the performance. However, in order to obtain information about cooking and cleaning, the following two questions were included in the questionnaire:

Who usually cooks in your household?

Who usually cleans in your household?

The answers were rated according to the person who usually cooked or cleaned of which there were two categories: (1) the person performs the task himself or herself or together with another person, and (2) the person does not perform or is not able to perform the task. The question concerning dressing, eating, daily washing, and bathing or sauna was:

Can you perform the following tasks yourself or do you need help?

There were four possible categorizations: (1) the person can perform the activity himself or herself without auxiliary means or without another person's help, (2) the person always needs auxiliary means when performing the activity, but he or she does not need another person's help, (3) the person nearly always needs another person's help to some extent in order to be able to perform the activity, and (4) the person always needs quite a lot of another person's help when performing the activity.[18]

Results of this study indicated that agreement between the questionnaire-based and the provider ratings was not very high for housework. In using dichotomous scales, the overall percentage of cases in which there was matching was 77 percent for cooking activities and 64 percent for cleaning activities. The levels of agreement between the questionnaire-based and the provider ratings were, however, high for the more basic self-care activities. In using quadritomous scales, the percentage of cases in which there was total agreement between these two measurements was 94 to 97 percent for the activities of dressing, eating, and daily washing. The more complex self-care activities, that is, bathing and sauna, showed a lower proportion of complete agreement than the three basic activities, 84 percent. Kivela[18] points out that the extent of the observer's earlier knowledge about the patient's performance and about the environment may have affected the results, as may the differences in the educational levels of the observers, although an attempt was made to measure the effect of their clinical background. It is evident, however, that self-report questionnaires and provider ratings agree very well in terms of self-care activities but not as well for cooking and cleaning activities.

• ARTHRITIS IMPACT MEASUREMENT SCALES (AIMS)

Meenan et al.[19] state that despite the multiple indices currently in use to evaluate the health status of people with arthritis, available methods still fail to provide reliable, valid, and comprehensive measures of the health of these patients. The major difficulty, they believe, is that these methods focus on physical health to the exclusion of mental and social well-being. As a disabling chronic disease, arthritis frequently produces serious limitations in multiple areas of function, and these measures are not able to assess such changes. As a result, they have developed the Arthritis Impact Measurement Scales (AIMS), which were designed to measure all three areas of human health: physical, emotional, social well-being.

The AIMS were constructed by building on two previously tested health status measures: Bush's Index of Well-Being and the Rand Health Insurance Study batteries. The Index of Well-Being is a behaviorally based scale that includes three function/dysfunction scales (mobility, physical activity, social activity) and a symptom-problem complex. The Rand approach combines the three behavioral components of the Index of Well-Being with psychologic scales for anxiety and depression. Both approaches have undergone extensive testing and refinement.[19]

One hundred arthritis patients were included in the study, and subjects were considered ineligible if their arthritis diagnosis was unclear or if they had any major comorbidity, such as other illnesses or medication use, that could impact on their health status. The AIMS instrument was self-administered either at the time of the clinic visit or at home. When completed, the questionnaire was given to the subject's physician who was asked to complete a three-item supplement indicating the doctor's opinion of the patient's functional level, recent arthritis activity, and number of affected joints.[19]

Analyses were directed toward measuring the scaling characteristics of the grouped items and examining the validity of the resulting scales. Related groups of questionnaire items were examined initially to determine the extent to which they met the characteristics of Guttman-format scales. In this type of scale, higher scores reflect more limitation (lower health status), and subjects at each scale level generally exhibit a similar pattern of limitation. Guttman scale scores were computed based on the total number of items failed, rather than using the rank of the highest item failed. This approach minimized the need to make assumptions about the probable direction of error in atypical response patterns.[19] Further data related to reliability and validity are discussed in Chapter 2.

The initial AIMS instrument consisted of demographic and health status items arranged into nine scale groups. The groups and the number of items in each were as follows: Mobility contained 5 items, Physical Activity 5, Social Activity 9, Social Role 7, ADL 5, Pain 5, Dexterity 5, Anxiety 8, and Depression 6. The other 11 items were related to health perceptions and overall estimates of functional status and arthritis severity. Sample questions in the categories of Social Activity, Anxiety, and Depression, which are integral components of attitudes toward chronic illness, included:

Social Activity
About how often were you on the telephone with close friends or relatives during the past month?
During the past month, about how often did you get together socially with friends or relatives?

Depression
During the past month, how often did you feel that others would be better off if you were dead?

How often during the past month did you feel that nothing turned out for you the way you wanted it to?

Anxiety

During the past month, how much of the time have you felt tense or "high strung"? How much of the time during the past month were you able to relax without difficulty? (p. 149)[19]

Individual health status items showed an impressive degree of disease impact in the study group. At least 25 percent of the subjects indicated difficulties with the vast majority of items, and a minimum of 5 percent had problems even with basic ADL items. The AIMS instrument was found to be easily completed by patients, the scales had a great deal of face validity and were easy to score in either Guttman or Likert format, and after deleting some questions due to confusion or low item-total correlation, all of the scales, with the exception of Social Activity, fulfilled a number of generally accepted criteria for reliability and scalability. The significance of the correlations held for both patient-generated and physician-generated health status proxies. Thus, the instrument was found to be practical, simple, and dependable and should prove useful for evaluating a wide variety of interventions in the area of arthritis. [19]

MEASURES OF ILLNESS BEHAVIOR

The concepts of illness behavior and the sick role have tremendous implications for public health programs, estimated needs for medical care, medical economics, and our understanding of health and illness in general. For example: What brings an "ill" person to a medical setting? What is the influence of various norms, values, fears, and expected rewards and punishments on how a symptomatic person behaves? What makes one person suffer in silence while another seeks immediate health care for the slightest discomfort? Are there systematic differences in illness behavior in given populations, and, if so, what effect would these differences have on the provision of educational and informational programs? All of these questions have been addressed in various research investigations through the use of three very important instruments: the Illness Behavior Questionnaire (IBQ), Dimensions of the Sick Role, and the Illness Self-Concept Repertory Grid.

DIMENSIONS OF THE SICK ROLE AND THE ILLNESS BEHAVIOR QUESTIONNAIRE (IBQ)

The term "illness behavior" refers to the ways in which symptoms may be differentially perceived, evaluated, and acted (or not acted) on by different kinds of people. Whether by reason of earlier experiences with illness, differential training in respect to symptoms, or otherwise, some people will make light of symptoms, shrug them off, and avoid seeking medical care; others will respond to the slightest twinges of pain or discomfort by quickly seeking such medical care as is available. [20,21]

▪ DIMENSIONS OF THE SICK ROLE

Kassebaum and Baumann[20] conducted research more than 20 years ago, using their test Dimensions of the Sick Role, to study the sick role and illness behavior in patients with chronic illness. It is important to discuss their research because their findings provided the foundation for the Illness Behavior Questionnaire (IBQ), which was later developed by Pilowsky and Spence in 1975.[22]

The test, Dimensions of the Sick Role, developed by Kassebaum and Baumann,[20] involved having patients with one or more primary diagnoses of chronic illness respond to 20 statements with stipulated response alternatives ranging from "strongly disagree" to "strongly agree" on a 7-point Likert-type scale. The method of factor analysis was selected for its advantage in permitting the subjects to cognitively group items. A scale was constructed for each factor, using the factor's most highly loaded items. Each respondent was given a sum score on each factor's scale. The distribution of scores for each factor scale was trichotomized into "high," "medium," and "low" categories.

Factor analysis yielded four factors. Although no two factors had their highest loadings supplied by the same items, nearly all items had some loading on each factor. Despite this overlapping, inspection of the highly loaded items on each factor indicated that among this sample of respondents, four distinct dimensions underlying sick role expectations could be observed: dependence, reciprocity, role performance, and denial. Sample questions on the Dimensions of the Sick Role included:

Factor 1: Dependence

    a. Illness makes a person a burden on other folks around him.
    b. The trouble with being ill is that you have to depend on other people.
    c. The most important thing for a sick person to understand is that he needs outside help because he cannot help himself.

Factor 2: Reciprocity

    a. People in general realize it is not the patient's fault that he is ill.
    b. While a woman is sick, people don't blame her for not managing the home the way she normally does.
    c. Most people do not blame a person for being sick.

Factor 3: Role performance

    a. People who are sick have a right to expect that others will help them.
    b. Often the only rest a busy person gets is when he is sick.
    c. When a person is sick, he usually isn't expected to hold a job.

Factor 4: Denial

    a. Many people act sicker than they are just in order to get sympathy.
    b. Most sickness is due to careless and wrong living habits.
    c. A person's health is his own responsibility just like any other part of his life.
    d. Most people do not understand the problems a sick person has in his life. (p. 20)[20]

Results of the investigation found that high scores on individual dimensions of the sick role varied with age, sex, ethnic origin, education, occupational category, and diagnosis. Chronic illness, the investigators suggested, may, therefore, be regarded as one subtype of the sick role, having special characteristics. Because of these characteristics, patients with chronic illness are likely to perceive the structure of the sick role along dimensions that differ from those perceived by patients with acute, temporary illness. Within the broad classification of chronic illness, they found that different diagnoses had different consequences for different kinds of people; for example, patients with arterio-scleritic heart disease (ASHD) were found to have almost double the number of high scores on the dimensions of dependence, reciprocity, role-performance, and denial as patients with diabetes. Diabetes patients were distinguished from patients with other diseases studied by their low level of denial. For this reason, the authors suggested further research into the concept of the sick role and illness behavior in terms of different types of illness, different social settings and different segments of the population.[20] The IBG later was developed to serve as a useful tool in such research efforts.

• ILLNESS BEHAVIOR QUESTIONNAIRE (IBQ)

In order to understand better the concept of illness behavior in relation to a specific symptom (in this case, pain), Pilowsky and Spence[22] conducted a research study with unselected patients referred to either the pain clinic or the psychiatric service of a large metropolitan hospital for the management of intractable pain. They developed the IBQ to determine the patient's attitudes and feelings about his or her illness, the patient's perception of the reactions of significant others in the environment (including doctors) to himself or herself and the illness, and the patient's own view of his or her current psychosocial situation. It is important to mention this questionnaire within the section on chronic illness measurements because of its potential for use with a variety of medical illnesses or symptoms and its importance in trying to understand how patients feel about their illness and symptoms.

The 52-item IBQ developed by Pilowsky and Spence[22] was administered to 48 men and 52 women with a mean age of 49.1 years. The commonest site of pain was in the back, followed by the head and the abdomen. The average length of time that patients had experienced pain was 7.4 years and ranged from 6 weeks to 60 years. There was no significant relationship between age and the duration of pain ($r = 0.12$). Fifty-five percent of the patients were judged to have only minor organic pathologic involvement, 25 percent moderate, and 20 percent major. Forty-two percent of the patients were judged to have mild impairment, 31 percent moderate impairment, and 27 percent marked impairment of customary functioning due to pain.

Responses to the IBQ (plus information concerning the patient's age, sex, and length of pain) were factor analyzed using the method of principal component analysis and rotated to orthogonal structure. Seven factors accounting for 63.3 percent of the variance were extracted. Items with loadings greater than 0.40 on these factors were used to construct seven subscales. Scoring was weighted arbitrarily in the direction of "abnormal" or "maladaptive" illness behavior such that a value of 1 was allotted to each "abnormal" response. The score on a particular scale is thus regarded as an index of the patient's relative position on the dimension of illness behavior reflected by the factor. High scores suggest maladaptive ways of perceiving, evaluating, or acting in relation to one's state of health.

The seven subscales and sample questions include:

1. Scale 1 (general hypochondriasis)
    a. If you feel ill and someone tells you that you are looking better, do you become annoyed?
    b. Are you more sensitive to pain than other people?
    c. Do you find that you get jealous of other people's good health?

2. Scale 2 (disease conviction)
    a. Does your illness interfere with your life a great deal?
    b. Do you find that you are bothered by many different symptoms?

3. Scale 3 (psychological versus somatic perception of illness)
   a. Do you ever think of your illness as a punishment for something you have done wrong in the past?
   b. Is your bad health the biggest difficulty of your life?

4. Scale 4 (affective inhibition)
   a. Can you express your personal feelings easily to other people?
   b. When you are angry, do you tend to bottle up your feelings?

5. Scale 5 (affective disturbance)
   a. Do you find that you get anxious easily?
   b. Do you find that you get sad easily?

6. Scale 6 (denial of problems)
   a. Except for your illness, do you have any problems in your life?
   b. Do you have any family problems?

7. Scale 7 (irritability)
   a. Does your illness affect the way you get on with your family or friends a great deal?
   b. Do you find that you get angry easily? (p. 64)[23]

The results of the numerical analysis showed six principal clusters of patients, each with definite illness behavior characteristics. Groups 1 through 3 had a relatively nonneurotic, reality-oriented attitude to illness as indicated by low scores on the first three scales. The symptom (pain) experience seemed part of what might be regarded as an adaptive reaction to stress but one which obscured all other aspects of the stress response. Groups 4 through 6 related more clearly to the syndrome of abnormal illness behavior. The symptom (pain) was interwoven with and was symptomatic of a personality disorder or an essentially maladaptive response to psychologic stress.[23]

· ILLNESS SELF-CONCEPT REPERTORY GRID

In an attempt to extend the use of the IBQ, Large[24] used a repertory grid technique that involved using various self-concepts as elements and concepts drawn from the IBQ as constructs. The expectation was that subjects scoring high on the disease conviction scale of the IBQ, since they presumably conceived of themselves as being ill, would similarly rate themselves toward the ill pole of the illness construct of the grid. Since illness is considered undesirable, one might expect a considerable difference on this construct between the patient's self-concept at the present time and his ideal self-concept. The patients with the greatest discrepancy between self and ideal-self concepts were hypothesized to have the most self-dissatisfaction and, therefore, would have the most motivation toward treatment and show the greatest improvement.

The grid was constructed using the following elements and bipolar constructs:

A. Elements
   1. As I am
   2. As I would like to be
   3. As others see me

    4. As my doctor sees me
    5. Like a "hypochondriac" or "neurotic"
    6. Like a physically ill person

B. Bipolar constructs and rating scales
    1. Worried about illness ("not at all" to "a great deal")
    2. Ill ("not at all" to "seriously ill")
    3. Emotionally distressed ("not at all" to "extremely distressed")
    4. Free in expressing positive and negative feelings to others ("bottle all feelings up" to "express all feelings regardless of consequences")
    5. Depressed ("not at all" to "so miserable that life is not worth living")
    6. Anxious ("not at all" to "panic stricken")
    7. Worried about problems apart from illness ("not at all" to "a great deal")
    8. Irritable ("not at all" to "ready to explode") (p. 282)[24]

Eighteen patients with chronic musculoskeletal pain were told that the purpose of the study was to gain some insight into their own views of themselves and their world and, therefore, they were being asked to complete a questionnaire. The repertory grids were then completed by each patient during an initial interview in which the subject was exposed to biofeedback. A second grid was completed at the final interview (posttrial), using identical elements and constructs. Thus, for each of the 18 subjects, two ratings of the grid were obtained, before and after exposure to the experimental and control conditions.[24]

The grids were analyzed by means of the principal component analysis devised by Slater for use with individual grids. This output provides measurements of the correlations and angular distances between constructs, the distances between elements and the principal components with loadings of the elements, and constructs on the first three components. In this study, the main focus of interest was the distance between element 1 (as I am) or "self" and element 2 (as I would like to be) or "ideal self," derived from the initial grid for each subject. The Spearman rank correlation coefficient was computed among three rankings: changes in pain scores calculated pretrial and posttrial, distances between elements 1 ("self") and 2 ("ideal self"), and correlations between electromyelogram (EMG) activity ratings and pain scores. The rank correlation between pain score changes and element 1–2 distance was $r = 0.43$, which was a significant rank correlation at alpha = 0.05. Thus, the greater the element 1–2 distance, the greater the decline in pain scores.[24]

The distance between elements 1 and 2 derived from the grids can be regarded as an expression of the discrepancy between self and ideal self concepts in these 18 subjects. The main finding was that there is a significant rank correlation between this measure and outcome as measured by total pain score change. The self/ideal self discrepancy might be construed as a measure of denial and resistance. An interesting finding of the study was that many of the subjects depicted themselves as being quite close to their ideal states on the grid, as could be seen by the fact that 11 patients had an element 1–2 distance that was smaller than expected. The smaller the self/ideal self discrepancy, the more satisfied the patient was with himself or herself and the more likely it is that he or she will not respond to biofeedback.[24]

Comparisons between the grids completed before and after the trial reflected changes in the element 1–2 distances, suggesting that this measurement is not stable over time and may be subject to treatment effects. Because the Illness Self-Concept Repertory Grid measures the more intrapsychic variables of self-concept, which may relate to denial and resistance, Large[24] believes that the grid could be used as an instrument to predict the optimum timing of treatment, that is, to predict when the patient is ready to respond to treatment. Further research with this grid, however, is suggested to ascertain its reliability as a prognostic tool in a variety of patients and diseases.

Closely related to the concept of illness behavior are beliefs about internal versus external control. Through comprehensive investigation of how patients with chronic illness feel about themselves, the world around them, and the relationship between the two, techniques can be tailored to individual expectancies to increase the possibility of a successful treatment outcome. The Health Locus of Control (LOC) Scale, Health-Specific Locus of Control Beliefs Questionnaire, and the Attribution Interview Schedule are three instruments that will aid in providing direction to research projects related to locus of control.

▪ HEALTH LOCUS OF CONTROL SCALE (LOC)

Social learning theory explains behavior potential in specific situations as a function of the expectancy that reinforcement will occur and the value of that reinforcement for the individual. Each time an individual's behavior is followed by the expected outcome, the individual's expectancy that the reinforcement is related to that behavior is increased. A history of reinforcements not related to individual effort results in the expectancy that reinforcements are not contingent on one's own behavior but dependent on an outside source.[25] Therefore, according to Rotter,[26] these two different reinforcement patterns lead to either the general expectancy that rewards are contingent on internal resources, such as effort, or the general expectancy that rewards are externally related to such things as luck, chance, fate, or powerful others. General expectancy is referred to as "locus of control."

One of the early scales used to measure generalized expectancies was the Rotter Internal-External (I-E) Locus of Control Scale.[27,39] This scale, although widely used, has often created contradictory findings because of its multidimensionality and limited predictive ability.[25] Wallston et al.[28] hypothesized that research predicting behavior in specific situations could profit from the use of more specific expectancy measures. Their research, therefore, was based on the assumption that a health-related locus of control scale would provide more sensitive predictions of the relationship between internality and health behaviors. The result of their research was the Health Locus of Control (LOC) Scale.

The LOC Scale[28] was developed using a 6-point, Likert-type format. An item pool consisting of 34 items written as face-valued measures of generalized expectancies regarding locus of control related to health was administered to 98 college students. Subjects also completed the Rotter I-E Scale and the Marlowe-Crowne Social Desirability Scale and provided demographic data. An item analysis was run, and 11 items were chosen for the final scale:

1. If I take care of myself, I can avoid illness. (internal direction)
2. Whenever I get sick, it is because of something I've done or not done. (internal direction)
3. Good health is largely a matter of good fortune. (external direction)
4. No matter what I do, if I am going to get sick I will get sick. (external direction)
5. Most people do not realize the extent to which their illnesses are controlled by accidental happenings. (external direction)
6. I can only do what my doctor tells me to do. (external direction)
7. There are so many strange diseases around that you can never know how or when you might pick one up. (external direction)
8. When I feel ill, I know it is because I have not been getting the proper exercise or eating right. (internal direction)
9. People who never get sick are just plain lucky. (external direction)
10. People's ill health results from their own carelessness. (internal direction)
11. I am directly responsible for my health (internal direction) (p. 581).[28]

The LOC Scale is scored in the external direction, with each item scored from 1 (strongly disagreed) to 6 (strongly agree) for the externally worded items and reverse scored for the internally worded items. It has a potential range of 11 (most internal) to 66 (most external). For the original scale, the mean was 35.57, and the standard deviation was 6.22. Alpha reliability of the 11 items chosen by specific criteria was 0.72. In addition, the LOC Scale did not reflect a social desirability bias as evidenced by alpha = −0.01 correlation with the Marlowe-Crowne Social Desirability Scale. Concurrent validity was evidenced by a 0.33 correlation ($p < 0.01$) with the Rotter I-E Scale for the original sample.[28]

To further test the new instrument, two studies were conducted to provide tests of the differential functional utility of the LOC Scale and the I-E Scale. Research has indicated that people who hold internal as opposed to external expectancies are more likely to assume responsibility for their health, particularly if they value health highly. Thus, such people should choose to expose themselves to more information about a given health condition than those with internal expectancies, who value health less or than those with external expectancies regardless of the value they place on health.[29] To test this theoretical assumption, Wallston et al.[28] conducted a study using 88 college students to determine the degree to which they sought information about hypertension. Results indicated a correlation between the I-E Scale and the LOC Scale of 0.25 ($n = 85$), indicating that the LOC Scale did, in fact, provide evidence of relationships between internal-external locus of control beliefs and health value beliefs that the I-E Scale was not able to identify. The results of this study have been replicated by Wallston et al.[30]

A second study used to test the LOC Scale involved the social learning theory that internals will be more likely to take steps to better their environmental condition than externals. It was hypothesized that subjects participating in a weight-reduction program that was consistent with their generalized expectancies would be more satisfied and more successful than subjects in a program inconsistent with their locus of control beliefs. This hypothesis was supported by the findings, which indicated a correlation between the I-E Scale and the LOC Scale of 0.46 ($n = 34$) and a test–retest reliability of the LOC Scale over an 8-week interval of 0.71.[28,30]

• HEALTH-SPECIFIC LOCUS OF CONTROL BELIEFS QUESTIONNAIRE

Whereas the LOC Scale provides an initial attempt to operationalize health-related locus of control beliefs, it is similar to the I-E Scale in that it is a generalized measure of expectancy as opposed to beliefs about specific behaviors. The authors of the LOC Scale have suggested that specific instruments should be developed to aid in better predicting particular behaviors in particular situations. This process was undertaken by Lau and Ware,[31] who attempted to make refinements in the instrument by developing the Health-Specific Locus of Control Beliefs Questionnaire. This questionnaire was constructed to measure a person's beliefs about self-control over health, provider control over health, chance health outcomes and general health threat, health care attitudes, health status perceptions, and value placed on health.

Lau and Ware[31] conducted exploratory studies out of which came 28 health-related locus of control items. Each item was worded as a statement of opinion (e.g., "There is little one can do to prevent illness.") and was associated with a seven-choice response scale ranging from "strongly agree" to "strongly disagree." Three weeks after the first administration, the subjects (college students in a psychology class), returned to fill out 68 items a second time to estimate reliability using a test–retest method. Internal consistency reliability was estimated using the alpha formula and data from all subjects. In the absence of agreed-upon criteria against which to judge the validity of the health-specific locus of control scales, another factor analysis was performed.[31]

The Health-Specific Locus of Control Beliefs Questionnaire as developed by Lau and Ware[31] has many similarities to the LOC Scale created by Wallston et al.[28] The content of items in the questionnaire's self-care, provider control, and chance scales is similar to the LOC Scale's internal, powerful other, and chance scales. However, Lau and Ware added a fourth dimension (general health threat) that appears to be independent of the others and has potential usefulness in health services research. In addition, Lau and Ware believe that each dimension in their questionnaire has been developed in a much more balanced manner, in terms of the direction of item wording, than other instruments.

The four scales in the Health-Specific Locus of Control Beliefs Questionnaire may be useful as dependent measures in the evaluation of interventions that attempt to alter beliefs about self-control and provider control over health. They may be useful also in distinguishing high-risk individuals who are unlikely to take personal responsibility for their own health from those who prefer to take more personal responsibility for their care. Outcomes may be better achieved by way of a good match between health-specific locus of control beliefs and treatment plans.[31]

▪ NAGY AND WOLFE'S COMPLIANCE TOOL

Another very important use of the construct of health locus of control can be found in the work of Nagy and Wolfe.[32] They conducted research, utilizing the health locus of control construct and the Health Belief Model, to predict compliance with medical regimens in chronically ill patients. They were testing the ability of Wallston's HLC Scale not only to predict a specific variable (compliance) but also to determine how well it could identify differences among specific diseases (adult-onset diabetes, hypertension, and pulmonary disease). Data for their study were collected from three groups of chronic disease patients: 52 adult-onset diabetic patients, 49 hypertensive patients, and 48 respiratory patients (emphysema, asthma, and bronchitis sufferers).

Two interviews were held, the first lasting 30 minutes to gather demographic information and information about value of health to the patient, perceived severity of illness, outlook on illness, experienced symptoms, satisfaction with clinic treatment, social support for treatment, and health locus of control beliefs. Three health locus of control scales were administered: the Internal Health Locus of Control Scale (measures a person's belief that health is a consequence of one's own actions and under personal control), the Chance Health Locus of Control Scale (assesses attributions of health status to chance factors), and the Powerful Others Health Locus of Control Scale (evaluates the person's expectations that health professionals or family affect one's health outcomes). The patients' perceptions of their medical problems were determined by using the following questions. All items were summed to form the symptoms index, with high scores indicating more symptoms:

1. Severity
   How would you describe the seriousness of your condition? (four response alternatives; high scores indicated perceived seriousness)

2. Outlook
   A. In the future, do you think your condition will probably improve, get worse, or remain the same? (five response alternatives)

    B. Do you think your condition will improve or remain the same as the result of treatment at this clinic? (four response alternatives; expected improvement was indicated by high scores)

3. Symptoms

Two sets of questions were used: one focused on the extent to which the patient's medical condition limited mobility, caused eating or sleeping problems, and prevented him from working or seeing others; the other set tapped the absence or presence of specific disease symptoms (disease specific) (p. 914–915).[32]

The second interview took place 6 months later and involved having the patient describe the medication and self-management procedures prescribed for him or her and the degree of compliance and then having the patient complete a two-page questionnaire about the patient's medication, self-management prescriptions, and compliance with treatment.[32]

Overall, Nagy and Wolfe[32] found a disappointing lack of relationship between the health locus of control scales and the compliance measures. However, they point out that recent studies with chronic disease patients have reported inconsistent findings. It is believed that the long-term, chronic nature of this population may account, in large part, for the tenuous relationships found between health control beliefs and compliance. Some studies on compliance involve patients just beginning treatment, whereas the patients in the Nagy and Wolfe study had been in treatment for an average of 17 years. Research has pointed out frequently that noncompliance increases with length of medical treatment. There is evidence also that health beliefs may be important initially but that other variables become more influential later. Thus, this study reemphasized the multidimensional nature of compliance and has suggested that cognitive variables in general, and health locus of control beliefs specifically play a limited role in determining compliance in chronic disease patients.[32]

• WEINER'S ATTRIBUTION MODEL

In response to the limitations of the HLC Scale, Weiner's Attribution Model has been used to study causal attributions for success and failure outcomes of chronically ill patients. Lowery and Jacobsen[33] conducted a study to compare arthritic, diabetic, and hypertensive patients, and Lowery et al.[34] focused only on patients with arthritis.

Attribution theory is concerned with the analysis of causal explanations, that is, how an individual ascribes a cause to an effect. According to the theory, such causal explanations are predictive of behavioral and emotional reactions of people to life events, both personal and interpersonal. The ultimate goal in a person's search for causal explanations, the "Whys" of life events, is management or control over the self or the environment.[34]

Weiner has found that causes most often given in response to achievement situations fall into three dimensions: (1) locus, whether the cause is internal or external to the person, (2) stability, whether or not the cause is changeable, and (3) control, whether the cause is under volitional control or is controlled by outside forces. The findings indicate that self-esteem is linked to the locus dimension, that is, when events are viewed as internally caused, people feel pride in positive events and shame in negative events. Expectancies are linked to the stability dimension, that is, if a person attributes success to a stable factor, expectations of success in similar future situations occur. The control dimension seems to be linked to feelings of helplessness and to interpersonal behaviors. Thus, construction of causal explanations and the characteristics of the causes, whether they promote loss of self-esteem, pessimism, and helplessness or their opposites, have been shown to have important motivational consequences. However, Weiner's research was conducted in academic situations, and the present exploratory research was conducted to test his theory in the nonacademic real-world situation of chronic illness.[33,34]

In relation to chronic illness, it is believed that situations of great importance involving possibility of loss or those that involve stress or unexpected outcomes are more likely to evoke causal questions than others. Some chronic illnesses, such as arthritis, have all of these elements, and since a direct causal link between previous events and the current condition is not always easily identified, the attributional question "Why" may occur. If Weiner's Attribution Model, which is based on achievement-related research, can be generalized to such real-life situations, knowing how patients answer the "Why" question may provide insight about their reactions to the illness.[33,34]

To test the use of Weiner's Attribution Model on patients with chronic disease, Lowery et al.[34] had 55 male rheumatoid arthritis patients from 29 to 85 years of age complete the Multiple Affect Adjective Checklist (MAACL), the Convery Index, and the Attributions Interview Schedule, in that order.

▪ MULTIPLE AFFECT ADJECTIVE CHECKLIST (MAACL)

The MAACL is self-administered and measures the three affects of anxiety, depression, and hostility. Test–retest reliability coefficients for the state measures are reported as low, which is expected, since moods vary from day to day. The test takes 5 to 10 minutes to complete.[35]

▪ ATTRIBUTIONS INTERVIEW SCHEDULE

The Attributions Interview Schedule, designed by the investigators,[34] began with an open-ended question:

1. With respect to your arthritis, have you ever thought about "Why me"?

2. If so, how did you answer it?

3. If not, please take a moment and think about it now.

Subjects were then asked to rate, as accurately as possible, the current success or nonsuccess of their treatment and to predict what its future success or failure might be. These ratings were made on a 4-point scale, with 1 as "not at all successful" and 4 as "very successful." In a separate questionnaire, physicians were asked to rate the current success of a patient's treatment.[34]

▪ CONVERY INDEX

Functional capacity was determined through the use of the Convery Index, an individual assessment by interview requiring approximately 15 minutes. This inventory consists of two parts: Daily Living Skills, such as feeding, and Mobility Skills, such as walking outdoors. Each item has a 7-point scale, which can be rated by an interviewer. Scores on the section for Daily Living Skills range from 0 (incapacitated) to 49 (able to perform all activities, including employment). Scores on Mobility range from 0 (totally dependent) to 56 (able to complete all activities under ordinary circumstances). Reliability evidence is given by Convery et al.[36] for interviewer concordance. Validity evidence is cited for correlation of the inventory with independent physician assessment.

Results indicated that although most arthritics constructed causes to explain their arthritis, some did not. The causes most often ascribed for the "Why me?" question fell within the external, stable, and uncontrollable dimensions, suggesting support for Weiner's theory if one defines the development of arthritis as a "failure" with respect to health. The arthritics' attribution of illness (or health failure) to a task difficulty (external and uncontrollable causes) supports the theory that people tend to ascribe failures externally and successes to effort (internal, stable, and controllable causes). What was not supported by this study was the idea that some blaming of self contributes to better outcomes in the illness situation, since there was no differentiation, in terms of estimates of treatment success or affect scores, between the groups.[34]

The most interesting finding was that those arthritics who did not ascribe causes in the response to the "Why me?" question were significantly more depressed, anxious, and hostile than those giving causes. This finding suggests that deciding "Why me?" may be an adaptive response to illness events.[34] In addition, it was demonstrated that arthritics who were less functional (i.e., have low scores in activities of Daily Living and Mobility) were significantly more depressed than other subjects.

Another study was undertaken by Lowery and Jacobsen[33] in which arthritic, diabetic, and hypertensive patients were compared to determine differences in perceived causes of successes or failures in illness, outcomes, and expectations between groups. Subjects were interviewed and asked to discuss the current general status of their disease. Patients were then asked to rate how well they were doing with their illness on a 4-point scale (1 = very well, 4 = not at all well). Because attribution theory is based on causes given for success versus failure, the scale was collapsed to two categories for analysis. Evidence for the validity of this measure of self-estimate of outcome was gathered from the subject's physicians, who provided an independent judgment of treatment success on the same type of 4-point scale. When the physician's ratings were collapsed to two categories of success and failure, the agreement between the two perceptions was 79 percent.[33]

The following procedure was then followed[33]:

A. Patients were asked an open-ended question on causal attributions for their success or failure:

Why do you think things have been going well?

Why do you think you're having problems?

B. After the open-ended question, the interviewers presented each patient with ten statements representing possible causes for disease outcome, to be rated on a 5-point scale (1 = not a cause, 5 = extremely important cause). The ten items were stated negatively (e.g., "I am not doing well because I am unlucky") for subjects who had initially rated their outcomes as failures:

1. I am doing well because I am lucky.
2. It's because of God that I am doing well.
3. I am doing well because my disease is fairly easy to control.
4. I am doing well because I get good advice from my doctor.
5. I am doing well because the drugs are making me better.
6. I am doing well because of other people helping.
7. I am doing well because I have been in a good frame of mind.
8. I have the type of body that responds well to treatment.
9. I am doing well because I do what I should to manage my disease.
10. I am doing well because I try to be healthy in every way (p. 84).[33]

C. After all items were rated, the patient was asked to agree or disagree with the following statement:
    Some people say that there is no real reason why they are doing well (or not well)—it's just happening.
D. Patients were asked about their expectations for their future outcome:
    In terms of the future, how do you expect your disease to do?
    The same 4-point scale used previously for the self-estimate of current disease outcome served also for the rating of the future. Again, the scale was collapsed to the two categories of success and failure for analysis.
E. Finally, descriptive information about the patient was gathered as well as information about treatment protocol and disease onset

When all data were collected, answers were scored on the basis of three dimensions: locus, stability, and controllability. Each dimension could receive from 1 to 3 points, depending on the answer, and each patient received three scores, one for each dimension. Interrater consistency was assessed for the dimensional scores by using analysis of variance to estimate reliability. The reliability coefficients for locus, stability, and control dimensions were 0.72, 0.86, and 0.89, respectively.[33]

Results of this study indicated that most patients readily reported causes for their illness outcomes, and these causes generally fell into the same dimensions as reported by Weiner: locus, stability, and controllability. An interesting finding that was similar to the earlier work done by Lowery et al.[34] was that some patients did not give a cause for their outcome. Further, in both the open-ended and closed-ended format the "don't know" answer was given significantly more often by those who perceived that they were failing than by those who perceived success with their illness. As seen in earlier research, chronically ill people who believe they are in trouble show different causal thinking patterns than those less troubled and tend to say "I don't know" or believe there is no reason for one's illness when asked about causal relationships.[33]

▪ CHRONICITY IMPACT AND COPING INSTRUMENT: PARENT QUESTIONNAIRE (CICI: PQ)

The CICI: PQ was developed in response to a perceived need by participants in a series of interdisciplinary conferences. It was thought that there was no satisfactory method for assessing the impact of chronic illness on families or measuring the outcome of intervention. Therefore, the CICI: PQ was developed to obtain parental perceptions of their child's chronic illness or disability and information on how parents cope with difficulties they encounter as a result of their child's condition. Thus, the instrument can be used by nurses to assist in the identification of needs of the families of chronically ill and disabled children. Also, it is hoped that the instrument could be used to measure the outcome of intervention strategies designed to meet the needs identified in the initial assessment.[37]

The instrument was developed following interviews with 63 mothers and fathers of children with either cystic fibrosis, biliary atresia, inherited metabolic disorders, hematologic disorders, spina bifida, juvenile diabetes mellitus, or osteogenesis imperfecta. The interview protocol made use of the critical incident technique, with critical incidents designed to elicit information about satisfying and problematic areas related to living with a chronically ill child and coping strategies used to solve identified problems.[37]

Parent interviews were tape-recorded and then transcribed to facilitate content analysis. Themes related to problems, satisfactions, resources, and coping strategies were analyzed. Situations and resources problematic for some parents were satisfactory for others; thus, the problems, satisfactions, and resources categories were included in a larger category—stressors. Subcategories of stressors included resources, knowledge, childrearing, family relationships, family adjustment, and management of the child's condition. The second major category, coping strategies used by parents to manage stressors, contained six subcategories: seeking behaviors, utilizing behaviors, managing stressors, modifying strategies, anticipatory planning, and helping and supporting others.[37]

Hymovich[37] then developed a closed-ended questionnaire that used the categories and subcategories described. Questions were organized into six sections, each designed to obtain information about stressors and coping strategies:

A. Your child (the child with the condition)

B. Yourself (parent completing the questionnaire)

C. Your spouse

D. Brothers and sisters

E. Hospitalization

F. Other

The instrument is self-administered and can be completed in approximately 20 minutes. For two-parent families, the author recommends that each parent independently complete the questionnaire.

The instrument went through several revisions to reduce redundancy and eliminate questions that were too specific to an age group or condition. Content validity was established by submitting the CICI: PQ to a clinical psychologist, three master's prepared registered nurses caring for families of children with chronic disorders, and a doctorally prepared nurse faculty member working with chronically ill adults. Hoyt's coefficient was used to determine internal consistency. Reliability for the stressor category was 0.94 and for the coping strategies 0.93. Further analysis of reliability and validity of the instrument is suggested by the author using a larger sample of parents of children with a wide variety of chronic conditions.[37]

Other Instruments

Instruments described in the Appendix fall within two categories: Tools to measure attitudes of patients with specific diseases

1. Hypertensive Interview Schedule
2. Respiratory Opinion Survey (RIOS)
3. Multiple Sclerosis Adjustment Scale

Tools to measure attitudes of patients with chronic diseases

1. Health-Related Hardiness Scale (HRHS)
2. Total Anxiety Scale
3. Social Readjustment Scale
4. Psychosocial Adjustment to Medical Illness (PAIS)
5. Coping with Chronic Illness: A self-appraisal device
6. Cantril's Self-Anchoring Striving Scale

These tools are different from those previously discussed in several ways: they tend to be less conceptual and more straightforward about attitudes toward chronic disease, they often are the only tools used in the study as opposed to the use of several tools, and although some were tested only on well subjects and others included well subjects, they all have many implications for use with patients with chronic disease.

APPENDIX. OTHER INSTRUMENTS

Name of instrument	Hypertensive Interview Schedule[38]
Dimensions, superordinate categories	This instrument is divided into three sections, with various subsections:

1. Measures of health perception
   a. Health status
      The patient is asked to put himself or herself on a 9-point scale of health: 1 = poorest health, 9 = best health.
   b. Presence of symptoms
      The patient is asked which of a list of 16 symptoms he or she has. Each symptom is given a score ranging from 1 (never) to 7 (always). Individual symptom scores are summed to produce a total score.
   c. Worry about health
      The patient lists his or her degree of worry about health on a 9-point scale ranging from 1 = no worry to 9 = most worried possible.
   d. Work absenteeism and illness days
      The patient estimates the number of days absent from work and illness days in the previous month.
2. Lifestyle
   a. Participation in physical and social activities
      The patient estimates the number of hours spent in an average week doing the above and the degree of difference from previous year's activities.
   b. Ability to participate
      Patient rates ability to participate in activities on a 9-point scale ranging from 1 = no participation to 9 = can do all activities.
   c. Self-care behaviors (list)
3. Problems and beliefs (list)

Target population	Testing was done on 100 adult hypertensives and 50 normotensive controls.
Method of administration	Interview format
Reliability and validity	For between-group comparisons, Yates' Chi-square test or Fisher's exact proportions test was used to assess nominal level data and the Mann-Whitney U-test was used for ordinal or interval level data. Kendall's tau was used to measure strength of association between pairs of variables. Analysis of covariance was used to test for differences between groups.
Utilization	To determine the effect of being treated for hypertension on health perception and lifestyle and the duration of any alterations after first being diagnosed

Name of instrument	Respiratory Opinion Survey (RIOS)[11]
Dimensions, superordinate categories	This questionnaire has 41 statements arranged in 7 clusters:

c1	Optimism (5 items)
c2	Negative regard (9 items)
c3	Specific internal awareness (4 items)
c4	External control (5 items)
c5	Psychologic stigma (5 items)
c6	Authoritarian attitudes toward illness and hospitalization (8 items)
c7	Unnamed triplet (3 items)

Target population	Testing was done on 78 adult asthmatic patients in a residential treatment program.
Number of items	41 statements arranged in 7 clusters
Method of administration	Self-report survey form
Scoring	A 5-point rating scale is used: 1 = strongly agree, 5 = strongly disagree. Subjects are asked to respond to each of the 41 statements in the seven clusters.

Reliability and validity	Internal consistency reliabilities were:

	First administration	Second administration
c1	0.73	0.80
c2	0.65	0.84
c3	0.49	0.68
c4	0.67	0.76
c5	0.64	0.82
c6	0.71	0.78

Test—retest reliabilities ranged from 0.64 (c2) to 0.79 (c5).

Utilization	To determine how directly, how subtly, and in exactly what directions attitudes influence the response to treatment. This will allow treatment programs to be tailored for maximum effectiveness and to focus efforts on changing the patient's attitudes in some crucial way.

Name of instrument	Multiple Sclerosis Adjustment Scale[39]
Dimensions, superordinate categories	This scale is used to identify the multiple sclerosis (MS) patient's capacity to maintain distress within manageable limits, to invest emotional concern and energy in non-MS areas, to reevaluate life values and priorities, and to maintain optimism and interest in the future.
Target population	Testing was done on 97 adult MS patients from an MS treatment center
Method of administration	Self-report
Scoring	Statements are scored in either a positive (good adaptation) direction or a negative (poor adaptation) direction on a Likert-type scale basis.
Reliability and validity	Reliability was found to be alpha = −0.79.
Utilization	To determine a chronic illness patient's ability to adapt to life with disease and exacerbations of the disease's course.

Name of instrument	Health-Related Hardiness Scale (HRHS)[40]
Dimensions, superordinate categories	Three categories are included in this instrument: 1. Commitment (15 items) 2. Challenge (15 items) 3. Control (18 items)
Target population	The scale was tested on 60 adult-onset diabetes, arthritis, or hypertension patients.
Number of items	The HRHS is a 48-item measurement
Method of administration	Self-report
Scoring	Items are scored on a 6-point Likert scale.
Reliability and validity	Testing found an alpha coefficient of 0.86. Internal consistency for the three subscales was: 1. Commitment: alpha = 0.74 2. Challenge: alpha = 0.84 3. Control: alpha = 0.82
Utilization	To determine direct and indirect relationships between the hardiness characteristics and physiologic and psychosocial adaptation to chronic illness

Name of instrument	Total Anxiety Scale[41]
Dimensions, superordinate categories	Patient is asked questions pertaining to his or her feelings about: 1. Death: fears of dying 2. Mutilation: fears of mutilation (as a result of the disease) 3. Separation: feelings of loneliness and loss 4. Guilt: feelings of moral disapproval and adverse criticism from others 5. Shame: criticisms coming from self and representing feelings of inadequacy and embarrassment 6. Diffuse: feelings of tension and vague fears; source is not immediately apparent

Target population	Initial subjects were 88 adult chronically ill patients who were interviewed once while hospitalized and again after discharge.
Method of administration	Interview format and tape recorded answers (with patient's knowledge)
Reliability and validity	Canonical correlation (CANONA) was applied to analyze relationships between each set of continuously measured variables (demographic factors, biographic factors, type of disability, handicap during hospitalization, goals during hospitalization, handicap in the community, goals set in the community, perceived gains, and patient's goal attainment) and the anxiety subscale scores.
Utilization	To examine the relationship between patterns of anxiety in patients with chronic illness and indices of rehabilitation in order to develop and assess postdischarge care services

Name of instrument	Social Readjustment Scale[42]
Dimensions, superordinate categories	Life events
Target population	The instrument was tested on 394 well subjects, but implications for chronically ill patients.
Number of items	43 life events are listed.
Method of administration	Self-report, paper and pencil test
Scoring	The subject rates each life event according to his or her perception of the degree of readjustment required by each event in a person's life.
Reliability and validity	All coefficients of correlation between discrete groups (Pearson's r) were above 0.90 (statistically significant) with the exception of the relationship between white and black subjects, which was 0.82. Kendall's coefficient of concordance (tau) for the 394 individuals was 0.477, significant at the $p = <0.0005$ level.
Utilization	To determine the psychological significance and emotions engendered in a particular patient by certain life events and to study the relationship between that event and the onset of medical illness

Name of instrument	Psychosocial Adjustment to Medical Illness (PAIS)[12,43]
Dimensions, superordinate categories	Seven independent domains: 1. Health Care Orientation 2. Sexual Relationships 3. Vocational Environment 4. Domestic Environment 5. Extended Family Relationships 6. Social Environment 7. Psychologic Distress (Items 3 and 4 provide an assessment of Role Function; items 5 and 6 provide an assessment of Social Support factors; item 7 looks at Intrapsychic Functioning.)
Target population	Testing was done with patients treated for Hodgkin's disease for at least 2 years and parents whose children had been treated for Hodgkin's disease or solid tumors. PAIS was later used with renal dialysis patients, lung cancer patients, cardiac patients, and hypertensives.
Number of items	45 multiple choice questions
Method of administration	Self-report questionnaire
Length of administration	20–30 minutes
Scoring	Rating is done on a 4-point Likert scale. Scores are summed for each domain and for the overall adjustment score.
Reliability	Interrated reliability coefficients were[a]: 1. Total scale score 0.83 2. Health care 0.70

3. Sexual	0.81
4. Vocational	0.62
5. Domestic	0.52
6. Family	0.33 (not significant)
7. Social	0.72
8. Psychologic	0.82

Validity
With an $r = 0.34$ significant at the $p < 0.05$ level, with df $= 35$, the intercorrelation matrix indicated that all dimensions were significant except for the Vocational (0.22) and Family (0.08) areas.

Utilization
To determine the outcome or impact of medical illness and its treatments on patients and their families

---

[a] Correlation coefficients above 0.50 considered statistically significant.

Name of instruments	Coping with Chronic Illness: A self-appraisal device[44]
Dimensions, superordinate categories	Six clusters of coping strategies were presented to the subject on six separate cards. Respondents were asked to rank the strategies from the one they were most likely to use (1) to that which they were least likely to use (6). The context and structure of the interview schedule, of which this request was a part, defined this request as referring to their illness and the implications it had for them. The clusters of strategies, with an example of a statement that would indicate use of that strategy, were:

1. Action: "I try to find out the cause of my problem."
2. Control: "I control my feelings."
3. Escape: "I cry, smoke, or eat."
4. Fatalism: "I accept that much of life is difficult."
5. Optimism: "Things usually work out fine."
6. Interpersonal coping: "I talk with friends about the problems."

Target population
The coping instrument was tested in 3 separate studies:

1. 92 chronically ill versus well subjects to determine differences in coping strategies—inhospital use only
2. 46 chronically ill subjects to determine differences in strategy preferences among patients with different types of chronic illness in different situations—inhospital and at-home use
3. Chronically ill patients only to determine associations between preferences for coping strategies and emotional reactions to chronic illness—inhospital and at-home use

Method of administration
Interview format

Reliability and validity
Overall reliability coefficient for a sample of 45 people with few stresses and relatively stable lives over 1 month was 0.70. Each cluster had a reliability score of:

1. Action	0.43
2. Control	0.30
3. Escape	0.30
4. Fatalism	0.50
5. Optimism	0.38
6. Interpersonal	0.54

Estimates of reliability over a shorter period of time (1 day) with a smaller sample ($N = 10$) have shown higher estimates; overall $r = 0.90$, with a range of 0.79–0.92 for the clusters.

Utilization
To determine the extent to which certain factors (demographic characteristics, lifestyles, illness roles, degree of disability, perceived handicap, and achievement of rehabilitation goals) are related to preferences for different coping strategies

Name of instrument	Cantril's Self-Anchoring Striving Scale[45]
Dimensions, superordinate categories	Cantril's Self-Anchoring Striving Scale is a 10-step ladder designed to assess a person's general sense of well-being at three points in time: past, present, and future. As described by Cantril, the scale was based on the premise that each individual's expression of concerns, values, and life perception can be used to establish top and bottom points of a self-defined measurement continuum. In this context, life satisfaction is viewed as the fit between present life experience and the best and worst possible life conditions. The best condition is identified in terms of highest aspiration; the worst as the greatest fear.
	The subject is asked to describe the best possible life for him or her and worse possible life. They are shown a drawing of a ladder with 10 rungs and told the top represents the best possible life and the bottom represents the worse life. They are to show where they now stand on the ladder; where were they 5 years ago; where will they be 5 years from now?
Target population	Model has been used in a variety of research projects to investigate life satisfaction of patients with chronic illness. Laborde and Powers[46] compared life satisfaction levels of patients undergoing hemodialysis and patients suffering from osteoarthritis. Brown et al.[47] compared patients with coronary artery disease with patients with COPD and also utilized measurements for disability and health locus of control.
Method of administration	Interview format
Scoring	Answers are coded into meaningful categories that make it possible to compare different groups.
Reliability and validity	Endpoints of the scale are self-defined, thus, the numerical ratings reflect individual criteria. Because of this, traditional notions of reliability may not be applicable to this type of scale. A rating by one person is not the same as a rating by another person. The extremes are entirely personal, and thus, the meaning of the endpoints remains relatively constant for a given individual over time, thereby minimizing error variance. Studies have reported test–retest reliability coefficient of 0.65 after administering Cantril's scale to 378 community residents over a 2-year period.[48]
	The face validity of the scale is supported by the overt relationship between the nature of the instrument and the phenomena under study, i.e., life satisfaction.
Utilization	Different chronic diseases differ in their impact on life satisfaction of the individuals involved. Further study is needed with a variety of diseases and populations to determine the effect of chronic illness.

REFERENCES

1. Bergner, M., Bobbitt, R.A., Carter, W.B., & Gilson, B.S. The sickness impact profile: Development and final revision of a health status measure. *Med Care,* 1981, *19*(8):787.
2. Brook, R.H., Ware, J.E., Davies-Avery, A., et al. Overview of adult health status measures fielded in Rand's health insurance study. *Med Care,* 1979, *17*(Suppl):(entire issue).
3. Linn, B.S., Linn, M.W., & Gurel, L. Cumulative illness rating scale. *J Am Geriatr Soc,* 1968, *16*:622.
4. Mahoney, R.I., & Barthel, D.W. Functional evaluation: The Barthel index. *Md State Med J,* 1965, *14*:61.
5. Wylie, C.M., & White, B.K. A measure of disability. *Arch Environ Health,* 1964, *8*:834.

6. Gauger, A.B., Brownwell, W.M., Russell, W.W., et al. Evaluation of levels of substance. *Arch Phy Med Rehabil,* 1964, *45:*286.
7. Katz, S., Ford, A.B., Moskowitz, R.W., et al. Studies of illness in the aged. The index of ADL: A standardized measure of biological and psychosocial function. *JAMA,* 1963, *185:*914.
8. Lawton, M.P., & Brody, E. Assessment of older people: Self-maintaining and instrumental activities of daily living. *Gerontologist,* 1969, *9:*179.
9. Linn, M.W., & Linn, B.S. The Rapid Disability Rating Scale-2. *J Am Geriatr Soc,* 1982, *30*(6):378.
10. Forsyth, G.L., Delaney, K.D., & Gresham, M.L. Vying for a winning position: Management style of the chronically ill. *Res Nurs Health,* 1984, *7*(3):181.
11. Kinsman, R.A., Jones, N.F., Matus, I., & Schum, R.A. Patient variables supporting chronic illness. *J Nerv Ment Dis,* 1976, *163*(3):159.
12. Morrow, G.R., Chiarello, R.J., & Derogatis, L.R. A new scale for assessing patient's psychosocial adjustment to medical illness. *Psychol Med,* 1978, *8:*605.
13. Linn, M.W. A rapid disability rating scale. *J Am Geriatr Soc,* 1967, *15:*211.
14. Sett, R.F. Simplified tests for evaluation of patients with chronic illness (cerebrovascular accidents). *J Am Geriatr Soc,* 1963, *11:*1095.
15. Carter, W.B., Bobbitt, R.A., Bergner, M., & Gilson, B.S. Validation of an interval scaling: The Sickness Impact Profile. *Health Serv Res,* 1976, *11*(4):516.
16. Pollard, W.E., Bobbitt, R.A., Bergner, M., et al. The Sickness Impact Profile: Reliability of a health status measure. *Med Care,* 1976, *14*(2):146.
17. Bergner, M., Bobbitt, R.A., Pollard, W.E., et al. The Sickness Impact Profile: Validation of a health status measure. Med Care, 1976, *14*(1):57.
18. Kivela, S-L. Measuring disability—Do self-ratings and service provider ratings compare? *J Chronic Dis,* 1984, *37*(2):115.
19. Meenan, R.F., Gertman, P.M., & Mason, J.H. Measuring health status in arthritis. *Arthritis Rheum,* 1980, *23*(2):146.
20. Kassebaum, G.G., & Baumann, B.O. Dimensions of the sick role in chronic illness. *J Health Human Behav,* 1965, *6*(1):16.
21. Mechanic, D. The concept of illness behavior. *J Chronic Dis,* 1962, *15:*189.
22. Pilowsky, I., & Spence, N.D. Patterns of illness behavior in patients with intractable pain. *J Psychosom Res,* 1975, *19*(4):279.
23. Pilowsky, I., & Spence, N.D. Illness behavior syndromes associated with intractable pain. *Pain,* 1976, *2*(1):61.
24. Large, R.G. Prediction of treatment response in pain patients: The illness self-concept repertory grid and EMG feedback. *Pain,* 1985, *21*(3):279.
25. Lowery, B.J. Misconceptions and limitations of locus of control and the I-E scale. *Nurs Res,* 1981, *30*(5):294.
26. Rotter, J.B. *Social learning and clinical psychology.* Englewood Cliffs, NJ: Prentice-Hall, 1954.
27. Rotter, J.B. Generalized expectancies for internal versus external control of reinforcement. *Psychol Monogr,* 1966, *80*(1):(entire issue).
28. Wallston, B.S., Wallston, H.A., Kaplan, G.D., & Maides, S.A. Development and validation of the Health Locus of Control (HLC) Scale. *J Consult Clin Psychol,* 1976, *44*(4):580.
29. Strickland, B.R. Internal-external expectancies and health-related behavior. *J Consult Clin Psychol,* 1978, *46*(6):1192.
30. Wallston, K.A., Maides, S., & Wallston, B.S. Health-related information seeking as a function of health-related locus of control and health value. *J Res Pers,* 1976, *10*(2):215.
31. Lau, R.R., & Ware, J.F. Refinements in the measurement of health-specific locus-of-control beliefs. *Med Care,* 1981, *19*(11):1147.
32. Nagy, V.T., & Wolfe, G.R. Cognitive predictors of compliance in chronic disease patients. *Med Care,* 1984, *22*(10):912.
33. Lowery, B.J., & Jacobsen, B.S. Attributional analysis of chronic illness outcomes. *Nurs Res,* 1985, *34*(2):82.
34. Lowery, B.J., Jacobsen, B.S., & Murphy, B.B. An exploratory investigation of causal thinking of arthritics. *Nurs Res,* 1983, *32*(3):157.

35. Zuckerman, M., & Lubin, B. *Manual for the multiple affect adjective check list.* San Diego, CA: Educational and Testing Service, 1965.
36. Convery, F.R., Minteer, M.A., Amiel, D., & Connett, K.L. Polyarticular disability: A functional assessment. *Arch Phys Med Rehabil,* 1977, *58:*434.
37. Hymovich, D.P. The chronicity impact and coping instrument: Parent questionnaire. *Nurs Res,* 1983, *32*(5):275.
38. Milne, B.J., Logan, A.G., & Flanagan, P.T. Alterations in health perception and life-style in treated hypertensives. *J Chronic Dis,* 1985, *38*(1):37.
39. Counte, M.A., Bieliauskas, L.A., & Pavlou, M. Stress and personal attitudes in chronic illness. *Arch Phys Med Rehabil,* 1983, *64*(6):272.
40. Pollock, S.E. Human responses to chronic illness: Physiologic and psychosocial adaptation. *Nurs Res,* 1986, *35*(2):90.
41. Viney, L.L., & Westbrook, M.T. Patterns of anxiety in the chronically ill. *Br J Med Psychol,* 1982, *55:*87.
42. Rahe, R.H., & Holmes, T.H. The social readjustment rating scale. *J Psychosom Res,* 1967, *11:*213.
43. DeVon, H.A., & Powers, M.J. Health beliefs, adjustment to illness, and control of hypertension. *Res Nurs Health,* 1984, *7*(1):10.
44. Viney, L.L., & Westbrook, M.T. Coping with chronic illness: Strategy preferences, changes in preferences and associated emotional reactions. *J Chronic Dis,* 1984, *37*(6):489.
45. Cantril, H. A study of aspirations. *Sci Am,* 1963, *208*(2):41.
46. Laborde, J.M., & Powers, M.J. Satisfaction with life for patients undergoing hemodialysis and patients suffering from osteoarthritis. *Res Nurs Health,* 1980, *3*(1):19.
47. Brown, J.S., Rawlinson, M.E., & Hilles, N.C. Life satisfaction and chronic disease: Exploration of a theoretical model. *Med Care,* 1981, *19*(11):1136.
48. Laborde, J.M., & Powers, M.J. Life satisfaction, health control orientation, and illness-related factors in persons with osteoarthritis. *Res Nurs Health,* 1985, *8*(2):183.

CHAPTER 17

Measuring Cancer Attitudes

Nancy Burns, R.N., Ph.D.

The word "cancer" generates in all of us a terror that we have difficulty defining. The illogical, unspoken, and often unrecognized attitudes or beliefs that lead to this intense emotion occur to some degree in everyone, regardless of their rationality, sophistication, or education. These attitudes or beliefs occur in cancer patients and their family members and also in health professionals and in the community at large.[1]

IMPACT OF ATTITUDES AND BELIEFS ON THE CANCER SITUATION

Our concern about the attitudes or beliefs about cancer comes from their impact on the cancer situation. The dictionary definition of *situation* is "a state of affairs of special or critical significance" and also "the aggregate of biological, psychological, and sociocultural factors acting on an individual or group to condition behavioral patterns."[2] Experiencing the risk of having cancer, the diagnosis of cancer, or of living through the event of having cancer or of a significant other having cancer is a state of affairs of critical significance affecting in a holistic way the behavioral patterns of the individual and those within the social environment of the individual. The phrase "cancer situation" describes this phenomenon, which affects not only the person with cancer but family members, social support systems, and health professionals providing care.

Decision making within the cancer situation is influenced by attitudes and beliefs. These decisions are made by patient/family units, society, and health professionals and may have a major impact on the healthiness of the response to the cancer situation. Because a major goal of nursing is to facilitate healthy responses, it is important to identify (1) situations in which unrealistically negative beliefs occur, (2) nursing activities that can modify beliefs, and (3) the impact of changed beliefs on healthy responses to the cancer situation.

Patient and Family Decisions

Patient and family decisions that are influenced by cancer beliefs may include decisions about lifestyles, self-examination, speed with which symptoms are reported to a health professional, decisions related to initiation of and adherence to treatment regimens, and decisions related to self-esteem, quality of life, and degree of hopefulness. Attitudes and beliefs leading to psychologic responses may also have a major impact on physiologic responses. If this is so, these beliefs to some degree may have an effect on functional capacity, length of life, and possibility of cure.

Societal Decisions

The social treatment of a person with cancer by his or her family, and of patient and family by the community, is related to beliefs about cancer. The loss of social support and the abandonment of the patient/family unit by the community, which often occur in the cancer situation, may have serious long-term consequences, not only for the person with cancer but also for the present and future mental health of family members. Negative attitudes in the community also influence our social and political systems. These negative attitudes have been helpful in obtaining funding for research. However, they also have led to problems related to rehabilitation programs, insurability, and employability. People who have had cancer are often labeled as "cancer patient" for the rest of their life, a stigmatized label that affects their view of themselves and their functioning within society.

Health Professional Decisions

The decisions of health professionals are influenced by their own negative beliefs. In a physical examination, signs and symptoms of cancer may be overlooked, minimized, or discounted. Lumps may be watched for months. Choices of referral sources and selection of appropriate treatments are related to beliefs about cancer. The relationship between the health professional and the client may be altered by beliefs about cancer.

If beliefs about cancer are more negative than warranted, nurses may provide physical care but not psychologic care, and rehabilitative strategies may not be considered. Personal closeness with the patient may be avoided. The nurse may remain unaware of the feelings and problems faced by the patient/family unit and thus deprive them of needed nursing care.

Choices about careers within the health professions are in many cases related to beliefs about cancer. These decisions are often made early in the professional career. Beginning student nurses had more negative beliefs about cancer than had any other group tested.[3] These beliefs became even more negative during the nursing school experience. Students reported avoiding selecting cancer patients to care for, feeling helpless to make a difference in the patient's status. Nursing staff on general medical-surgical units were perceived by students to be providing only minimal care to cancer patients. Few students had clinical experiences on oncology units. Nursing faculty seemed to avoid clinical contact with cancer patients and tended to limit the number of hours of classroom content related to cancer nursing. These behaviors clearly influence career decisions by the new graduate.

BELIEFS, ATTITUDES, AND VALUES: A THEORETICAL PERSPECTIVE

Beliefs, attitudes, and values are related ideas but are not the same. Most theorists make clear distinctions among the three. According to Rokeach,[4] beliefs reflect an individual's perception of reality. Scheibe[5] proposes that beliefs allow the person to make inferences about what expectations he or she can have in a given situation. Thus a belief reflects what a person expects to happen in the external world in a given situation. Beliefs often develop during childhood, tend to be unconscious, and cannot be directly observed. Therefore, beliefs must be measured using indirect means.[4] Jung[6] saw beliefs as part of the collective unconscious and thus acquired from one's culture and also influencing one's culture. Antonovsky[7] considers beliefs as important factors that influence people's sense of coherence and thus their state of health. Caplan[8] thinks that beliefs are important in determining whether a person responds in an effective or ineffective way to a crisis situation.

Rokeach[4] sees attitudes as emerging from the belief system. Attitudes involve the joining together of several beliefs. Attitudes are more likely to be conscious and, therefore, can be obtained by direct measurement.

A value is defined by Rokeach as a special type of belief that is an abstract ideal about ideal ways of behaving and ideal goals of life. For example, values would be involved in determining what beliefs a nurse "should" have about cancer. It would be possible, then, to compare the ideal belief with the actual belief.

Ajzen and Fishbein[9] have developed a theory of reasoned action, which suggests relationships among beliefs, attitudes, intentions, and behavior. They believe that humans are rational rather than driven by uncontrollable desires and that behavior is carefully reasoned as opposed to automatic. They propose that beliefs (that a certain behavior will lead to a certain outcome) lead to attitudes about that behavior. Attitudes about the behavior lead to intentions to perform a specific behavior. Intentions are highly predictive of the actual behavior of an individual.

MEASUREMENT OF BELIEFS AND ATTITUDES

Measurement of beliefs and attitudes about cancer is in the initial stages of development. Few tools exist, and those that have been developed have not yet been used in large numbers of studies. Existing tools need further work to develop validity and reliability. There is not yet a generally accepted conceptual definition within the body of knowledge of the most critical elements of beliefs or attitudes that need to be measured. Therefore, each scientist has operationalized the concept using somewhat different criteria.

Potential Studies

Researchers might be interested in using available tools in clinical situations to describe more clearly beliefs existing within the cancer situation or to determine the impact of a nursing treatment on beliefs. It is important to determine if it is possible for nursing interventions to modify beliefs and if the change identified is short term or long term. We must determine also whether modifying beliefs significantly affects patient/family outcomes. In some cases, cancer belief or attitude tools may be used in conjunction with instruments measuring other phenomena. Correlational studies are needed to examine the relationship of cancer beliefs to other variables of interest within the cancer situation. The development of studies specifically designed to examine further the validity and reliability of existing tools will make a major contribution. Studies from which theory about cancer beliefs and attitudes can be developed are badly needed.

Selection of a Belief or Attitude Tool

Initial measurement strategies used open-ended interviews to determine beliefs about cancer.[10,11] Other early studies about cancer attitudes used stimulus stories followed by questions.[12] More recently, a qualitative research approach with symbolic interaction theory as the framework has been used by Dodd et al.[13] and by Kesselring et al.[14] to examine cancer attitudes in other countries. Questions related to knowledge about cancer, hopelessness, and self-esteem have been used in many studies to indirectly reflect cancer attitudes. Direct examination of beliefs and attitudes is more recent.

The selection of a tool for use in a study involves decisions related to how well the tool measures all the dimensions of attitudes or beliefs about cancer, the established validity and reliability of the tool, time required to administer the tool, ease in completing and scoring the tool, and the complexity of required data analysis. The researcher must consider whether it is desirable within the study to examine attitudes or beliefs. It is also important to determine if the tool fits conceptually with the researcher's perception of cancer beliefs or attitudes and the theoretical framework of the study.

American Cancer Society Studies

The initial studies into attitudes about cancer were generated by the American Cancer Society, which conducted national surveys in 1948, 1964, and 1979. The 1964 survey by Horn and Waingrow[15] indicated that 38 percent of those surveyed thought that the patient was not likely to tell people he had cancer, 12 percent indicated that they would not be willing to work next to someone who had cancer, 12 percent did not believe cancer was curable, and 6 percent believed that cancer was contagious. The percentage of people with these views had decreased since the 1948 survey.

The 1979 survey was conducted by Lieberman Research, Inc.[16] This study indicated that people continue to experience a considerable degree of fearfulness and anxiety about cancer. Forty-nine percent agreed that the word "cancer" itself scared them. Thirty-seven percent believed that cancer was the worst thing that could happen to a person. Thirty-six percent considered cancer to be a death sentence for most people. Twenty percent skipped over news stories about cancer. Sixteen percent did not believe a cure for cancer will ever be found. Sixteen percent stated that if they had cancer, they would prefer not to know about it. Nine percent would feel uncomfortable working next to someone who had cancer. In 1981, the tool was used to examine attitudes of black Americans toward cancer through EVAXX, Inc., a black-owned evaluation organization.[17] The study indicated that black Americans underestimate the prevalence of cancer and think it unlikely that they will get cancer. They are pessimistic about the curability of cancer. They are far less likely than whites to hear about cancer in the mass media, in organizations, or from relatives or friends. The tool used for these surveys has not been published but is available through the American Cancer Society.

▪ CANCER ATTITUDE INVENTORY

In 1968, Hohloch and Coulson[18] published a report of the development of a tool to measure attitudes of nursing students toward cancer. A conceptual framework of attitude change by Sherif et al.[19] was used as a basis for development of the tool. To construct the tool, tape-recorded interviews were held with colleagues in the nursing school. Key words and phrases were extracted from these interviews. Other statements were taken from the experiences and insights of the researchers. Contrasting statements about the same issue were developed. Eighty-six statements were submitted to a panel of judges, who selected 36 statements to comprise the tool. This strategy provided content validity. Test–retest reliability is reported at 0.96. A Likert-type scale is used to obtain responses to the statements, which are then weighted to develop a profile of responses for each subject.

▪ CRAYTOR'S ONCOLOGY NURSING QUESTIONNAIRE

In 1968, Craytor began work on a questionnaire to identify attitudes and learning needs of nurses working with cancer patients in order to develop appropriate continuing education programs.[20] The questionnaire was designed to survey attitudes about various nursing activities in caring for the cancer patient, such as:

Helping patient come to terms with the fact that he has cancer

Dealing with your own feelings about cancer

Giving physical care

Teaching early detection of cancer

Nurses are asked to respond in two ways to each item: (1) the importance of the activity and (2) how successfully the activity is carried out.[5] Craytor has used the questionnaire in three studies over a 10-year period. The tool has been modified as cancer nursing skills have changed.

In addition to the questionnaire, an Activity Vector Analysis (AVA) technique was used to identify (1) the nurse's perceptions of the typical hospital patient, (2) the ideal cancer nurse, (3) the ideal patient, (4) the nurse's self-perception, and (5) the typical cancer patient. The tool used 81 nonderogatory adjectives commonly used to describe human behavior. A card including each of the 81 adjectives is developed for each of the five perceptions listed. Subjects are asked to check the words they would use to describe each of the five perceptions. The adjectives were grouped for analysis into the four primary vectors of (1) aggressiveness, (2) sociability, (3) emotional control, and (4) adaptability. The number of adjectives checked and the specific adjectives checked provide a personality description. Correlational analysis can be used to compare pairs of personality descriptions.

▪ HALEY CANCER ATTITUDE SURVEY

In 1968, Haley et al.[21] developed a tool to measure the attitudes of medical school students. The tool was developed from 600 statements that expressed attitudes toward cancer and the care of cancer patients. From these statements, a preliminary form, with 33 questions, was developed and given to 163 physicians, 89 medical students, and 13 laymen. Responses were examined using factor analysis, from which three dimensions of cancer attitude were identified: "(a) attitudes toward the patient's inner resources to cope with serious illness such as cancer (CAS I); (b) attitudes toward the value of early diagnosis and aggressive treatment (CAS II); and attitudes toward personal immortality and preparation for and acceptance of death (CAS III)" (p. 501).[22]

A new sample of 94 physicians was used to develop the tool further. Correlational analysis of the new data led to the subdivision of CAS II into two subscales: CAS IIa, early diagnosis, and CAS IIb, aggressive treatment. The instrument used a 9-point Likert-type scale with responses ranging from "strongly disagree" to "strongly agree." Scoring used −4 for "strongly disagree," 0 for "no opinion," and +4 for "strongly agree." Completion of the instrument requires approximately 15 minutes.

Examples from the survey are:

Any psychologic stress on a patient should be avoided.

A physician can be so discouraged by the low cure rate of cancer that he will not feel the need to do routine "cancer tests," especially when he is so busy working with sick patients.

Aggressive treatment of cancer frequently subjects the patient to illness, pain, and expense without much actual benefit to him.

The dying patient has to be kept happy, since he has nothing to look forward to.

Validity and reliability data are not clearly reported on the instrument. Face validity and content validity can be inferred from the tool development process. Initial steps toward construct validity are obtained through factor analysis and the formation of clearly defined factors. However, no report is given of the constancy of the factors across samples. Reliability data are not reported.

The tool was used in a study reported by Haley et al. in 1977.[22] The tool was not revised at that time, and validity and reliability information are not discussed in the paper. In 1981, the tool was revised by Blanchard et al.[23] Twenty-seven new items were added to address changes in medical practice and modifications in the doctor–patient relationship that had occurred in medical practice since the original development of the tool. The structure of the original tool was kept intact, and the new items were added to the end of the instrument. Using only the original 33 questions, Blanchard's study failed to replicate the original factor structure reported by Haley. Responses showed a high degree of variability, and only 50 percent of the variance could be explained even when using eight factors. In 1982, Cohen et al.[24] used the revised tool in a comparative study of the responses of cancer patients, medical students, medical residents, physicians, and medical cancer educators. The sample was purposely selected to allow comparison with Haley's original sample. However, factor analysis apparently was not performed on the new data, and, therefore, no additional information is provided related to the validity of the original factor structure.

▪ CANCER ATTITUDES QUESTIONNAIRE

Hoffmeister[25] developed the Cancer Attitudes Questionnaire in 1976 as part of a funded research project. Items for the questionnaire were selected from attitudes people were presumed to have toward cancer. Subsets of questions were developed relating to each identified attitude. A 5-point Likert-type scale was used to obtain responses to the questions. The response alternates were: "agree completely," "agree mostly," "not sure" or "depends on the situation," "disagree mostly," and "disagree completely."

To develop the tool, both professional and nonprofessional groups and individuals were asked to respond to the questionnaire. This included groups employed in hospitals, nursing homes, and other professions. Data analysis included computation of the item means, variances, and frequency distributions. Those items that had minimal variability were excluded. Cluster analysis was used to determine which groups of questions clustered together. Each cluster of questions was combined into a score for that measure according to convergence analysis, which ensures that scores are computed for a person on a measure only if the responses to the questions that make up a measure are reasonably consistent.

Frequency distributions were conducted on the scores of various variables and measures. Pearson correlations were conducted between the measures and demographic variables. Chi-square tests and one-or two-way analysis of variance were conducted between selected variables and scores on the questionnaire. Results were not assumed to be significant unless they had a probability of occurrence due to chance of 1 in 1000 or less.

Three items of the questionnaire were eliminated because over 90 percent of the responses were similar. Four clusters were identified from the remaining questions: Fatalism, Cancer Phobia, Optimism, and Stigma. Correlations between scores on the clusters were in the expected directions.

Examples from the questionnaire include:

A cancer diagnosis means a person is going to die.

A person who gets cancer will always be sick.

If I get cancer, other people would not want to be around me.

Reliability: Test–retest information was gathered from a group of 47 nurses attending a series of lectures. The initial test was given before the first lecture. The retest was given 1 week later before the second lecture. Hoffmeister reported the computation of difference scores and *t*-tests for related groups to examine test–retest reliability. Although he reports that none of the differences were significant, no specific test–retest values were reported.[25]

Validity: According to Hoffmeister, cluster characteristics of the measures indicate that the clusters are valid from the standpoint of internal consistency.[25] The cluster characteristics are also suggested to reflect face content validity of the various subgroups of questions.

The questionnaire contains 21 items. Completion requires 5 to 10 minutes. The tool is not published but is available for a small fee, which includes data analysis using cluster analysis techniques.*

The instrument has been used in a published study by Nielsen et al.[26] designed to evaluate the effectiveness of a course for nurses caring for cancer patients in community hospitals. The data from the study were compared to Hoffmeister's original data. The pretest scores of the study group were comparable to Hoffmeister's group. No apparent effort was made to reexamine the validity and reliability of the instrument on the study data.

▪ BURNS' CANCER BELIEFS SCALES

The Burns' Cancer Beliefs Scales were developed between 1977 and 1981 as part of a doctoral dissertation.[27] A concept analysis of cancer beliefs was performed, with essential elements being obtained from the literature and personal experience. A semantic differential format was used to develop an instrument. Therefore, each item is considered a separate scale. The semantic differential was designed to measure meaning. It tends to capture the affective component of meaning rather than factual meaning. It uses strategies similar to word association used by psychotherapists to reflect the unconscious. Thus the significance of the responses go far beyond the simple dictionary definition of the word used in the instrument. It provides a link with the unconscious belief structure of the individual. The intensity of the response and the forming of groupings of scales that are correlated can give a much clearer reflection of an experience or thought that often cannot be expressed directly.

The instrument was first tested on 13 family members of cancer patients participating in a family support group. Then four groups were selected to test the instrument: American Cancer Society volunteers, high school teachers, beginning nursing students, and members of a Baptist church. It was hypothesized that the American Cancer Society volunteers would

---

*Questionnaires can be ordered from Dr. J. Hoffmeister, Test Analysis and Development Corporation, 2400 Park Lake Drive, Boulder, CO 80301; (303) 666-8651.

score highest, high school teachers and beginning nursing students would have moderate scores, and the Baptist church members would score lowest. The total sample was 153 persons. Analysis of variance was used to test the hypotheses. American Cancer Society volunteers scored highest, and beginning nursing students had the lowest scores. The group scores showed a statistically significant difference at the 0.001 level.

To further develop the instrument, factor analysis was performed using a sample of 767 subjects. Three distinct factors emerged and were labeled, Fear of the Cancer Situation, Hopelessness, and Stigma. Correlations between the factor scores and other variables of interest were examined. Weights on the items in each factor are available, and normative values, such as means and other statistical data, are available for each scale from examination of a sample of 767 subjects.

The Burns' Cancer Beliefs Scales contain 23 semantic differential scales consisting of bipolar adjectives or descriptive terms associated with beliefs about cancer. Each opposing set of descriptive terms is placed at opposite ends of a 7-point scale. Instructions for completing the scale are included on the instrument form. Individuals are instructed to respond quickly with their initial gut reaction to the descriptive terms by marking one space on each scale.

Examples of the scales are:

Punishment		_____	_____	_____	_____	_____	_____	_____		No punishment
Body mutilation		_____	_____	_____	_____	_____	_____	_____		No body changes
Alienation		_____	_____	_____	_____	_____	_____	_____		Belonging

The most negative response on some of the scales is on the right side to diminish the probability of global scoring by the respondent.

Administration of the instrument is fairly simple and should take only 5 or 10 minutes. Participants should be instructed to respond quickly and spontaneously with as little thought as possible to each item. Completion of the tool can generate emotional responses in patients and family members; therefore, it is recommended that a health professional be present at the time the tool is used with these groups.

Scoring is performed by rating the most negative response as 1 and increasing each space by 1 to the most positive response, which is rated as 7. The lowest possible score is 23, and the highest possible score is 161. Increased insight can be obtained by calculating factor scores for each of the three factors.

Reliability: Internal consistency had been examined through use of the alpha coefficient. In various samples ($n = 153$, $n = 58$, $n = 43$) alpha coefficients for factors range from 0.76 to 0.91. These statistics indicate an acceptable level of internal consistency for the tool.

Validity: Content validity has been developed through the literature review and concept analysis. The instrument was reviewed by family members of cancer patients, nurses practicing oncology, and nursing doctoral students and revised based on their suggestions.

Construct validity has been examined through the use of factor analysis. The grouping of the concepts that form the scales leads to the formation of a higher construct defined by the factor. The factors of the Burns' Cancer Beliefs Scales have remained relatively consistent across samples (*N. Burns, unpublished data*), adding to its construct validity. Factor structure has been examined further using a sample of 767 subjects, providing factorial validity.

Concurrent validity is obtained by administering the tool to a sample of people concurrently with other instruments that are thought to measure the same concept. Hoffmeister's

Cancer Attitudes Questionnaire[25] and Beck's Hopelessness Scale[28] were administered with the Burns' Cancer Beliefs Scales to a sample of 58 subjects to examine concurrent validity. Factor scores of Beck's scale and Hoffmeister's questionnaire were correlated with factor scores of Burns' scales, using a Pearson product moment correlations. All three factors of Burns' scales correlated significantly beyond the 0.001 level with the factors of Hoffmeister's questionnaire. The pessimism factor in Beck's scale correlated beyond the 0.001 level of significance with all factors of Burns' scales. Correlations of Beck's other two factors (factor 2, Loss of Motivation, and factor 3, Future Expectations) with Burns' factors and Hoffmeister's clusters indicated no significant correlations. Beck's two factors apparently measure a phenomenon not related to cancer attitudes and beliefs. The results of the correlations indicate concurrent validity for both Burns' scale and Hoffmeister's questionnaire.

Divergent validity was examined by correlating the three factors on Burns' scale with the Cancer Optimism Cluster in Hoffmeister's questionnaire. The two scores were significantly negatively correlated, suggesting divergent validity.

The instrument has been used in a masters thesis study by Clarke[29] comparing beliefs of nursing students toward cancer in adults and cancer in children. Comparisons were made between individual scale items. However, the results have not been published. The thesis was supervised by Virginia Hagemann, Ph.D., at the University of Missouri—Columbia and completed in July 1984. The instrument is currently in use by a number of researchers who have studies in progress.†

• CROEN AND LEBOVITS CANCER ATTITUDES QUESTIONNAIRE

In 1984, Lebovits et al.[30] published a paper describing the development of the Cancer Attitudes Questionnaire, expressing concern about the validity and reliability of Haley's tool and the lack of other published tools to measure cancer attitudes. Initial development involved review of the literature and examination of both published and unpublished tools. A pool of 200 items expressing attitudes about cancer was developed. These statements were narrowed down to 28 items, which were categorized by the researchers into seven attitudinal dimensions. The number of items in each dimension ranged from 3 to 6. Items within a dimension were worded so that 50 percent of them were expressed negatively and 50 percent positively. A 6-point Likert scale was used, with a forced choice (no option of selecting an undecided or neutral response).

Examples of the questions are:

A patient's attitude influences the course of cancer disease.

The physician should allow almost nothing to interfere with an aggressive approach to treating the cancer patient.

Cancer patients managed on an outpatient basis are as productive and capable in their occupations as anyone else.

It is unfair to tell terminally ill cancer patients that there is hope of recovery.

Construct Validity: An expert panel of judges consisting of three psychologists and three medical educators was asked to categorize the 28 items into the seven dimensions developed

†Information on the instrument can be obtained by writing Nancy Burns, R.N., Ph.D., Professor of Nursing, University of Texas at Arlington, School of Nursing, Box 19407, Arlington, Tx 76019.

by the researchers. On 25 of the items, there was at least 84 percent agreement. A factor analysis to determine construct validity was then conducted to further evaluate the seven dimensions. The factor analysis agreed 74 percent with the researcher's categories and 77 percent with the panel of judges.

Reliability: Repeated measures ANOVA was used to determine interrater reliability. An alpha coefficient of 0.96 was obtained. This indicates a high degree of internal consistency within the instrument.

Instrument Modification: A pilot test was conducted using 75 first-year medical students. The tool was revised to adjust for skewedness in some scales and readministered to a second sample of 151 students and a third sample of 159 students. Factor analysis was again performed, and factors were determined and named. Factor analysis revealed five factors that explained 42 percent of the variance. Cronbach alpha indicated reliabilities of the factors ranging from 0.55 to 0.79. Based on these reliabilities and the factor loadings, the tool was again modified. A "candor" scale was omitted, and items were redefined to be included on different dimensions within the tool in keeping with the factor analysis. The factors were named (1) Importance of patient–family attitudes, (2) Importance of physician attitudes toward patient and treatment, (3) Pessimism, (4) Outpatient functioning, and (5) Team treatment. Item to factor loadings and item to scale correlations are presented as well as reliability analyses.

The instrument was used in a study reported in the same paper[30] examining the effect of an elective course in oncology on the attitudes of medical students. Because of its recent development, the tool has not been used in other published studies. The authors express the need for further development of the tool, particularly using larger and more varied samples.

• NURSES' CANCER ATTITUDE QUESTIONNAIRE

In 1984, Whelan[31] reported the development of a questionnaire examining attitudes toward cancer that was modified from one developed earlier by Davison.[32] The questionnaire was used to compare attitudes toward cancer of nurses in the United States and in England. The instrument, containing 14 multiple choice questions, is published in its entirety in the article by Whelan.[31] No validity or reliability data are offered.

• FANSLOW'S CANCER ATTITUDES INSTRUMENT

In 1985, Fanslow published a study using an instrument on cancer attitudes developed during her dissertation research.[33] The tool was developed by combining items in the American Cancer Society questionnaire and items in Craytor's Oncology Nursing Questionnaire. The questionnaire consists of 49 items. The first 15 items address attitudes about skills in cancer nursing, and the last 34 items address cancer-related myths and knowledge of disease process and treatment. Responses to the questions are indicated on a Likert scale ranging from 1 to 5, with 5 indicating the most positive response and 1 the most negative response. An increase in the total score is expected to reflect a more positive attitude toward cancer. Fanslow proposes that positiveness of scores is related to the nurse's ability to effectively care for cancer patients and their families and to satisfactory knowledge about cancer, its treatment, and effective symptom management.

Items used in the questionnaire include:

As a nurse I am able to:
    Deal with the side effects of treatment for cancer
    Listen to the cancer patient.

My personal beliefs and attitudes about cancer are:
    Even with early detection cancer cannot be cured.
    If I got cancer I'd rather not know about it.

Internal consistency of the questionnaire is satisfactory, with an alpha of 0.9 for the skill portion and 0.7 for the knowledge portion. The instrument has face validity obtained through review by three oncology nurse specialists. It was piloted on faculty in a school of nursing to obtain content validity (*J. Fanslow, personal communication*). The questionnaire was used by Taub[34] for her masters thesis, which was chaired by Dr. Pamela Watson and completed in May 1986 at Boston University. Taub's study includes further examination of the validity and reliability of the instrument.‡

▪ YASKO AND POWER'S CANCER ATTITUDE SURVEY

Yasko and Power developed an attitude survey that was used initially in a National Cancer Institute-funded study in 1977 by Donovan et al.[35] (*J. Yasko, personal communication, November 1987*). It was then further developed in Power's masters thesis at the University of Pittsburgh, supervised by Yasko.[36] To develop the survey, all available tools were sought and examined. As is traditional in questionnaire development, many items from previous questionnaires were used in their existing form to develop the tool. Additional items were developed by Yasko and Power. The tool contains 38 items using a forced choice Likert-type scale with possible responses of 1 (completely disagree), 2 (somewhat disagree), 3 (somewhat agree), 4 (completely agree).
    Examples of items are:

Caring for persons with cancer is usually more demanding for the nurse than caring for persons with other illnesses.

Caring for persons with cancer is usually depressing for nurses.

Persons with metastatic cancer should not receive additional treatment.

Yasko reports a reliability of 0.80 for the instrument. Additional studies will examine validity.‖

SUMMARY

Few instruments are available to measure attitudes and beliefs about cancer. Some of the instruments have not been easily accessible, since they were not widely distributed through a

---

‡Further information on the instrument can be obtained from Julia Fanslow, R.N., Ed.D., Associate Professor, School of Nursing, Pacific Lutheran University, Tacoma, WA 98447; (202) 535-7672.
‖ For further information on the tool, contact Joyce Yasko, R.N., Ph.D., Room 367, Victoria Building, University of Pittsburgh, School of Nursing, Pittsburgh, PA 15261.

major publication. All available instruments need further development of validity and reliability. Attitudes and beliefs appear to be an important dimension of the cancer situation, which needs to be more clearly understood. Adding this information to the current body of knowledge has the potential of enhancing prediction and control and thus leading to more effective measures for nursing interventions in the psychosocial dimension of cancer.

REFERENCES

1. Burns, N. *Nursing and cancer.* Philadelphia: Saunders, 1982.
2. Stein, J. *The Random House dictionary of the English language.* New York: Random House, 1967, p. 1333.
3. Burns, N. Development of the Burns' Cancer Beliefs Scales. *Proceedings of the American Cancer Society Third West Coast Cancer Nursing Research Conference,* American Cancer Society, August 4–5, 1983, Portland, Oregon.
4. Rokeach, M. *Beliefs, attitudes and values.* San Francisco: Jossey-Bass, 1968.
5. Scheibe, K.E. *Beliefs and values.* New York: Holt, Rinehart, and Winston, 1970.
6. Read, H., Fordham, M., & Adler, G. (Eds.). *The collected works of C.G. Jung.* New York: Pantheon Books, 1960.
7. Antonovsky, A. *Health, stress, and coping.* San Francisco: Jossey-Bass, 1979.
8. Caplan, G. *Support systems and community mental health.* New York: Grune & Stratton, 1976.
9. Ajzen, I., & Fishbein, M. *Understanding attitudes and predicting social behavior.* Englewood Cliffs, NJ: Prentice-Hall, 1980.
10. Geer, S., Morris, T., & Pettingale, K.W. Psychological response to breast cancer: Effect on outcome. *Lancet,* 1977, 2:785.
11. Mitchell, G.W., & Glicksman, A.S. Cancer patients: Knowledge and attitudes. *Cancer,* 1977, 40:61.
12. Sloan, R.P., & Gruman, J.C. Beliefs about cancer, heart disease, and their victims. *Psychol Rep,* 1983, 52:415.
13. Dodd, M.J., Chen, S., Lindsey, A.M., & Piper, B.F. Attitudes of patients living in Taiwan about cancer and its treatment. *Cancer Nurs,* 1985, 8(4):214.
14. Kesselring, A., Dodd, M.J., Lindsey, A.M., & Strauss, A.L. Attitudes of patients living in Switzerland about cancer and its treatment. *Cancer Nurs,* 1986, 9(2):77.
15. Horn, D., & Waingrow, S. What changes are occurring in public opinion survey? *Am J Public Health,* 1964, 54:431.
16. *A basic study of public attitudes toward cancer and cancer tests.* Unpublished research report conducted for the American Cancer Society by Lieberman Research, Inc., May 1979.
17. Black Americans' attitudes toward cancer and cancer tests: Highlights of a study. *CA,* 1981, 31(4):212.
18. Hohloch, F.J., & Coulson, M.E. Developing an attitude inventory. *J Nurs Ed,* 1968, 7:9.
19. Sherif, C.W., Sherif, M., & Nebergall, R.E. *Attitudes and attitude change.* Philadelphia: Saunders, 1965.
20. Craytor, J.K., Brown, J.K., & Morrow, G.R. Assessing learning needs of nurses who care for persons with cancer. *Cancer Nurs,* 1978, 1(3):211.
21. Haley, H.B., Juan, I.R., & Galen, J.F. Factor-analytic approach to attitude scale construction. *J Med Educ,* 1968, 43:331.
22. Haley, H.B., Huynh, H., Paiva, R.E.A., & Juan, I.R. Student attitudes toward cancer: Changes in medical school. *J Med Educ,* 1977, 52:500.
23. Blanchard, C.G., Ruckdeschel, J.C., Cohen, R.E., et al. Attitudes toward cancer: I. The impact of a comprehensive oncology course on second-year medical students. *Cancer,* 1981, 47:2756.
24. Cohen, R.E., Ruckdeschel, J.C., Blanchard, C.G., et al. Attitudes toward cancer: II. A comparative analysis of cancer patients, medical students, medical residents, physicians and cancer educators. *Cancer,* 1982, 50:1218.

25. Hoffmeister, J. *First year evaluation results: Test development information, oncology nursing project (#1-CN-65185),* June 21, 1976.
26. Nielsen, B., Hyman R.B., & Abruzzese, R.S. Designing cancer nursing courses for community hospitals. *Cancer Nurs,* 1979, *2:*109.
27. Burns, N. *Evaluation of a supportive-expressive group for families of cancer patients.* Unpublished Dissertation, Denton, Texas Woman's University, 1981.
28. Beck, A., Weissman, A., Lester, D., & Trexler, L. The measurement of pessimism: The Hopelessness Scale. *J Consult Clin Psychol,* 1974, *42:*861.
29. Clark, L. *Attitudes of nursing students toward cancer in children and adults.* Unpublished Masters Thesis, University of Missouri—Columbia, July 1984.
30. Lebovits, A.H., Croen, L.G., & Goetzel, R.Z. Attitudes towards cancer: Development of the Cancer Attitudes Questionnaire. *Cancer,* 1984, *54:*1124.
31. Whelan, J. Oncology nurses' attitudes toward cancer treatment and survival. *Cancer Nurs,* 1984, *7*(5):375.
32. Davison, R.L. Opinion of nurses on cancer, its treatment and curability—A survey among nurses in Public Health Service. *Br J Prev Sociol Med,* 1965, *189:*24.
33. Fanslow, J. Attitudes of nurses toward cancer and cancer therapies. *Oncol Nurs Forum,* 1985, *12*(1):43.
34. Taub, J. *Attitudes of nurses toward oncology based knowledge and oncology related nursing skills: A replication of the Fanslow Study.* Unpublished masters thesis, Boston University, May 1986.
35. Donovan, M., Yasko, J., Wolpert, P., & Fedak, M. *Cancer Attitude Survey.* University of Pittsburgh National Cancer Institute Contract 1-CN-55186-07, 1977.
36. Power, K. *A comparison between two teaching methods on home care nurses' attitudes toward cancer.* Unpublished Masters Thesis, University of Pittsburgh, 1986.

PART III

Instruments for Assessing Clinical Problems

Part III

Instruments
for Assessing
Clinical Problems

CHAPTER 18

Measuring Nausea and Vomiting

Patricia H. Cotanch, R.N., Ph.D.

The symptoms of nausea and vomiting occur with relatively common frequency in psychiatrically, neurotically, and physically ill patients. Nausea and vomiting, sometimes collectively described as upper gastrointestinal distress, are a common side effect from many different kinds of pharmacologic agents.[1] Despite the relative frequency of the occurrence of nausea and vomiting in patients, literature on the subject is sparse.[2] The paucity of published literature may be due to the fact that the symptoms of nausea and vomiting are usually self-limiting and seldom life threatening.[3] A review of the literature by Penta et al.[4] showed that there was more published research on nausea and vomiting and on the efficacy of antiemetics in 1 year (31 studies published in 1980–1981) than in the previous 20 years (26 studies from 1960–1979). All of the recent work on assessment of nausea and vomiting has been done by health professionals associated with the field of oncology. There is little doubt that the increased interest in the occurrence of nausea and vomiting has come from the prevalence and severity of the side effects associated with cancer chemotherapy and other cancer treatments. Although health professionals in the oncology field have been the trailblazers of nausea and vomiting research, it is very possible that researchers in other health care areas will be able to use the information to improve the quality of life of patients affected with disorders in which the symptoms of nausea and vomiting are likely to occur.

At present, nausea and vomiting are among the most troublesome and most frequently encountered side effects of chemotherapy. Not only does the chemotherapy produce a variety of direct toxic effects on the body, including anorexia, nausea, and vomiting, but frequently patients experience these problems in anticipation of treatment through conditioned responses. As chemotherapy regimens become more aggressive in dosage and type of drug combination, both the direct (postchemotherapy) and the anticipatory effects of nausea and vomiting become progressively worse. Severe nausea and vomiting not only add psychologic stress to patients undergoing chemotherapy but also subject patients to nutritional deficits, dehydration electrolyte imbalance, weakness, and disruption in lifestyle. Many patients view the treatment and resulting discomfort as being worse than the disease and are reluctant to subject themselves to repeated courses of treatment. As a consequence, some patients terminate or seriously delay potentially curative treatment and thereby choose possible death from cancer rather than continue treatment. The side effects of nausea and vomiting could thus be considered a potentially fatal toxicity if the patients' disease is responsive to chemotherapy.[5]

Considering the negative impact of this side effect on patients, it is appropriate that considerable effort is being placed in the development and assessment of better pharmacologic and nonpharmacologic methods for controlling chemotherapy-related nausea and vomiting. As stated earlier, there has been a dramatic increase in the number and types of scientific investigation carried out to determine better ways to control the side effects of nausea and vomiting. Unfortunately, attention to improving assessment of nausea and vomiting has not kept pace with development of interventions to alleviate the symptoms. Only very recently have investigators given attention to more accurate measurement and assessment of the symptoms of nausea and vomiting.

SELECTING A MEASURING INSTRUMENT

Several aspects must be considered in selecting an appropriate measuring instrument for qualifying and quantifying nausea and vomiting. Some of the key issues to be addressed in the assessment of nausea and vomiting are:

1. How soon after the symptoms begin is the assessment made (in chemotherapy-related nausea and vomiting, a decision has to be made about how soon after treatment the assessment is made)
2. Definition of response terms
3. Issue of self-reporting versus observer-rated assessment
4. Usefulness of both direct and indirect assessment of nausea and vomiting
5. If combining nausea and vomiting responses to an overall measure is justified
6. The need to include measures of anticipatory nausea and vomiting
7. Measures that can determine accurately both the intensity and the unpleasantness of the side affects

An excellent review by Morrow[5] expertly addresses many of these issues. This chapter is an update on the issues addressed by Morrow. It includes examples of the most recent specific measuring tools used to assess nausea and vomiting, particularly the different types of instruments that have been used to quantify and qualify the occurrence, amount, intensity, and duration of nausea and vomiting as side effects of cancer treatment.

The information is presented in a format that follows the chronologic order of how nausea and vomiting have been assessed over the past 15 years. The logical growth and development of this area of assessment has proceeded from a simple counting method to the possibility of high technologic hardwiring of the human gut. It is hoped that increased familiarity with the tools now available will further research in the areas of nausea and vomiting in order to (1) better evaluate the incidence of the side effects, (2) evaluate the effectiveness of antiemetic intervention, and (3) formulate more accurate assessment tools.

METHODS AVAILABLE

The assessment of nausea and vomiting is still an evolving area of clinical research. As more information is obtained on measurements of nausea and vomiting, new issues arise that reveal inherent difficulties in quantifying these untoward objective and subjective experiences. Researchers need to maintain a suitable balance of obtaining accurate data about the side effect while not overstressing the patient or taxing the clinical environment or focusing too much attention on the side effect. Indeed, the latter may increase the incidence of the side effect because of associative learning or conditioned responses that can occur in patients experiencing drug-related nausea and vomiting.

Measurement of vomiting has been reported by simply counting the number of emetic episode and expressing them in absolute number or obtaining a mean score per time unit (e.g., X/hour) for a defined period of observation. This measurement was used in an investigation in which the change in the mean number of hourly episodes of nausea and/or vomiting was recorded for a period of 8 hours.[6] Measurements obtained in this manner accurately reflect the objective finding of vomiting, but the assessment of nausea (a subjective experience) is difficult, if not impossible, to quantify by direct observation. In addition, the patient must be under continuous observation by an investigator or be trusted to deliver an accurate self-report when this method of data gathering is used.

Nausea and vomiting have been assessed by grouping the number of emetic and nausea episodes according to predefined criteria and then labeling the degree of severity of the side effect (e.g., a scale from 0 to 4).[7] This method is sometimes used when fairly consistent patterns of nausea and vomiting are likely to occur. It requires a self-report format.

Investigators have developed guidelines for rating the severity of nausea and vomiting in order to compare responsiveness to antiemetic agents. An example of such grading is "none" (no nausea or vomiting, no antiemetic needed), "moderate" (nausea and vomiting requiring antiemetics but controllable), and "severe" (uncontrolled nausea and vomiting that interferes with performance of daily activities).[8]

• DUKE DESCRIPTIVE SCALE (DDS)

The Duke Descriptive Scale (DDS) (Table 18–1) is a nausea and vomiting grading scale ranging from grades 1 to 4 that includes intensity, severity, and impairment in patient activity levels, which has been used by several investigators.[9,10] This scale was selected for a relaxation antiemetic study because it was a method of rapid data collection and included an activity level. There was one major limitation with the DDS. The highest grade (grade IV) had a low ceiling of 10 emetic episodes for a 24-hour period. Consequently, patients who actually had an increase in emetic episodes are evaluated as unchanged [i.e., 15 emetic episodes (grade IV) during the next course of drugs]. Of course, the low ceiling of the DDS also conceals an improvement in the number of emetic episodes.

ADVANCES IN MEASURING INSTRUMENTS

A group of investigators has reported an exploratory pilot study that has identified three separate functional entities of the emetic process, labeled the lag, peak, and residual phases.[11] These authors have formulated a measuring scale in which each functional entity is operationally defined by a 5-point interval scale incorporating the emetic response, frequency of vomiting, and intensity of episodes. The scale is currently being tested for reliability and clinical usefulness.[11]

TABLE 18–1. DUKE DESCRIPTIVE SCALE (DDS)

A. Nausea grades I to IV
  I = None
  II = Mild, activity not interfered with
  III = Moderate, activity interfered with
  IV = Severe, bedridden with nausea for more than 2 hours
B. Vomiting grades I to IV
  I = No vomiting 24 hours after chemotherapy
  II = Mild, vomiting less than five times in the 24 hours after chemotherapy
  III = Moderate, 5–10 times in the 24 hours after chemotherapy
  IV = Severe, more than 10 times in 24 hours, patient bedridden, possible dehydration
C. Response will be graded as follows:
  CR (complete response) = No nausea or vomiting
  PR (partial response) = Grade II–III, nausea and vomiting
  NR (no response)   = Grade IV, nausea and vomiting
D. Source of response data
  PI   = Patient interview
  NO = Nurse observation
  HCT = Other health care team

• MORROW ASSESSMENT OF NAUSEA AND EMESIS (MANE)

One of the most complete nausea and vomiting assessment tools was developed by Morrow.[5] The Morrow Assessment of Nausea and Emesis (MANE) is a self-report Likert scale that asks questions about nausea and vomiting separately. Using this scale, an investigator can obtain data on onset, intensity, severity, and duration for prechemotherapy and postchemotherapy nausea and vomiting. Figure 18–1 gives examples of questions on MANE.

• VISUAL ANALOG SCALES

The use of Visual Analog Scales to measure nausea and vomiting in children[12] and adults[13] has been reported. Visual Analog Scales were first investigated as a method of quantifying the subjective feeling of pain.[14] The scale uses a 10 cm vertical or horizontal line with opposite descriptors at each end (e.g., "worst nausea ever," "no nausea at all"). The patient places a mark on the line indicating the degree of nausea. Investigators who have used Visual Analog Scales with children have incorporated the scale into a sketch of a thermometer (Fig. 18–2), and the children color in their degree of nausea, pain, or whatever is being measured.[12] The Visual Analog Scale is an easy method of quantifying the subjective experience of patients; it is therefore a useful tool for attempting to measure nausea.

• TURSKY PAIN PERCEPTION PROFILE (PPP)

At Duke University we are investigating currently the use of psychophysical scaling in order to measure perception of both the intensity and the reactive component (unpleasantness) of

These questions will ask about NAUSEA. NAUSEA is feeling sick to your stomach; VOMITING is actually throwing up.

The word "treatment" will refer to any drugs you are given here or take home.

I have experienced nausea: (please circle one)

1. during or after every treatment
2. after many of my treatments
3. after only about half my treatments
4. rarely after a treatment
5. never after a treatment

When I have NAUSEA after a treatment, it usually lasts ____ hours.

I would describe NAUSEA as:

1. very mild
2. mild
3. moderate
4. severe
5. very severe
6. intolerable

The NAUSEA is usually the worst:

1. during treatment
2. 0–4 hours after treatment
3. 4–8 hours after treatment
4. 8–12 hours after treatment
5. 12–24 hours after treatment
6. 24 or more hours after treatment
7. no time is any more severe than any other time

Figure 18–1. A section of the Morrow Assessment of Nausea and Vomiting (MANE).

the emetic experience.[15] The psychophysical scaling method of measuring perception was first investigated in the United States by Tursky et al. when they used the technique to assess patients' perception of pain.[16] We have adapted the Tursky Pain Perception Profile (PPP)[16] to assess the changes in intensity and unpleasantness of nausea in a study.

The PPP uses a sophisticated psychophysical scaling technique to evaluate the qualitative and quantitative aspects of the experience that is being measured. Heretofore, attempts to measure changes in the emetic experience have used verbal reports, verbal rating scales (descriptors or numbers), and a Visual Analog Scale. These measures have the following deficiencies: (1) distances between responses on verbal rating scales, although unknown, are assumed to be equal, (2) responses to the Visual Analog are influenced by various biases and preconceptions, and (3) responses measure only a single aspect (intensity) of a multidimensional phenomenon. The use of psychophysical scaling to record each patient's quantitative and qualitative judgments and reactions to a number of discrete symptom variables can be of considerable value because it eliminates these deficiencies.

Psychophysical scaling has the major advantage of measuring how "unpleasant" the emetic experience is for the patient. All effective antiemetic drugs have sedative or mood-altering properties that produce an altered state of consciousness. Behavioral interventions

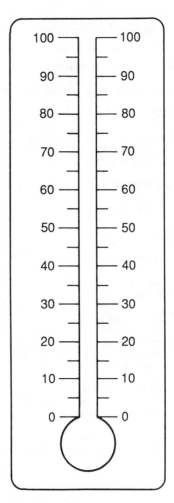

This is a thermometer, just like the ones we use to tell how hot or cold something is. But this thermometer measures how much nausea you have. At the bottom is zero—no nausea at all. At the top is 100—the most nausea you could feel. Use this red pen and fill in how much nausea you felt during the chemotherapy.

Figure 18—2. Device used as Visual Analog Scale for measuring nausea in children.

also induce altered states of consciousness for control of nausea and vomiting. Investigators who have used behavioral intervention have found some decrease in anticipatory and post-chemotherapy nausea and vomiting as well as lower physiologic arousal and decreased emotional distress, as measured by various standardized psychologic tests.[17-22] These studies note that many patients who have learned relaxation skills "feel better" about chemotherapy procedures and say that behavioral interventions were "helpful" even if nausea and vomiting persist. However, these studies, as well as studies that use drug intervention quantitatively and qualitatively, measure only change in the intensity of nausea and vomiting. The "feeling better" response, if it is reported, is stated as an anecdote. According to Tursky, misconceptions about the effectiveness of a treatment can occur when the treatment is aimed at modifying psychologic reactions to a symptom (or side effect), but the assessment techniques for evaluating outcomes measure only the intensity of the symptom. This is important, since mood-altering drug or behavioral interventions used to treat symptoms of disease or side

---

PURPOSE: To teach a method you can use to measure your nausea

Step 1: Assigning numbers to lines that are different lengths.
Example:
If we assign the number 50 to a line this long,

_____

What number would you assign to a line this long?

_____

Step 2: Assigning numbers and lines of different lengths to words describing the unpleas-antness of nausea.
Example:
The following is a list of words that describe the unpleasantness of nausea:
Distressing
Tolerable
Awful
Bearable
Miserable
Not unpleasant
Agonizing
If we assign the number 50 to the word "distressing" and draw a line this long
_____ to indicate a "distressing" level of nausea, what number and how long a line would you assign to the following words? (Fill in the answer)

Word	Number	Line Length
1. Tolerable		
2. Awful		
3. Bearable		
4. Miserable		
5. Not unpleasant		
6. Agonizing		

Step 3: What word best describes the unpleasantness of your nausea at this time?

(Please write the word)

Figure 18-3. Example of psychophysical scaling methodology to assess nausea in patients.

effects related to treatment may manifest their therapeutic effect primarily by increasing the patient's tolerance or altering his or her perception thereof. A complete description of psycho-physical scaling methodology has been reported by Tursky.[16] Figure 18-3 is an abbreviated example of how the scaling technique is used to assess nausea in patients.

▪ RHODES INDEX OF NAUSEA AND VOMITING (INV)

Another instrument that measures separately the patient's perception, intensity, and duration of nausea and vomiting has been reported. Rhodes et al. were the first to conduct a study to determine the validity of a self-report measure of nausea and vomiting.[23] The Rhodes Index of Nausea and Vomiting (INV) was compared to an adapted version of McCorkel and Young Symptom Distress Scale (ASDS). Both the INV and ASDS use a Likert self-report method. Reliability estimates of less than 0.83 were obtained using the split-half procedure. Construct and concurrent validity were assessed comparing family members' ratings to chemotherapy patients' ratings and yielded a correlation of $r = 0.87$. The investigators reported that both tools (the INV and ASDS) were a reliable and valid measure of posttreatment nausea and vomiting.[23]

Electrophysiologic Measurements

Electrophysiologic equipment to measure electrical disturbances in the stomach and intestine caused by chemotherapy has been used in animals. Using this method, one investigator demonstrated disturbances in electrical impulses produced by cisplatin in the stomach and small intestine of dogs and the anti-arrhythmic effects of metoclopramide thereon.[24]

If feasible, electrophysiologic measurements could be an important means of studying the physiologic relationships of gastrointestinal activity, the perception of nausea, and the act of vomiting in patients. Measurement of intrathoracic and intraabdominal venous pressure (not yet performed in humans) may also become a useful tool for distinguishing vomiting from retching and other components of the emetic process.[25]

SUMMARY

Research on chemotherapy-related nausea and vomiting is only now receiving adequate attention. To date, techniques used to measure nausea and vomiting have been simple and direct. Clinical trials now involve multiple antiemetics and behavioral interventions to abate the side effect. We need to have accurate measurements of nausea and vomiting if the results of the clinical trials are to be applied to various patient population. Although progress has been made from the simple counting of emetic episodes to more sophisticated measurements, such as various functional entities of the emetic process and application of psychophysical scaling, much remains to be learned about the various aspects of measuring the emetic experience, many questions remain unanswered.

REFERENCES

1. *Physicians' Desk Reference* (39th ed.). Oradell, NJ: Medical Economics Co., 1985.
2. Cleghan, R., and Brown, W. Psychogenicity of emesis. *Can Psychiatry Assoc J,* 1964, *9*(4):299.
3. Hill, O. Psychogenic vomiting. *Gut,* 1968, *9*:348.
4. Penta, J. Poster, D., & Bruno, S. The pharmacologic treatment of nausea and vomiting caused by cancer chemotherapy: A review. In J. Laszlo (Ed.), *Antiemetics and cancer chemotherapy.* Baltimore: Williams & Wilkins, 1983, p. 53.
5. Morrow, G. Assessment of nausea and vomiting: Past problems, current issues and suggestions for future research. *Cancer,* 1984, *53*(10):2267.
6. D'Souza, D., Reyntjens, A., & Thornes, R. Domperidone in the prevention of nausea and vomiting induced by antineoplastic agents. A three-fold evaluation. *Curr Ther Res,* 1980, *27*(3):384.
7. Moertel, C., & Reirtemeire, R. Controlled clinical studies of orally administered antiemetic drug. *Gastroenterology,* 1969, *57*(3):262.
8. Wilcox, P., Fetting, J., Nettesheim, K., & Abeloff, M. Anticipatory vomiting in women receiving cyclophosphamide, methotrexate, and 5-FU (CMF) adjuvant chemotherapy for breast carcinoma. *Cancer Treat Rep,* 1982, *66*(8):1601.
9. Laszlo, J., Lucas, V., Hanson, D., et al. Levonantradol for chemotherapy-induced emesis: Phase I-II oral administration. *J Clin Pharmacol,* 1981, *21*(8,9):515.
10. Cotanch, P. Relaxation training for control of nausea and vomiting in patients receiving chemotherapy. *Cancer Nurs,* 1983, *6*(4):277.

11. Scott, D., Donahue, D., Mastrovito, R., & Hokes, T. The antiemetic effect of clinical relaxation. Report of an exploratory pilot study. *J Psychosoc Oncol*, 1983, *1*(1):71.
12. LeBaron, S., & Zeltzer, L. Behavioral treatment for control of chemotherapy-related nausea and vomiting in children and adolescents with cancer. *Pediatr Res*, 1982, *16*(4):208A.
13. Fetting, J., Grochow, L., Folstern, M., et al. The course of nausea and vomiting after high-dose cyclophosphamide. *Cancer Treat Rep*, 1982, *66*(7):1487.
14. Scott, J., & Huskisson, E. Graphic representation of pain. *Pain*, 1976, *2*(2):175.
15. Cotanch, P., Hockenberry, M., Herman, S. Self-hypnosis as antiemetic therapy in children receiving chemotherapy. *Oncology Nursing Forum*, 1985, *12*(4):41.
16. Tursky, B., Jammer, L., & Friedman, R. The pain perception profile: A psychophysical approach to the assessment of pain report. *Behav Ther*, 1982, *13*:376.
17. Burish, T.G., & Lyles, J.N. Effectiveness of relaxation training in reducing the aversiveness of chemotherapy in the treatment of cancer. *J Behav Ther Exp Psychiatry*, 1979, *10*(4):357.
18. Burish, T.G., & Lyles, J.N. Effectiveness of relaxation training in reducing adverse reactions to cancer chemotherapy. *J Behav Med*, 1981, *4*(1):65.
19. Redd, W.H., & Andresen, G.V. Conditioned aversion in cancer patients. *Behav Ther* 1981, *4*(2):3.
20. Redd, W.H., & Andrykowski, M.A. Behavioral intervention in cancer treatment: Controlling aversion reactions to chemotherapy. *J Consult Clin Psychol*, 1982, *50*(6):1018.
21. Morrow, G.R., Arseneau, J.C., Asbury, R.F., et al. Anticipatory nausea and vomiting in chemotherapy patients. *N Engl J Med*, 1982, *306*(1):431.
22. Morrow, G.R., & Morrell, C. Behavioral treatment for anticipatory nausea and vomiting induced by cancer chemotherapy. *N Engl J Med*, 1982, *307*(2):1476.
23. Rhodes, V., Watson, P., & Johnson, M. Development of reliable and valid measures of nausea and vomiting. *Cancer Nurs*, 1984, *7*(1):33.
24. Akwari, O., The gastrointestinal tract in chemotherapy-induced emesis: A final common pathway. *Drugs*, 1983, *25*(1):18.
25. Laszlo, J. Methods for measuring clinical effectiveness of antimetics. In J. Laszlo (Ed.), *Antiemetics and cancer chemotherapy*. Baltimore: Williams & Wilkins, 1983, p. 43.

CHAPTER 19

Measuring Bowel Elimination

Linda Bartkowski-Dodds, R.N., M.S.

Various methodologies and instruments have been developed that provide quantitative data for human bowel function. Early attempts in the objective evaluation of elimination were by simple questioning. However, wide differences in health status among populations, absence of dietary considerations, and reliance on patient recall of defecation performance resulted in questionable data.[1]

By the mid-1960s, research into the effects of diet on bowel performance precipitated the development of measurement tools and techniques for quantifying frequency of defecation, stool consistency, stool wet weight, and intestinal transit time.[2-9] Further studies of gastrointestinal motility produced methods for quantifying intraluminal pressures within the alimentary tract.[10-14] Focusing on these parameters, numerous studies were performed on normal subjects and those with elimination problems.

Other investigators have developed questionnaires and surveys that have provided subjective data describing attitudes and behaviors related to elimination and evaluating bowel patterns among various populations.[15-18] Depending on study objectives and the population under investigation, however, both subjective and objective dimensions may need to be measured as they relate to the concept of elimination.

Because bowel function can be affected by neurophysiologic, psychologic, and cultural conditions, a comprehensive approach to the measurement of the concept of elimination must include all such parameters. Bowel function not only will vary among subjects with different underlying conditions but also can vary in the same subject at different times. Instrument selection, therefore, is critical, and it is generally believed that a thorough study will require the use of more than one instrument.

Instruments that result in quantitative data provide objective measures of bowel function, but interpretations are limited by the normal variability of colonic function[19] and the influence of multiple variables.[20] In contrast, instruments that result in qualitative data (descriptive data) provide subjective measures that attempt to identify various bowel patterns or describe the concept of elimination per se. Choice of instruments will be determined ultimately by research goals, populations under study (normal versus abnormal bowel function), number of subjects, and resources available.

OBJECTIVE SCALES YIELDING QUANTITATIVE DATA

Objective measures can be categorized according to the parameters considered relevant to the investigation of bowel function. The following instruments and methodologies have been used to investigate both normal subjects and those with problems of elimination, for example, bowel syndromes, megacolon, diverticulitis, Crohn's disease, constipation related to medications, and diarrhea associated with enteral feedings.

Bowel Transit Time

Methods that have been used to measure gut transit time may be classified as radiologic, colorimetric, particulate, chemical, and isotopic.

▪ RADIOLOGIC MEASURES

Hinton et al., developed a simple technique using radiopaque pellets of barium-impregnated polyethylene.[2] A known number of pellets are swallowed, usually 20, and the disappearance of the pellets from the gut or the appearance of the pellets in the stool is observed by serial radiographs. Results are expressed as the time taken for the passage of the first and of 80 percent of the markers. Recovery rate using 30 subjects was 99.3 percent. Replicate studies were performed providing only descriptive data, with variability in transit time up to 2 days in the same subject. Comparison studies with other markers, again using descriptive data only, were difficult to assess because of the inherent differences in the various methods. For instance, radiopaque pellets were compared to glass beads and were shown to have a shorter mean transit time; it was believed that this was probably because of the high specific gravity of the beads as compared to that of the pellets. Comparisons with chemical markers were less than optimal, since some of the chemical was found in the urine as well as the stool.

Paylor et al., used Hinton's method for measuring intestinal transit time while studying the effect of bran on intestinal transit and found reproducibility poor, with variability in transit times even in the same subject.[4]

In an attempt to provide more accurate and reproducible data, Cummings et al. compared mean transit times (MTT) using radiopaque pellets in two different ways and compared this to Hinton's method of 80 percent excretion as an expression of transit time (80% TT).[3] MTT was measured using a constant amount of marker fed to subjects over a period of weeks (MTT-C) and again measured by giving single doses of similar markers to the subjects (MTT-S). The MTT-S method was found to be preferable to the 80% TT if a single dose technique was used. The MTT-S correlated more closely with the MTT-C ($r = 0.87$) than did the 80% TT ($r = 0.78$) and gave a value for transit that is more physiologic. Although the MTT-C method provided more information about transit in individuals (data that reflect the way residue passes through the gut, i.e., colon), it can be tedious and is not suitable for studies on an epidemiologic scale.

Although it has limitations, an alternative method for measuring transit time through the gut was developed and tested by Cummings and Wiggins.[5] It requires the collection of only one stool after 4 days of ingestion of markers. It is suitable for use in epidemiologic studies on an outpatient basis. This method compared favorably with MTT-C (r = 0.78, $p < 0.001$) and

MTT-S ($r = 0.94$, $p < 0.001$) and proved a satisfactory alternative method for validating transit techniques. Once transit times begin to exceed 4 days, its accuracy falls off, and it would not be suitable for studying the constipated patient.

▪ COLORIMETRIC MEASURES

Various dyes have been used to mark stool and then calculate passage through the intestinal tract. The simplicity makes this method especially attractive, and it has been used in a variety of research settings.[21–23] Two widely used dyes are brilliant blue 100 mg/capsule and carmine 500 mg/capsule. Dosing usually requires three capsules per each experimental day. Transit time is computed as the time from ingestion of the marker until most of the color has appeared in the feces. This requires daily stool collection and careful examination of the stool, which may lend itself to misinterpretation.

Rogers et al. compared the use of radiopaque pellets and dye in measuring bowel transit time and, after rigorous analysis of variance, concluded that the two methods gave identical information. [23]

Colorimetric measures provide mouth-to-anus transit time but cannot provide data about passage through the different parts of the gastrointestinal tract. They would, therefore, be limited in usefulness when studying the diseased colon or other bowel disorders to ascertain segmental function. They lend themselves well to the study of diarrhea, since the specific gravity of radiologic markers may affect the transit time in the diarrheal stool.

▪ PARTICULATE MEASURES

Particulate measures are tedious and require complex and careful analysis of stool specimens. Furthermore, complete recovery can be seriously altered by stool adsorption of the reagent secondary to dietary fiber composition. Polyethylene glycol (PEG) can be ingested by subjects (1 g doses) after dilution in water and then analyzed in stools with a spectrophotometer. The use of PEG as a transit time measure was compared to other standard measures, including dyes, pellets, and isotopes.[21] Mean recovery for 242 doses was 85.3 ± 12.6 percent. Low recovery was attributed to binding of PEG by stool components. A separate analysis of MTT values from all markers revealed no significant differences in transit time estimates among marker types.

▪ CHEMICAL MEASURES

One of the major limitations of the use of radiopaque pellets is that total excretion may not represent pool sizes and turnover rates of unexcreted intestinal content. Thus, pellet excretion may not have any significant relationship to the usual clinical descriptions of bowel habits. Patients may report daily bowel movements, but pool sizes could be very large and turnover small, that is, a large proportion of the colonic contents may not be excreted for long periods.[7]

Since chemical markers are incorporated into the food intake, their excretion can indicate the completeness of stool collections and permit corrections for variations in fecal flow. Chromic oxide (Cr-203) has been used widely in humans since 1947 for these purposes, since it is nontoxic, readily measurable in the feces, and appears to be completely unabsorbable.[7] Subjects are given chromic oxide 60 mg tablets with meals, not to exceed 300 mg/day. Fecal collections are pooled and stored at 4°C until the collection period is completed. Although measurements demonstrated reliability (replicate demonstrations showed a coefficient of variation of 2.8 percent ± 1.5 percent), analysis is time consuming.[8]

Thus, Dick reported on the use of cuprous thiocynate as a continuous marker for feces that is insoluble under physiologic conditions but could be decomposed by relatively mild chemical treatments.[6] The marker is administered with each meal, with a total daily dose of 1 g; stools are collected and stored and then analyzed for copper content. Analysis requires the addition of nitric acid followed by atomic absorption spectroscopy. Copper recovery over 79 four-day periods on 14 subjects was 99.7 percent. Although not statistically analyzed, a histogram comparing the recoveries of cuprous thiocyanate to barium sulfate and chromium oxide demonstrated a higher percentage of recovery with cuprous thiocyanate.

In an investigation into the effects of fiber on bowel function, Wrick et al. compared various markers for transit time, one of which was Cr (III) mordanted onto isolated bran fiber, and found no significant differences in transit time estimates between CR (III) and PEG or radiopaque pellets.[21] Chromium-mordanted bran is prepared and placed into capsules, each dose providing 35 to 45 mg Cr, and ingested daily. Fecal Cr recovery is assessed by atomic absorption spectrophotometry. Complete stool collection is required, and a lengthy preparation procedure for spectroscopy is necessary.[21] Mean fecal Cr recovery from 244 doses of Cr-mordanted bran was 84 ± 16.9 percent. Incomplete conversion to chromic oxide (during preparation for spectroscopy) and marker overlap between testing periods were explanations offered by these investigators for results lower than 100 percent. Apparently, the cellulose within the mordanted bran altered the colonic microflora so that there was a microbial interaction with the mordant, which somehow influenced the recovery of Cr. This limitation needs to be considered with subjects who may have slow turnover of intestinal pool.

▪ ISOTOPIC MEASURES

Isotopic measures have the advantage of quantifying transit rates separately through the small and large intestines, whereas other transit time measures are suitable for total mouth-to-anus assessments only. Hansky and Connell first used Cr-51 to investigate transit times by labeling sodium chromate (Na_2CrO_4).[9] A gelatin capsule filled with 0.5 g of chromic oxide with an activity of 1 to 2 microcuries (μCi) is swallowed by the subject, and a scintillation counter permits quantification according to the amount of Cr-51 present in stools. A mean percentage recovery of radioactivity of 83.5 percent was demonstrated, but more important, this technique permits quantitative measurement of the rate of passage of the maximum bulk of the marker.

Waller used Cr-51 as a marker while investigating small and large bowel transit times in subjects with constipation and diarrhea.[24] Other markers were used concurrently, but comparative statistical analysis was not performed. Transit times for all markers were similar. However, Cr-51 provided differential measurements for colonic function in diarrheal and constipated states that would not have been ascertained using standard measures and would be useful when investigating segmental gastrointestinal transit.

Stool Consistency

▪ PENETROMETER CONE

A quantitative technique for assessing stool consistency has been devised by Exton-Smith et al. that uses a penetrometer cone, which is lowered until it is touching the stool, released, and then allowed to penetrate the stool for 5 seconds.[25] Distance of penetration is measured in units of 0.1 mm. Several readings are taken along the column of the stool and are averaged. The total range of penetrometer readings was 0 to 240, with a mean of 80.6 for hard stools and 128.9 for soft stools. Further work is being carried out to refine the method and to establish a normal range of values.

▪ STOOL ASH ANALYSIS

In a clinical study assessing lactose intolerance with tube-fed patients, Walike and Walike found that stool ash analysis validated subjective ratings of stool consistency made by nurse-clinicians.[15] Stool content was analyzed for sodium, potassium, percentage of fat, nitrogen, phosphate, percentage of ash, and wet and dry weight. Stool weight, percentage of water, and sodium were significantly higher with the lactose-containing diet and correlated nicely with stool consistency ratings.

Frequency of Defecation
Since self-reporting has been considered unreliable by most investigators, Hinton et al. devised a collection technique that provided accurate measurements of frequency as well as a convenient way to transport specimens to the laboratory for further analysis.[2] This method continues to be used today with a few minor alterations. It basically entails the use of a polythene bag that is suspended over the toilet and collects the specimen while allowing the urine to pass freely. The plastic bag is then sealed with a rubber band and inserted into a specimen cup and labeled with the appropriate information. Assuming subject compliance, this method should provide objective, quantifiable data about stool frequency.

Stool Wet/Dry Weight and Volume
Numerous investigations have shown that dietary constituents, medications, and colonic function will affect fecal characteristics.[10,11,19,23] Statistical analysis of fecal measurements often includes the calculation of coefficients of variation for each subject for each measurement. Statistical comparisons of these measures to other variables (transit time, dietary fiber, medications) are then determined to further explore any relationships.[19] Although no special instruments for measuring these parameters are described in the literature, techniques for such assessments are clearly delineated.[19]

Gastrointestinal Motility Measures

▪ MANOMETER

Various invasive measures have been used for quantitatively assessing the motility of the alimentary tract. Early studies using miniature balloons connected through polyethylene tubing to a metal capsule optical manometer of high sensitivity provided intraluminal pressure readings in both normal patients and those with dysfunctional conditions.[10,11] The same technique has been used to compare the effects of codeine and senna on the motor activity of the left colon.[12] Any type of cardiovascular, respiratory, or somatic movement will affect the tracings and can interfere with accurate interpretations. An assessment of colonic activity is given by the product of the total duration of activity and the mean amplitude of the slow waves. Analysis for observer error initially produced a mean standard deviation of ± 3.2 percent. This was considered to be too great an error, and therefore the standard deviations of duplicate analyses were calculated and the mean of these standard deviations was ± 1.8 percent ($p = 0.01$).

▪ THERMISTOR PROBE

Kagawa-Busby et al. studied the effects of diet temperature on the tolerance of enteral feedings and evaluated gastric motility and intragastric temperature by inserting a nasogastric feeding tube with a thermistor probe for recording temperature and a polyethylene cannula for pressure recordings.[14] No reference was made to establishing validity or reliability of the instruments used. Observation periods were predetermined and identical for all subjects; thus, analysis of observer error was not relevant. However, this does not exclude the possibility of misinterpretation of readings by omission.

SUBJECTIVE SCALES YIELDING QUANTITATIVE DATA

Elimination studies frequently attempt to measure the effects of certain variables (diet, medications, bowel diseases) on stool consistency and require the quantification of subjective data. A previously mentioned study was conducted by Walike and Walike, who assessed stool consistency among tube-fed patients on lactose-containing versus lactose-free diets. Descriptive ratings were performed by nurse-clinicians and validated by concurrent stool ash analysis.[15] Descriptive parameters were plotted against time and categorized between both diets (Fig. 19–1).

To evaluate the effectiveness of dioctyl sodium sulfosuccinate as a prophylactic measure in preventing constipation among hospitalized patients, Goodman et al. used a scale for grading stool consistency.[16] Six descriptive categories were used. Examples are:

A = watery
B = soft-formed, normal stool
C = watery, hard-formed stool

The scales used by Walike and Walike and by Goodman et al. offer ways to categorize stool consistency. However there was no mention of interrater reliability or validity testing by

	DIET								
	LACTOSE-FREE					LACTOSE-CONTAINING			
Watery						XX	XXX	XX	
Liquid						XX		X	
Very loose, semiliquid	X			X				XX	XXX
Loose, very soft		X	X						
Day	2	4	6	8	10	2	4	6	8	10

Figure 19–1. Comparison of stool frequencies and consistencies on two diets for one subject. Each X represents one stool.

either group of investigators. It is apparent that criteria selection will vary for a given population; that is, stool characteristics for subjects with tube-fed diets will differ from those of subjects who may be at risk for constipation. This makes establishment of a standardized scale for measuring stool consistency difficult and emphasizes the importance of selecting appropriate criteria for the population under study.

SUBJECTIVE SCALES YIELDING QUALITATIVE DATA

▪ ANDERSSON ET AL. SCALE

Andersson et al. developed a scale for evaluating bowel habits while investigating the effects of dietary restriction of fat and the use of antidiarrheal agents after bowel resection in patients with Crohn's disease.[17] The bowel habits were evaluated according to the following scale:

Satisfactory or good	Three or less bowel movements/24 hours, usually after breakfast and causing no social inconvenience
Fair	Four to six movements/24 hours, mostly in relation to meals and with minor inconvenience
Poor	Seven or more bowel movements/24 hours, considerable social inconvenience and/or incapacity for work

▪ DROSSMAN ET AL. QUESTIONNAIRE

Using a broader approach, Drossman et al. developed a brief, self-administered questionnaire to identify bowel patterns among the general population.[18] The questionnaire contained several areas of inquiry for comparative analysis and provided demographic data as well as information about subject attitudes and behavior related to bowel function. Based on their responses to questions about stool frequency, abdominal pain, or awareness of changes in bowel patterns, subjects could be classified into several categories. Examples are:

Category A. Alternating bowel function.	Subject responded affirmatively to questions about loose, frequent stools alternating with hard, infrequent stools, and similar questions.
Category B. Abdominal pain.	Included in this category were subjects with more than six episodes of lower abdominal pain in the last year under various circumstances, such as abdominal pain relieved by bowel movement, loose stools associated with pain.

Criteria selection for each category was based on reports from other investigations into dysfunctional bowel syndromes and were both objective and subjective. Subject attitudes regarding bowel dysfunction were assessed by such questions as:

Does stress affect your bowel pattern?
    never
    sometimes
    always

Do stresses lead to abdominal pain:

never
sometimes
always

The instrument allows the researcher to identify by questionnaire a range of bowel patterns in the general population and to categorize subjects into groups with specific types of bowel dysfunction. It was administered to 789 subjects, and the results were in agreement with data reported from other investigations into comparable bowel patterns.

SUMMARY

From the investigations of various researches, it becomes apparent that the use of several measures will be necessary in order to obtain data that will accurately reflect the concept of elimination and human bowel patterns. Furthermore, considering the normal variability of colonic function, interpretations of these data will need to reflect the dynamic status of this basic human process.

Although early studies relied mostly on self-reporting and one-dimensional measures, more recent investigations have revealed the multifaceted aspects of human bowel function and have developed measures to realize its accurate evaluation.

REFERENCES

1. Godding, E.W. Physiological yardsticks for bowel function and the rehabilitation of the constipated bowel. *Pharmacology,* 1980, *20*[Suppl 1]:88.
2. Hinton, J.M., Lennard-Jones, J.E., & Young, A.C. A new method for studying gut transit times using radioopaque markers. *Gut,* 1969, *10*(10):842.
3. Cummings, J.H., Jenkins, D.J.A., & Wiggins, H.S. Measurement of the mean transit time of dietary residue through the human gut. *Gut,* 1976, *17*(3):210.
4. Payler, D.K., Pomare, E.W., Heaton, K.W., & Harvey, R.F. The effect of wheat bran on intestinal transit. *Gut,* 1975, *16*(3):209.
5. Cummings, J.H., & Wiggins, H.S. Transit through the gut measured by analysis of a single stool. *Gut,* 1976, *17*(3):219.
6. Dick, M. Use of cuprous thiocyanate as a short-term continuous marker for feces. *Gut,* 1969, *10*(5):408.
7. Davignon, J., Simmonds, W.J., & Aherns, E.H. Jr. Usefulness of chromic oxide as an internal standard for balance studies in formula-fed patients for assessment of colonic function. *J Clin Invest,* 1968, *47*:127.
8. Bolin, D.W., King, R.P., & Klosterman, E.W. A simplified method for the determination of chromic oxide when used as an index substance. *Science,* 1952, *116*(5):634.
9. Hansky, J., & Connell, A.M. Measurement of gastrointestinal transit using radioactive chromium. *Gut,* 1962, *3*(2):187.
10. Connell, A.M. The motility of the pelvic colon. Part I. *Gut,* 1961, *2*(2):175.
11. Connell, A.M. The motility of the pelvic colon. Part II. *Gut,* 1962, *3*(4):342.
12. Waller, S.L. Comparative effects of codeine and senna on the motor activity of the left colon. *Gut,* 1975, *16*(5):407.
13. Meunier, P., Rochas, A., & Lambert, R. Motor activity of the sigmoid colon in chronic constipation: Comparative study with normal subjects. *Gut,* 1979, *20*(12):1095.
14. Kagawa-Busby, K.S., Heitkemper, M.M., Hansen, B.C., et al. Effects of diet temperature on tolerance of enteral feedings. *Nurs Res,* 1980, *29*(5):276.

15. Walike, B.C., & Walike, J.W. Relative lactose intolerance. *JAMA,* 1977, *238*(9):948.

16. Goodman, J., Pang, J., & Bessman, A.N. Dioctyl sodium sulfosuccinate—An ineffective prophylactic laxative. *J Chronic Dis,* 1976, *29*(1):59.

17. Andersson, H., Bosaeus, I., Hellberg, R., & Hulten, L. Effect of a low-fat diet and antidiarrheal agents on bowel habits after excisional surgery for classical Crohn's disease. *Acta Chir Scand,* 1982, *148*(3):291.

18. Drossman, D.A., Sandler, R.S., McKee, D.C., & Lovitz, A.J. Bowel patterns among subjects not seeking health care: Use of a questionnaire to identify a population with bowel dysfunction. *Gastroenterology,* 1982, *83*(3):529.

19. Wyman, J.B., Heaton, K.W., Manning, A.P., & Wicks, A.C.B. Variability of colonic function in healthy subjects. *Gut,* 1978, *19*(2):146.

20. Slavin, J.L., Sempos, C.T., Brauer, P.M., & Marlett, J.A. Limits of predicting gastrointestinal transit time from other measures of bowel function. *Am J Clin Nutr,* 1981, *34*(10):2111.

21. Wrick, K.L., Robertson, J.B., Van Soest, P.J., et al. The influence of dietary fiber source on human intestinal transit and stool output. *J Nutr,* 1983, *113*(8):1464.

22. Kelsay, J.L., Behall, K.M., & Prather, E.S. Effect of fiber from fruits and vegetables on metabolic responses of human subjects: Bowel transit time, number of defecations, fecal weight, urinary excretions of energy and nitrogen and apparent digestibilities of energy, nitrogen and fat. *Am J Clin Nutr,* 1978, *31*(7):1149.

23. Rogers, H.J., House, F.R., Morrison, P.J., & Bradbrook, I.D. Comparison of the effect of drugs upon some commonly used measures of bowel transit time. *Br J Clin Pharmacol,* 1978, *6*(6):493.

24. Waller, S.L. Differential measurement of small and large bowel transit times in constipation and diarrhea: A new approach. *Gut,* 1975, *16*(5):372.

25. Exton-Smith, A.N., Bendall, M.J., & Kent, F. A new technique for measuring the consistency of feces. A report in the elderly. *Age Ageing,* 1975, *4*(1):58.

CHAPTER 20

Measuring Pain

Deborah B. McGuire, R.N., Ph.D.

DEFINITIONS OF PAIN

Pain is such an individual subjective experience that its measurement has long been a challenge for researchers. Indeed, even a satisfactory definition of pain has remained elusive. Sternbach called pain "(1) a personal, private sensation of hurt; (2) a harmful stimulus which signals current or impending tissue damage; (3) a pattern of responses which operate to protect the organism from harm" (p. 12).[1] Melzack and Casey emphasized that pain was a sensory experience with motivational and affective properties.[2] Merskey and Spear described pain as an unpleasant experience primarily associated with actual tissue damage, described in such terms, or both.[3]

Because of these many definitions of pain and the complexity of pain as a phenomenon, the International Association for the Study of Pain (IASP) developed a list of pain terms and definitions.[4] Pain was defined as "an unpleasant sensory and emotional experience associated with actual or potential tissue damage, or described in terms of such damage" (p. S217).[4] This definition encompassed pain of pathophysiologic and psychologic origin and also accounted for the sensory, affective, and motivational aspects of the experience.

Melzack and Wall believe that an accurate definition of pain cannot be formulated.[5] They view the word pain as representing a "category of experiences" that are unique, have different causes, and are characterized by different sensory and affective dimensions.[5]

PERCEPTION AND EXPERIENCE OF PAIN

Although the dispute over definitions of pain may not be resolved entirely, the crucial point to remember when attempting to measure pain is the highly subjective and unique nature of the experience. The IASP and many individual authors have recognized the importance of viewing pain from the vantage point of those who are experiencing it.[3,4,6,7]

Two concepts related to the subjectivity of the pain experience are important in individuals' responses to pain. "Threshold" refers to the point at which pain is first experienced, that is, the lowest level of potentially injurious sensation that produces a report of pain. Tolerance is the point at which an individual reports pain to be so intense that it can no longer be tolerated. These two pain response parameters are generally measured in studies of laboratory-induced pain and have little relevance in clinical pain.

Traditionally, there have been two opposing schools of thought on the nature of pain, both based on Descartes' seventeenth century notion that pain was an alarm system designed to signal injury of the body. The specificity theory proposed that pain was a specific entity, similar to sight or smell, with its own peripheral and central components. Specific pain receptors in the skin were thought to project to a specific pain center in the brain. The pattern theory proposed that there were no specific fibers or endings, but the nerve impulse pattern for pain was produced by stimulation of nonspecific receptors. Several versions of the pattern theory were developed, some stressing the intensity of the painful stimuli as the critical determinants of pain and others emphasizing a central summative mechanism.

Several people in the twentieth century developed a new concept of pain in which the perception of pain was determined by factors, such as personality, previous experience, and culture.[8,9] In 1965, Melzack and Wall challenged the adequacy of the specificity and pattern theories to provide a satisfactory general explanation of the phenomenon of pain and proposed the now classic gate control theory of pain.[10] The theory postulated that pain phenomena were determined by the interactions among three spinal cord systems. First, peripheral stimulation sent nerve impulses to the substantia gelatinosa in the dorsal horn of the spinal cord, where these cells modulated the afferent impulses (the gate control mechanism). Second, the afferent patterns in the fibers of the dorsal column acted as a central control trigger that activated selective brain processes, which in turn influenced the modulating gate control properties of the substantia gelatinosa. Third, central transmission cells in the dorsal horn activated neural mechanisms believed to be responsible for the perception of and response to pain.

The gate control theory helped to explain many puzzling aspects of the phenomenon of pain and placed emphasis on the sensory and emotional components of pain perception. Although some of the proposed components of the theory have not been documented experimentally, there appears to be universal acknowledgment of the importance and value of the theory in guiding pain research and the clinical management of pain.[11] Even Melzack and Wall believe that the gate control theory is not the "final truth" about pain, but they point out that a satisfactory alternate theory has yet to be devised.[5]

Following the introduction of the gate control theory, a new conceptual model of pain, comprised of three dimensions, was developed by Melzack and Casey.[2] The selection and modulation of incoming pain sensations in the neospinothalamic projection system were the basis for the sensory/discriminative component of pain. Subsequently, the brain reticular formation and limbic systems became involved in aversive drive and affective reactions to pain, forming the motivational/affective component of pain. Finally, higher central nervous system or central control activities were involved in the pain experience and response. These activities were primarily cognitive functions that acted selectively on sensory processes and/or motivational mechanisms. The influences of present and past experiences were believed integral to the cognitive activities. Thus, the pain experience was believed to be a function of the interaction of all three of these determinants. These notions gradually evolved into a concept of pain that was multidimensional in nature.

In summary, pain initially was considered by many researchers to be a purely sensory phenomenon. Later researchers recognized both sensory and reactive (emotional) components.[6,9] Then Melzack and Casey described sensory/discriminative, motivational/affective, and cognitive components.[2] Finally, Ahles et al. described pain as a multidimensional experience consisting of physiologic, sensory, affective, cognitive, and behavioral aspects.[12] Although their conceptualization involved cancer-related pain, it certainly appears to have applicability to many situations of clinical pain.

TYPES OF PAIN

Pain can be arbitrarily categorized in a number of ways, but two commonly used methods are according to duration and cause. A primary distinction can be drawn between pain that is caused by experimental procedures in the laboratory and pain that is caused by various organic processes (usually termed clinical pain). Researchers in the field of pain have long disagreed about whether these two types of pain are directly comparable.[13] It seems to be generally agreed that experimental and clinical pain are not truly synonymous, however, since the former is transient and controllable and the latter may be persistent and uncontrollable. An indepth discussion of the issues surrounding this controversy can be found in a recent article by Wolff.[14]

The focus of this chapter is on the measurement of clinical pain for research purposes. A distinction based on duration can be made. Acute pain is pain associated with tissue damage that begins to decrease as the tissues heal. It is generally of short duration, that is, days to weeks. Examples of acute pain are incisional discomfort following a surgical procedure, cholecystitis, and the unpleasant sensations that follow hitting one's thumb with a hammer.

Chronic pain, on the other hand, is generally described as a pain state that persists for 6 months or more. Real or impending tissue damage may or may not be a factor in chronic pain. Examples include inflammatory joint or degenerative disk disease, postherpetic neuralgia, and persistent cancer pain.

Some authors have developed subcategories of acute and chronic pain.[15,16] For example, acute pain may become subacute (or limited) in cases of prolonged healing, such as a crushing musculoskeletal injury. Acute pain may also be recurrent (or intermittent), such as migraine headaches or sickle cell crisis. Chronic pain can be divided into subcategories as well. Chronic pain due to cancer is sometimes called intractable pain. Another variant of chronic pain is persistent or chronic benign pain, such as low back pain or neuralgias.

PROBLEMS IN MEASURING PAIN

Regardless of the type of clinical pain one wishes to measure, a variety of problems will be encountered. Viewing the experience of pain from the subjective stance of the sufferer is the first major problem. Adequate measurement of pain may be hindered by individuals' differing perceptions of and responses to pain. Thus, patients who are experiencing pain are simply not comparable, even when their pain has the same etiology. Additionally, their verbal reports of pain are not readily verifiable, and particular measures of pain may mean different things to different people. Finally, health professionals may differ in their responses to people with pain, occasionally underestimating or overestimating its severity.[17,18] Despite these multiple problems with viewing pain subjectively, pain remains an individual experience that is variable (dependent on many factors) and private yet consistent within each individual. It is important in measuring clinical pain that this perspective be acknowledged.

A variety of clinical and personal issues influence the measurement of pain as well. The type of pain experienced by the individual according to duration and/or cause is one important factor, as is the therapy employed for the pain. A number of specific patient characteristics, such as educational level, nature of physical illness, presence of affective disorders,[19] age, [20-22] motor coordination, visual ability, and ethnic background,[23] will influence the measurement of pain in a particular patient population. Situational factors can create problems for the researcher or clinician who is attempting to measure pain. Examples include the actual physical environment, health personnel, or the presence or absence of family or friends.

A third problem that occurs in measuring pain is the limited number of available instruments that are quantifiable, reliable, and valid. The lack of quantifiable instruments is bothersome to many researchers. Some have attempted to develop measures of clinical pain that, although subjective, can be quantified through a variety of experimental pain procedures used to match estimates of clinical pain sensations and verbal subjective judgments.[24] These sensory matching techniques, as they are called, are based on psychophysics.[25-27] Since sensory matching techniques have not been used extensively in the measurement of clinical pain, they are not discussed here.

Many researchers use ordinal level Likert-type or interval level visual analog scales in their attempts to measure and quantify pain, but the validity of such instruments in measuring the total experience of pain may be questioned. Reliability of particular tools across groups, settings, and time periods may not be established adequately, thus limiting their use to appropriate samples only.

A final problem in measuring clinical pain in the conduct of pain research is a multitude of ethical issues, addressed in some detail by Sternbach.[28] Particularly problematic in experimental research is the infliction or manipulation of pain, which occurs as part of the normal design of such studies. In the clinical arena, other issues arise. The researcher must balance his or her goal of increasing our knowledge of pain and its management with the potential for coercion, physical harm, mental harm, or breach of human dignity. The procedures of any study involving pain, including and especially the measurement of pain, must observe all accepted standards for the rights and protection of human subjects.

The discussion of tools for measuring pain in this chapter is limited to those that have been developed or used to measure clinical pain in adults. Reviews of instruments available to measure pain in children may be found elsewhere.[21,22] Since pain is a multidimensional experience, instruments are classified according to the dimensions they measure.[2,12]

For each tool, the discussion includes the dimension(s) of pain it measures, a description, available reliability and validity data, examples of situations in which it has been used, recommendations for appropriate use in a research context, and advantages and disadvantages.

The overall focus of the chapter is on the use of these instruments for measuring pain in a clinical research setting rather than assessing pain in the clinical practice setting. It is acknowledged, however, that many of the tools are highly appropriate for use by the clinician in assessing and managing pain.

AVAILABLE TOOLS

Sensory/Discriminative Dimension

Scales are the most commonly used tools to measure the sensory dimension of pain. There are many types of scales available, but the variable generally measured by all of them is pain intensity. Occasionally, investigators will use scales to measure degree of pain relief rather than pain intensity (e.g., "no relief" to "complete relief").[29]

• VERBAL DESCRIPTOR SCALES

Verbal Descriptor Scales (VDS) measure pain intensity, a major component of the sensory/discriminative dimension of pain. They usually consist of three to five numerically ranked words:

```
_____1   None
_____2   Mild
_____3   Moderate
_____4   Severe
_____5   Unbearable
```

The number corresponding to the word chosen can be used to analyze the data on an ordinal level.

The forerunner of VDS appears to have been Keele's Pain Chart, originally devised to assess responses to analgesics over a 24-hour time period[30]:

```
Agony
Severe
Moderate
Slight
Nil
_____
AM   2   4   6   8   10   12   14   16   18   20   22   24
```

Thus, the pain chart is a time–intensity curve. Keele established the reliability of the chart by administering it repeatedly to patients with various painful medical conditions. He assessed the validity of the chart by administering it to patients with known painful conditions, such as angina or peptic ulcer disease, and observing increases and decreases of pain on the time–intensity curve in relation to physical activity, treatment, and other factors. More recently, researchers have used simple word descriptor lists rather than an entire pain chart, although Keele makes a good case for the usefulness of the Pain Chart in clinical and experimental research.[31] Melzack's Present Pain Intensity Scale (PPI) on the McGill Pain Questionnaire is an additional type of VDS commonly seen in the literature[32]:

```
_____0   No pain
_____1   Mild
_____2   Discomforting
_____3   Distressing
_____4   Horrible
_____5   Excruciating
```

Few authors using VDS, however, have discussed reliability and validity, but most would agree that an individual's subjective rating of the intensity of pain using word descriptors probably is a valid measurement.

Keele used the Pain Chart to assess patients' responses to drugs and other therapy in many conditions, including postoperatively, in angina, in cancer, and in peptic ulcer disease.[30,31] Kruszewski et al. used a 5-point VDS to assess discomfort in surgical patients who received dorsogluteal injections while in various positions.[33] Appropriate uses of the Pain Chart or simple VDS would include assessment of responses to therapy in patients with these conditions as well as others, provided the investigator limited the variable measured to pain intensity.

Verbal Descriptor Scales have the advantages of brevity, ease of administration and completion, ease of scoring, and applicability to many types of patients and to acute or chronic pain. The data produced are probably reliable and valid. On the other hand, the word descriptors on a VDS may artificially categorize the intensity of pain and may not reflect accurately an individual's real sensory experience. Furthermore, recent studies have indicated that the category words on a VDS do not divide the perceptual continuum of pain into equal segments and may lack sufficient sensitivity to measure pain intensity.[34]

▪ VISUAL ANALOGUE SCALES (VAS)

Visual Analogue Scales (VAS) were first developed approximately 60 years ago to measure a variety of subjective phenomena,[35] but the reference cited by most researchers who use VAS is that of Clarke and Spear.[36] In pain research, VAS are generally used to measure the intensity of pain. The VAS usually consists of a line 10 cm long with verbal anchors at either end:

```
          _____
No pain                                         Pain as bad as it
                                                could possibly be
```

The patient is asked to place a mark through the line at the point that best describes how much pain is experienced at that particular moment. The VAS is called a Graphic Rating Scale (GRS) if descriptive words are placed along the line[37]:

```
          _____
No pain      Mild      Moderate      Severe   Pain as bad as it
                                              could possibly be
```

Interval level data are obtained on visual or graphic scales by measuring from the left end of the scale to the mark made by the patient. Price et al. have validated the use of VAS as ratio scale measures in chronic and experimental pain.[38] VAS are considered more sensitive measures of pain intensity than VDS because they have a straight line continuum rather than categorical responses. One report, however, found no differences in sensitivity when comparing these scales.[29]

Many researchers using VAS have discussed reliability/validity issues in their published reports. Revill et al. used a VAS with ten women in labor and demonstrated reliability on repeated measurements ($r = 0.95$, $p < 0.001$).[39] Similarly, Clarke and Spear found the VAS reliable and sensitive to changes in the self-assessment of well-being.[36] Although Maxwell did not study pain, he found that individuals rating sound volumes had more sensitive and accurate ratings on a VAS than did different subjects, suggesting that using VAS to compare groups might not produce reliable measures across the different groups.[35] Dixon and Bird, in studying eight people, demonstrated that subjects' ability to reproduce a set of marked scales within a given time period was often inconsistent, suggesting that estimation of the same sensation could be placed at different points on the scale over time.[40] Carlsson found that in patients with chronic pain, a regular VAS was less sensitive to bias than a comparative VAS (e.g., a scale in which the anchor words are defined in terms of pain relief).[41] Although these reliability data are somewhat varied and conflicting, validity of the VAS seems to have been assumed, as with the VDS. However, subjective ratings of pain intensity may be considered reasonably valid regardless of the scale used.

VAS have been used to measure pain intensity in a variety of patients, including women in labor,[39] people with cancer,[42] people with arthritis, and others. Appropriate use of the VAS would encompass any group of patients with acute or chronic pain, provided such use was restricted to the measurement of pain intensity. The evaluation of treatment outcomes, particularly pharmacologic interventions, is a popular application of VAS in clinical research.

VAS are easy to administer and score, an advantage in clinical research where time may be limited. Additionally, since VAS are considered to produce interval level data, parametric statistics may be used in analysis. VAS have several disadvantages. Although it does not appear to matter whether the VAS are horizontal or vertical in format,[43] some people have difficulty conceptualizing a sensory phenomenon, such as pain intensity, in a straight line continuum. They may place their marks near the anchor words, yielding data of questionable reliability and validity. Scott and Huskisson believe that patient access to previous scores is important in obtaining accurate subsequent measures when administering the VAS repeatedly, since previous ratings can be used for comparison.[44] Careful instructions to individuals using a VAS to rate pain intensity are imperative to proper understanding and use of the scale.

Comparisons of Scales. Since both VDS and VAS measure pain intensity, many researchers have compared the two in terms of sensitivity, reliability, validity, ease of administration and patient use, and patient preferences. Correlations ranging from 0.81 to 0.89 ($p = 0.01$ to 0.001) between VDS and VAS were found in several studies.[29,45–48] When Wallenstein compared scores from one population of patients to another, he found a high degree of reliability in the obtained measures and no obvious or consistent response effects due to sex or age.[47]

Studies of different forms of VDS and VAS have been performed as well. Scott and Huskisson[46] compared six different VAS and GRS to a simple VDS. They concluded that a horizontal VAS and a horizontal GRS with the descriptor words placed along the length of the line

No pain	Mild	Moderate	Severe	Pain as bad as it could possibly be

produced more uniform distributions, were more sensitive to perceived pain intensity, and were easier for patients to use.

Reading[49] compared the PPI scale from the McGill Pain Questionnaire,[32] a 10-cm VAS, and a 10-point horizontal numerical scale with anchor words of none–mild–moderately distressing–very distressing–unbearable in patients with episiotomy pain. He found wide variability in the distribution of ratings as well as in agreement between scale differences over time and subjective comparisons. His correlations between the VAS and VDS were significant ($r = 0.57$ to 0.71), although lower than those reported elsewhere. Reading's conclusions were that insufficient psychometric analyses of scales had been done and that the efficacy or usefulness of such scales may vary according to the characteristics of patients and settings in which they were employed.

Downie et al. examined the validity of VAS and VDS by comparing them to one another as well as to a 0 to 100 Numerical Rating Scale (NRS).[50] All the scales correlated well and had similar loadings on a factor analysis, leading the investigators to conclude that the scales probably measured the same variable (i.e., pain intensity). They expressed preference for the 0 to 100 NRS because it offered more choices than the VDS and was less confusing than the VAS.

Kremer et al. asked patients to express their preferences when using a VAS, an NRS, and a five-adjective adaptation of Melzack's PPI.[51] The results indicated that most patients preferred the five-adjective scale, and all were able to complete it. The VAS had an 11 percent failure rate, and the NRS had a 2 percent failure rate. Thus, in certain circumstances, a VDS, such as Melzack's PPI, may be more reliable.

Littman et al.[29] assessed a VDS, a VAS, and a verbal pain relief scale in 1497 patients with a variety of acute and chronic types of pain (postoperative, cancer, orthopedic, renal colic) who were receiving analgesics. They reported that all three measures correlated well ($r = 0.89$ to 0.93) but that there were no consistent differences in sensitivity between the verbal and analog scales; in fact, the verbal pain relief scale was slightly more sensitive than the other two. They concluded that choice of scale may not be critical and should be dictated by the particular measurement situation.

In summary, the results of these comparative studies indicate that the scales discussed are useful for measuring perceived pain intensity and, in general, correlate reasonably well. Their reliability is relatively well established, but any researcher using such scales must consider the individual characteristics of both patients and settings before choosing specific scales. For example, the VAS may be too abstract for patients with severe acute pain, lower educational levels, or impaired motor coordination. In such instances, a VDS may be easier to use and may produce more reliable data.

Affective/Evaluative Dimension

Instruments that measure the affective/evaluative dimension of the pain experience generally include the sensory dimension (usually pain intensity) and a subjective or reactive component. Such tools are an attempt to measure more of the total pain experience than simply intensity.

▪ TWO-COMPONENT SCALE

Probably the earliest tool developed to measure the affective/evaluative dimension of pain was Johnson's Two-Component Scale.[52-54] She separated pain into a sensory component and a reactive component, each measured on a separate scale. Subjects experiencing experimentally induced pain were asked to rate the physical sensation on a 0 to 100 scale and the distress caused by the sensation on a scale labeled "slightly distressing," "moderately distressing," "very distressing," and "just bearable." The distress scale lacked a "none" or "not distressing" category.

The researchers reported that high pain intensity (physical sensation) ratings were not always accompanied by high distress ratings. They did not, however, discuss the psychometric development of the scale and did not present any reliability or validity data.

Although the scale was developed to measure experimentally induced pain, the researchers suggested that it might be useful in measuring clinical pain, particularly when evaluating the effect of pharmacologic interventions. Wells used the Two-Component Scale to assess the effects of relaxation on postoperative pain and distress.[55] Although subjects who received relaxation training reported less distress, their pain intensity ratings were similar to those of the control group. Wells did not address any psychometric aspects of the scales in either the method or discussion sections. Because of the simple format and short time required for the administration of the scale, it could be used with almost any type of clinical pain. It might be especially useful in helping the researcher determine how much a given level of physical sensation distressed an individual. On the other hand, caution in interpreting the data from the scale would be advisable, since its reliability and validity are unclear. Concurrent evaluation of these psychometric parameters would certainly provide valuable information about the appropriateness of the Two-Component Scale for measuring clinical pain.

▪ TURSKY'S PAIN PERCEPTION PROFILE (PPP)

Tursky devised three sets of adjectives to measure the intensity, sensory, and reactive components of pain in a tool called the Pain Perception Profile (PPP).[56,57] The intensity list included 15 words, such as excruciating, very intense, strong, moderate, and weak. The sensory list contained 13 words, such as piercing, shooting, burning, cramping, and stinging. The reactive list consisted of 11 words, such as agonizing, unbearable, miserable, unpleasant, and bearable. Subjects selected one word from each list.

Tursky developed his lists and tested them with 56 college undergraduates who did not have clinical pain.[56] No reliability or validity data pertinent to people with clinical pain were presented or discussed. The goal of Tursky's work was to enable patients to scale pain by magnitude estimation, that is, in equal interval stimuli, as compared to a standard pain stimulus. He felt that magnitude estimation had two advantages over categorical scaling as described under VDS: (1) it imposed fewer constraints on reponses, and (2) it enabled investigators to test the validity of responses with known reliable interrelationships.

Turksy's PPP has not been used very frequently in clinical research. Andrasik et al. used the intensity and reactive lists for headache pain in 30 patients, finding support for the validity of the two-component approach.[58] They found that patients' ratings on intensity adjectives correlated well with a numerical scale (0 = no headache, 5 = extremely intense headache). Ahles et al. used the lists to measure pain in 40 cancer patients, but did not comment on their psychometric properties.[12] Urban et al. used the same lists of the PPP with a sample of 42 chronic pain patients.[59] They found that most patients were able to scale pain reliably on the intensity but not on the reactive dimension. The value of Tursky's PPP is not clear in the measurement of clinical pain, but more exploration of its usefulness is needed.

Cognitive/Behavioral Dimension

Instruments that measure the cognitive/behavioral dimension of pain include such variables as spatial and temporal aspects of pain and specific or general behaviors exhibited by people with pain.

Cognitive Measures

▪ TIME ESTIMATION OF PAIN MAGNITUDE

Bilting et al. attempted to use patients' estimates of time as a measure of pain magnitude, based on the underlying assumption that pain has spatial (or intensity) and temporal properties.[60] In the experiment, a group of pain patients and a control group were asked to estimate the duration of certain amounts of time. It was hypothesized that an increase in time estimation would correlate roughly with increasing pain intensity. For each participant, the deformation of time was expressed as the difference between the average values of estimated and real time. Pain patients perceived a particular time period as significantly longer ($p < 0.001$) than did controls; their distortion of time correlated ($r = 0.88$) with a clinical assessment of pain severity. These findings are very preliminary, emanating from one study with a sample of 35 pain patients (or unreported diagnoses) and 40 controls. Weeks[61] urged evalutation of the reliability and validity of the tool against established measures of pain.

▪ PAIN CHART

Margoles developed a Pain Chart, a two-dimensional graphic account to be used by patients in reporting subjective components of their pain.[62] Specifically, the chart consists of drawings of the body or body parts on which the patient can draw in the location of pain as well as its sensory aspects (e.g., red to indicate burning, green for cramping). The chart has a temporal component, since it can be used over time to report increases, decreases, or sensory changes in pain. Margoles did not present reliability or validity data on the Pain Chart but emphasized that it was used to record the patient's subjective perceptions. He developed the chart originally for use in orthopedic patients, but it could easily be extended to patients with other painful medical or surgical conditions. Margoles cautioned that the pain chart was a "non-specific, adjunctive diagnostic tool" but that it lent itself well to a variety of studies in pain treatment. For certain patient populations, it seems to offer promise and needs further evaluation.

Behavioral Measures

Acute Pain

• HANKEN ET AL. PAIN RATING SCALE

A person who is experiencing acute pain may have observable behaviors and physiologic parameters that can be measured and recorded. Hanken et al. used six such parameters to develop a Pain Rating Scale to evaluate attention directed toward pain, anxiety, verbal statement of degree of pain, skeletal muscle response, characteristics of respiration, and amount of perspiration.[63,64] An example is depicted below:

> Skeletal muscle response:
> Patient is: _____very restless _____markedly restless _____slightly
> restless _____very slightly restless _____quiet

Although the researchers reported reasonably good agreement in their reliability assessments, they did not give correlation values. They examined construct validity by analyzing 289 nurse observations of 70 patients. A correlation matrix of the six parameters indicated positive relationships ($r = 0.44$ to 0.71) between attention, anxiety, stated degree of pain, and skeletal muscle response. Factor analysis with an unspecified method of rotation showed the first factor to be composed of attention directed toward pain and stated degree of pain, both of which had the highest factor loadings.[64]

Chambers and Price later modified this Pain Rating Scale by deleting respiration and adding scales for sounds made by the patient, nausea, muscle tension, and facial expression.[65] They did not, however, give any reliability or validity data for the revised instrument except to comment that correlations between total scores and scores for verbal report of degree of pain ranged from $r = 0.66$ to $r = 0.87$. Bruegel used the revised scale to measure postoperative pain and reported evidence of validity because pain scores were positively correlated ($r = 0.38$) with amount of analgesic.[66]

Hanken and McDowell developed the original scale to measure acute postoperative pain.[64] Bruegel used the revised version similarly,[66] and Chambers and Price used it to measure acute, chronic, and progressive pain.[65] The revised scale may be most appropriate for samples with acute pain, since the items deal with indicants of acute pain. Patients with chronic pain may not manifest the same indicants. Potential uses of the scale include assessment of response to a wide variety of interventions.

The revised scale is advantageous when compared to other scales because it is multidimensional, focusing on anxiety, attention paid to pain, and physiologic parameters. Additionally, its observational and subjective nature make it easy to administer and score. The disadvantages are questionable construct validity, applicability only to acute pain, and an administration time of 5 to 15 minutes.[67]

• BEHAVIORAL INDEX FOR THE ASSESSMENT OF LABOR PAIN

Bonnel and Bourneau[68] developed a Behavioral Index for the Assessment of Labor Pain. In 100 primiparous women, respiratory modifications, motor responses (e.g., grasping with hands), and agitation were measured on a cumulative 5-point scale in which higher numbers indicated more behavioral manifestations of pain. For example, a patient scoring a 1 displayed increased respiratory rate or amplitude during contractions, whereas a patient scoring a 2 displayed the same plus signs of tension, such as grasping of sheets or someone's hand.

Ratings were made by obstetricians or midwives and were compared to patients' self-ratings of their present pain intensity to investigate the validity of the method. Global scores obtained over the entire labor period were significantly correlated ($r = 0.88$, $p < 0.001$), as were scores from different phases of labor (cervical dilations of 3, 5, 7, and 10 cm) ($r = 0.30$ to 0.50, $p < 0.01$ to 0.001). Additionally, interrater reliability was reported as good, since mean behavioral scores recorded by two observers were not significantly different. Overall, the investigators concluded that their index was valid if correspondence between its observational measures and subjects' self-reports was considered. They cited a need for further evaluation of the tool, however, in relation to physical parameters of labor progression and to the notion of behavioral ratings as a potential index of self-control behaviors during labor.[68] This tool appears to have potential usefulness in studies involving labor pain.

Chronic Pain

• FORDYCE ET AL. PAIN DIARY

Fordyce et al. developed a diary form for home recording of chronic pain that measures physical activity, medications, and pain intensity.[69] The form contains space for hour by hour recording over a 24-hour time period of (1) whether an individual is sitting, standing, walking, or reclining, (2) the kind and amount of medications used; and (3) ratings of pain on a 0 (no pain) to 10 (intolerable pain) scale. Time spent performing certain activities can be calculated so that functional impairment is assessed, particularly in relation to consumption of pain medication and to intensity of pain.

• FOLLICK ET AL. PAIN DIARY

Fordyce et al. reported no reliability or validity data,[69] but Follick et al. did address these issues in their evaluation of a daily activity diary for chronic pain patients.[70] Their form was used by patients to record various postures and activities, the use of pain relief measures, time spent in pain relief activities, and the use of analgesics. Patient self-reports were compared to spouse observations and, in the case of postures and activities, to an automated electromechanical device. Follick et al. found that reliability coefficients for categories of daily activity were positive ($r = 0.44$ to 0.89) and significant ($p = 0.05$ to 0.01), as were the correlations between patient and spouse ratings on certain variables, including time spent on standing, walking, lying down, pain intensity, and pill counts. Additionally, correlations between patient reports of lying down and electromechanical monitor measurements were high ($r = 0.94$, $p < 0.01$).

▪ UNIVERSITY OF ALABAMA–BIRMINGHAM (UAB) PAIN BEHAVIOR SCALE

Some researchers question the accuracy of patient self-reports, believing that people may overreport or underreport their activities.[71] As a result, methods for the direct observation of pain behaviors have been developed.[72,73] Richards et al. developed the University of Alabama–Birmingham (UAB) Pain Behavior Scale to objectively assess ten pain-related behaviors: verbal vocal complaints, nonverbal vocal complaints, time spent lying down, facial grimaces, standing posture, mobility, body language, use of visible supportive equipment, stationary movement, and medication.[73] Richards et al. cited good interrater reliability for the scale ($r = 0.95$, $p < 0.01$) and good test–retest reliability ($r = 0.89$, $p < 0.01$). The researchers had difficulty assessing the scale's validity adequately, since there were few other measures to compare it to.

The UAB Pain Behavior Scale[73] and Fordyce's tool[69] have been used in chronic pain. They are simple and easy for either health personnel or patients to use. The UAB Scale in particular appears very reliable. Both instruments could be used in clinical research to evaluate treatments, but they may be of more help to the clinician who is assessing pain than to the researcher who is trying to obtain precise measurements of pain.

▪ BEHAVIORAL DYSFUNCTION INDEX (BDI)

One final behavioral measure of chronic pain is the method to assess pain from head and neck cancer developed by Keefe et al.[74] Six quantitative areas were evaluated: motor pain behaviors, specific painful activities, general activity level, pain-relieving methods, pain medication intake, and weight loss. For motor pain behaviors, observers recorded occurrence/nonoccurrence of four specific behaviors (guarded movement, grimacing, rubbing, sighing) while patients sat, stood, walked, reclined, rotated their heads left and right, swallowed, and coughed. For the remaining five areas, data were collected through structured interview.

A Behavioral Dysfunction Index (BDI) was developed as a composite measure for each patient based on responses during observation and to interview questions. The scores ranged from 0 to 6 with 0 = no dysfunction, 1–3 = mild to moderate dysfunction, and 4–6 = extreme dysfunction. Although Keefe et al. did not discuss specifically the reliability or validity of their method, they indicated that increased BDI scores were positively and significantly ($p < 0.05$) related to pain ratings on a 0 to 10 numerical scale (0 = no pain, 10 = pain as bad as it can be). Although developed as a clinical assessment tool and needing further psychometric evaluation, this method could be used for research purposes. A major disadvantage, however, would be the time and skill required to administer the questions.

Multiple Dimensions

The instruments described thus far are limited in their ability to measure the total experience of pain since they are restricted to one or two dimensions. Several tools have been developed over the past decade or so to measure pain from a multidimensional standpoint.

• MCGILL PAIN QUESTIONNAIRE (MPQ)

The McGill Pain Questionnaire (MPQ) originated in 1971 with the work of Melzack and Torgerson, who grouped words to describe pain and scaled them along an intensity dimension.[75] They found that the words fell into classes and subclasses describing dimensions other than intensity, for example, affective and evaluative aspects of pain. The full version of the MPQ was published in 1975 by Melzack.[32] The dimensions measured by the MPQ include location of pain, pattern of pain over time, sensory, affective, evaluative, and miscellaneous components of pain, and intensity. Other individual patient characteristics that can be assessed on the full version of the MPQ include diagnosis, drug intake, pain and medical history, therapy, personal history, factors increasing or decreasing pain, effects on sleep, sexual activity, and work, least and worst pain, and other factors.

An abbreviated version of the MPQ (Fig. 20–1) is used commonly for both clinical and research purposes. The short version consists of four parts. One part has drawings of the human body on which a person indicates the location of pain. A second part consists of 20 lists of word descriptors (ranging from two to six words each), used to measure the sensory, affective, evaluative, and miscellaneous dimensions of pain. Patients select only words that describe their pain. A third part of the questionnaire is used to assess the pattern of pain (e.g., brief, transient, intermittent, continuous), and a fourth part measures present pain intensity (PPI) on a scale ranging from 0 (no pain) to 5 (excruciating pain).

The scoring method for the MPQ provides three major indices of pain. The Total Pain Rating Index (PRI-T) is a sum of the rank value of words chosen from the lists. In each list, the first word (implying the least pain) receives a value of 1, the next word a 2, and so on. In addition, the 20 lists are subdivided into four groups (Fig. 20–1), each yielding a subindex of pain (lists 1–10 PRI-sensory, 11–15 PRI-affective, 16 PRI-evaluative, 17–20 PRI-miscellaneous). Although rank values are generally summed to obtain scores on the PRI indices, Melzack et al.[76] described a technique to convert these to weighted-rank values to avoid loss of information about relative sensitivity of words chosen. The second major index is the Number of Words Chosen (NWC) from the 20 lists, which is not commonly analyzed in using the MPQ. The final major index is the Present Pain Intensity (PPI), or the number–word combination selected from the 0 to 5 scale. The PRI scores and PPI yield data that can be analyzed statistically.

Melzack considered the MPQ a "rough instrument",[32] and since its introduction in 1975, many other people have conducted studies to examine its reliability and validity. Reliability and consistency of the MPQ across many groups of subjects have been demonstrated repeatedly, including cancer patients,[77,78] people with experimentally induced pain,[79] and patients with a variety of medical and surgical diagnoses.[32]

The MPQ has been explored with respect to several major kinds of validity. Construct validity of the three major dimensions of the questionnaire (sensory, affective, and evaluative) has been supported in a series of factor analytic studies of patients with low back pain,[80,81] dysmenorrhea,[82] chronic benign pain,[83] arthritis,[84] and others.[85] Concurrent and predictive validity have been established by investigators studying dental pain,[86] dysmenorrhea,[82] laboratory pain,[87] headache,[88] and others.[89] Finally, the ability of the MPQ to discriminate among groups of patients has been examined in acute and chronic pain,[90] different types of toothache pain,[91] and different pain syndromes.[92–94] Reading et al. attempted to replicate the construction of the MPQ word lists using multidimensional scaling and cluster analysis.[95] Their results indicated considerable similarity to the 20 word lists in the original tool but also provided evidence for reducing the number of lists to 16. In another study, Turk et al.[96] confirmed the three dimensions of the MPQ through factor analysis but found that the dimensions were

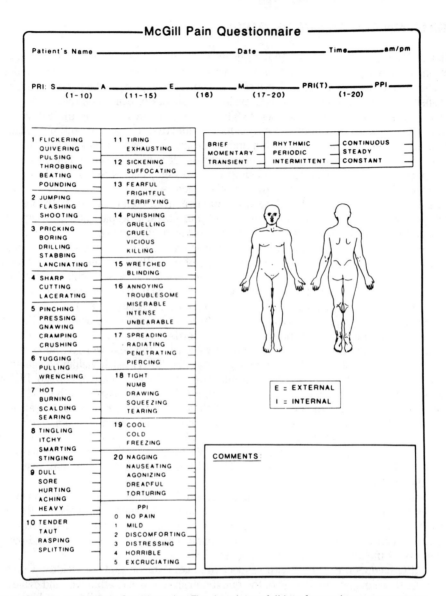

Figure 20—1. McGill Pain Questionnaire. The descriptors fall into four major groups: sensory, 1 to 10; affective, 11 to 15; evaluative, 16; and miscellaneous, 17 to 20. The rank value for each descriptor is based on its position in the word set. The sum of the rank values is the Pain Rating Index (PRI). The Present Pain Intensity (PPI) is based on a scale of 0 to 5. *(From Melzack. In Melzack,* Pain measurement and assessment, *1983. Courtesy of Raven Press.)*

highly intercorrelated and did not display discriminant validity. They recommended the use of only the PRI-T score in assessing pain. The area obviously needs further exploration in the clinical research setting.

From this large body of work, it can be seen that the MPQ is a reliable and valid multidimensional measure of pain that can be used in a large variety of patient groups with different types of pain. It is indisputably one of the most adequate and versatile instruments currently available for measuring pain. Appropriate uses of the MPQ in clinical research include descriptive studies of characteristics of pain caused by different disease processes, evaluations of pharmacologic and other interventions, simple baseline or ongoing assessments of pain, and clarification of differences and similarities among various types of pain.

The MPQ is not without disadvantages, however. It may not be easy to use in all clinical settings, since it is relatively long and complex. It can require intense concentration from respondents and up to 30 minutes for completion. Some of the word descriptors may be difficult for some patients to understand. Scoring the MPQ takes several minutes, so despite the instrument's obvious advantages, careful deliberation should precede a decision to use it in clinical research.

▪ DARTMOUTH PAIN QUESTIONNAIRE (DPQ)

The Dartmouth Pain Questionnaire (DPQ) was developed as an adjunct to the MPQ.[97] The DPQ consists of four objective measures (pain complaints, somatic interventions, impaired functioning, and remaining positive aspects of function) and one subjective measure (changes in self-esteem since onset of pain), all of which address essential items of pain assessment, according to Corson and Schneider, that are not covered by the MPQ.[97] The section on self-esteem, for example, asks patients to rate how they feel now compared to how they felt before having pain:

> Tense or anxious:
> 2 Much Worse/1 Slightly Worse/0 Same/1 Slightly Better/2 Much Better

The items from each section are incorporated onto a single page that can be self-administered easily by patients in 20 to 40 minutes. Initial evaluations were conducted with 297 patients with a variety of disorders and 92 terminal cancer patients. Although preliminary data from test–retest procedures are on small samples, reliability appears to be satisfactory. Both reliability and validity need more study, but the instrument clearly has potential for research purposes.

▪ CARD SORT METHOD

Reading and Newton developed the Card Sort Method as a multidimensional alternative to the MPQ.[98] They believed that their instrument was easier, shorter, and faster to administer. Patients are asked to sort 30 cards with paired adjectives describing sensory, affective, temporal, and evaluative aspects of pain, choosing the words that describe their pain. Among eight possible sorting patterns, only four are internally consistent, allowing a judgment of reliability through examination of the resulting patterns.

The technique was tested initially in 213 patients, yielding a high rate of consistent responses. Validity was assessed by comparing the patients' subjective reports of pain with behavioral indices, such as consumption of analgesics. Carroll has shown preliminary evidence of reliability and validity for the method.[99] Reading and Newton studied women with intra-uterine device-related pain or primary dysmenorrhea,[98] whereas Carroll studied patients with acute postoperative pain.[99]

The instrument could be used in a descriptive or evaluative manner in a variety of clinical research situations, including assessment of therapeutic interventions. The card-sorting task takes approximately 5 minutes and appears to be relatively easy for most patients. Scoring is more time consuming, however, and the smaller number of words than the MPQ may limit pain descriptions to some extent. The Card Sort Method is intriguing and potentially very useful, but additional psychometric work is needed.

▪ BRIEF PAIN INVENTORY

Another multidimensional instrument for measuring pain, also modeled after the McGill Pain Questionnaire, is the Wisconsin Brief Pain Questionnaire,[100] now known as the Brief Pain Inventory (BPI).[101] It is a survey instrument constructed to measure pain caused by cancer and other diseases, such as rheumatoid arthritis or chronic orthopedic problems. Items on the BPI address pain history, etiology, intensity, location, quality, and interference with activities. For example:

> Please circle the one number that describes how, during the past week, pain has interfered with your:
> Walking ability: 0   1   2   3   4   5   6   7   8   9   10
>   Does not   Completely
>   interfere   interferes

Daut et al. have demonstrated respectable test–retest reliability over short periods of time.[100] The validity of the tool was assessed through use in cancer patients. Differences in severity of pain were found in patients with (who had more pain) and without (who had less pain) metastatic disease. Additionally, ratings of interference with activities increased as severity of pain increased, and the number of patients receiving narcotic analgesics increased as severity ratings increased. Finally, when used in different diseases, it was found that intercorrelations among pain measures differed, suggesting that the BPI was sensitive to different pain characteristics.

The BPI could be used for measuring pain in cancer and other conditions. It appears most useful for surveys of patients where fairly superficial information is needed. It is short, easily understood, and designed for self-administration. The initial reliability and validity data suggest that the BPI is promising as a research instrument.

▪ VISUAL ANALOG SCALES (AHLES)

Several investigators have attempted to develop streamlined multidimensional measures by using Visual Analog Scales. In a sample of 40 cancer patients, Ahles et al.[102] compared VAS ratings of pain, depression, and anxiety to scores on standardized instruments, such as the MPQ, Turksy's PPP, a numerical (0–5) scale for pain, the Beck Depression Inventory, the State-Trait Anxiety Inventory, and the Symptom Checklist-90.

The VAS for pain correlated significantly with all the pain measures ($r = 0.30$ to 0.92, $p = 0.01$ to 0.001). The VAS for depression was significantly correlated (p values not reported) with both the Beck ($r = 0.51$) and the depression subscale of the Symptom Checklist-90 ($r = 0.41$), but the VAS for anxiety was not correlated with any standard measures of anxiety. Although the VAS for pain and depression appear useful in measuring clinical cancer pain and are certainly quick and easy, further work on these scales in additional patients is needed.

▪ MEMORIAL PAIN ASSESSMENT CARD (MPAC)

Fishman et al.[103] took a similar approach in developing the Memorial Pain Assessment Card (MPAC) for the evaluation of cancer pain and pain relief. The MPAC consists of an 8 and ½ by 11 inch card containing VAS measuring pain relief, pain intensity, and mood, and an adaptation of Tursky's pain adjectives rating scale. For example:

MOOD SCALE

Worst mood_____Best mood

The card is folded in the middle so that the four sides can be presented separately and quickly to patients.

In a study of 50 hospitalized cancer patients, Fishman et al. found strong correlations between the VAS pain and adjective rating scales and the MPQ ($r = 0.36$ to 0.45, $p = 0.005$ to 0.001). The VAS pain relief scale did not correlate with these measures but appeared related to the VAS mood scale ($r = 0.57$, $p < 0.001$). Finally, the VAS mood scale was correlated at varying degrees of significance with several subscales and the total score from the Profile of Mood States ($r = 0.31$ to -0.47, $p = 0.02$ to 0.001) as well as with the Hamilton ($r = -0.41$, $p = 0.005$) and Zung ($r = -0.44$, $p = 0.001$) Depression Scales. The researchers suggested that the VAS mood scale was a compound measure of experience characterized by confusion, anxiety, and lack of vigor that could be labeled general psychologic distress. The MPAC is short, simple, easy to administer and score, and may be used for a variety of clinical research purposes. Although it offers promise, it is clear that further studies of its reliability and validity are needed to substantiate its use in both cancer and other types of pain.

▪ HEADACHE SCALE

The Headache Scale is a tool developed to provide an assessment of both the subjective quality and the intensity of headache pain.[104] In a pilot study, 40 headache sufferers were asked to select adjectives descriptive of their headaches from the MPQ and to include additional descriptors as well. As a result, 30 words were incorporated into the scale, each with a 0 to 3 point scale for ranking. For example:

Splitting: Not at all   Mildly   Moderately   Severely

The Headache Scale was then tested in 150 headache-prone patients who rated the intensity, presence of symptoms, and pain quality of their most recent headache by responding to each adjective in terms of absence or intensity with which it was experienced. Additionally, an overall headache intensity scale of 0 = no headache to 5 = excruciating headache was used. Cluster analyses of the adjective data yielded five sensory clusters describing pain as aching, sharp, tight, autonomic, and dull and two affective clusters labeled discomfort and anxiety/depression. Evidence for content validity was provided by the selection of two thirds of the 30 adjectives by 50 percent of subjects, whereas evidence for concurrent validity was provided by strong correlations between total pain and the intensity scale ($r = 0.55$, $p < 0.001$). Sensory and affective scale scores were also highly correlated with total pain ($r = 0.77$ to 0.96, $p < 0.001$). Hunter's results suggest that the Headache Scale may be a useful tool for measuring pain, but as she herself recommends, replication in various headache populations is needed, as is further work on validity and reliability.

▪ WEST HAVEN-YALE MULTIDIMENSIONAL PAIN INVENTORY

A multidimensional instrument for measuring clinical pain is the West Haven-Yale Multidimensional Pain Inventory (WHYMPI). This tool was based on cognitive/behavioral theory and was designed specifically for patients with chronic pain.[105] The WHYMPI consists of 52 items divided into three parts: perceived pain intensity and impact of pain on various aspects of life, perceptions of others' responses to pain and suffering, and involvement in common daily activities. Each part contains a number of 6-point or 7-point scales on which patients record their responses. For example, in Part II, a patient would rate on a 6-point scale (0 = never, 6 = very frequently) the frequency with which others responded to his display of pain and suffering with a particular behavior.

Item analysis and psychometric assessment of the WHYMPI scales were conducted in 120 chronic pain patients. Kerns et al.[105] described in some detail their statistical procedures and results, and only a brief summary is presented here. Reliability and stability were assessed by coefficient alphas for internal consistency (0.70 to 0.90) and Pearson product moment correlations for test–retest reliability (0.62 to 0.92). Factor analytic techniques were used to devise and confirm the utility of the scales within each part of the WHYMPI. Finally, factor analysis was used to document the construct validity of the tool. From this initial study, the WHYMPI appears to be reliable and valid for the assessment of pain-related problems in a chronic pain population. Administration time is 15 to 30 minutes. Cross-validation is needed in other patient populations, since the initial sample was mostly male veterans of the United States Armed Services. Documentation of the tool's utility is needed in clinical research studies as well.

CONSIDERATIONS IN SELECTING A TOOL

When considering the instruments available for measuring pain, the researcher must be deliberate in selection. Information given in Table 20–1 may help in the decision process. The overall objective is to achieve useful and reliable data in the most expedient and sound manner possible. Several factors are important in the selection process.

The research question or goal is a prime consideration. The tool must mesh with the researcher's measurement goals. For example, a survey of the prevalence of pain in a specific sample of patients obviously would require a different tool than the evaluation of a therapeutic intervention for pain.

The dimension(s) of pain the researcher wishes to measure is the next factor to be considered. Once the researcher has decided on specific dimensions of the pain experience, the selection of instruments is narrowed considerably (Table 20–1).

The type of pain the study sample has is a third consideration. Tools designed for and used only in acute pain would probably be inappropriate for patients with chronic pain. It is especially important for the researcher to assess previous uses of the instrument she or he is interested in using.

The nature of the patient population to be studied is an extremely important factor to consider in the selection process. Many individual characteristics, such as educational level, visual and hearing ability, motor coordination, diagnosis, type of pain, clinical environment,

TABLE 20–1. TOOLS FOR MEASURING PAIN

Dimension/Tools	Advantages	Disadvantages
Sensory/discriminative		
Verbal Descriptor Scales (VDS)	Brief, easy, versatile	Possible artificial categorization of pain or inaccurate reflection of sensory experience
Visual Analog Scales (VAS)	Same as VDS but may be more sensitive	Possible difficulty with conceptualizing pain as a line; confusing for some patients
Affective/evaluative		
Johnson's Two-Component Scale	Brief, easy, versatile	Unclear reliability/validity
Tursky's Pain Perception Profile (PPP)	Unclear	Unclear reliability/validity
Cognitive		
Time Estimation of Pain Magnitude	Evaluates temporal property	Unclear reliability/validity
Pain Chart	Location and sensory properties	Unclear reliability/validity
Behavioral		
Acute pain		
Pain Rating Scale	Simple, easy, multidimensional	5–15 minutes long, unclear reliability/validity
Behavioral Index for the Assessment of Labor Pain	Simple, easy	Unclear reliability/validity
Chronic pain		
Pain Diary	Comprehensive	Subjective, may be unreliable
University of Alabama-Birmingham (UAB) Pain Behavior Scale	Comprehensive, objective	Unclear reliability/validity
Behavioral Dysfunction Index (BDI)	Comprehensive, head and neck cancer pain	Unclear reliability/validity, time consuming
Multidimensional		
McGill Pain Questionnaire (MPQ)	Versatile, reliable, and valid	Time consuming, may be confusing to some patients
Dartmouth Pain Questionnaire (DPQ)	Adjunct to MPQ, provides additional data	Unclear reliability/validity
Card Sort Method	Easier, briefer than MPQ	Unclear reliability/validity
Brief Pain Inventory (BPI)	Brief, simple self-administered, comprehensive	Unclear reliability/validity
Visual Analog Scale (Ahles)	Brief, easy	Unclear reliability/validity VAS-anxiety
Memorial Pain Assessment Card (MPAC)	Brief, easy	Unclear reliability/validity
Headache Scale	Specifically for headache, easy to administer/score	Unclear reliability/validity
West Haven-Yale Multidimensional Pain Inventory (WHYMPI)	Comprehensive, chronic pain	Unclear reliability/validity

and other factors, can influence a patient's ability to complete specific instruments. For example, the use of a long and complex instrument would be inappropriate in a sample of hearing-impaired people with severe acute pain. A simple, short pain intensity scale might be a better choice.

Ease of administration and scoring are a fifth important consideration in the selection process. The burden on the patient is of primary concern, particularly since the patient is in pain. Time and effort for the patient must be minimized to the greatest extent possible. The burden on the researcher is of secondary importance but certainly should not be ignored. A long complicated interview tool, for example, would be inappropriate when the researcher may only have 10 or 15 minutes with each subject.

A final consideration, and one of the most critical, is the available reliability and validity data of tools the researcher is considering. A careful evaluation of the data should be made before final selection, since this will ensure that the researcher is aware of the benefits and limitations of using a particular instrument in a given sample of subjects.

SUMMARY

Although compromises will inevitably have to be made by the researcher, a careful and deliberative selection process will help to ensure that the researcher obtains reliable and valid data that will assist in answering the research question. Given the long and painstaking process of instrument development, it may be more expedient for the researcher to use a tool that has been developed and assessed psychometrically. As can be seen in Table 20–1, many instruments need further validation. The repeated use of such instruments, with careful attention to psychometric issues, will help to refine and improve existing tools, resulting in better measures of clinical pain.

REFERENCES

1. Sternbach, R.A. *Pain: A psychophysiological analysis.* New York: Academic Press, 1960, p. 12.
2. Melzack, R., & Casey, K.L. Sensory, motivational, and central control determinants of pain: A new conceptual model. In D. Kenshalo (Ed.), *The skin senses.* Springfield, IL: Chas. C Thomas, 1968, p. 423.
3. Merskey, H., & Spear, F.G. *Pain: Psychological and psychiatric Aspects.* London: Balliere, Tindall, and Cassell, 1967.
4. International Association for the Study of Pain. Pain terms: A current list with definitions and notes on usage. *Pain* [Suppl], 1986, *3*:S216.
5. Melzack, R., & Wall, P.D. *The challenge of pain.* New York: Basic Books, 1982.
6. Beecher, H.K. *Measurements of subjective responses. Quantitative effects of drugs.* New York: Oxford University Press, 1959.
7. Benoliel, J.Q., & Crowley, D.M. The patient in pain: New concepts. In *Proceedings of the National Conference on Cancer Nursing.* New York: American Cancer Society, 1973, p. 70.
8. Beecher, H.K. Pain in men wounded in battle. *Ann Surg,* 1946, *123*:96.
9. Hardy, J.D., Wolff, H.G., & Goodell, H. *Pain sensations and reactions.* Baltimore: Williams & Wilkins, 1952.
10. Melzack, R., & Wall, P.D. Pain mechanisms: A new theory. *Science,* 1965, *150*(3699):971.
11. Weisenberg, M. Pain and pain control. *Psychol Bull,* 1977, *84*(5):1008.
12. Ahles, T. A., Blanchard, E.B., & Ruckdeschel, J.C. The multidimensional nature of cancer-related pain. *Pain,* 1983, *17*(3):277.

13. Wolff, B.B. Laboratory methods of pain measurement. In R. Melzack (Ed.), *Pain measurement and assessment*. New York: Raven, 1983, p. 7.
14. Wolff, B.B. Measurement of human pain. In J.J. Bonica (Ed.), *Pain*. New York: Raven, 1980, p. 173.
15. Agnew, D.C., et al. A taxonomy for diagnosis and information storage for patients with chronic pain. *Bull LA Neurol Soc*, 1979, *44*:84.
16. Meinhart, N.T., & McCaffery, M. *Pain: A nursing approach to assessment and analysis*. Norwalk, CT: Appleton-Century-Crofts, 1983, p. 198.
17. Davitz, J.R., & Davitz, L.L. *Inferences of patients' pain and psychological distress: Studies of nursing behaviors*. New York: Springer, 1981.
18. Rankin, M.A., & Snider, B. Nurses' perceptions of cancer patients' pain. *Cancer Nurs*, 1984, *7*(2):149.
19. Kremer, E.F., & Atkinson, J.H. Pain language as a measure of affect in chronic pain patients. In R. Melzack (Ed.), *Pain measurement and assessment*. New York: Raven, 1983, p. 119.
20. Eland, J.M. The child who is hurting. *Semin Oncol Nurs*, 1985, *1*(2):116.
21. Jeans, M.E. The measurement of pain in children. In R. Melzack (Ed.), *Pain measurement and assessment*. New York: Raven, 1983, p. 183.
22. Patterson, K.L., & Klopovich, P.M. Pain in the pediatric oncology patient. In D.B. McGuire & C.H. Yarbro (Eds.), *Cancer pain*. Orlando, FL: Grune & Stratton, 1987, p. 259.
23. McGuire, D.B. The multidimensional phenomenon of cancer pain. In D.B. McGuire & C.H. Yarbro (Eds.), *Cancer pain*. Orlando, FL: Grune & Stratton, 1987, p. 1.
24. Gracely, R.H. Subjective quantification of pain perception. In B. Bromm (Ed.), *Pain measurement in man: Neurophysiological correlates of pain*. Amsterdam: Elsevier, 1984, p. 376.
25. Clark, W.C. Pain sensitivity and the report of pain: An introduction to Sensory Decision Theory. *Anesthesiology*, 1974, *40*:(3)272.
26. Gracely, R.H. Psychophysical assessment of human pain. In J.J. Bonica, J.C. Liebeskind, & D.G. Albe-Fessard (Eds.), *Advances in pain research and therapy*, Vol. 3. New York: Raven, 1979, p. 805.
27. Stevens, S.S. *Psychophysics: Introduction to its perceptual, neural, and social aspects*. New York: Wiley, 1975.
28. Sternbach, R.A. Ethical considerations in pain research in man. In R. Melzack (Ed.), *Pain measurement and assessment*. New York: Raven, 1983, p. 259.
29. Littman, G.S., Walker, B.R., & Schneider, B.E. Reassessment of verbal and visual analogue ratings in analgesic studies. *Clin Pharmacol Ther*, 1985, *38*(1):16.
30. Keele, K.D. The pain chart. *Lancet*, 1948, *2*:6.
31. Keele, K.D. The temporal aspects of pain: The pain chart. In R. Melzack (Ed.), *Pain measurement and assessment*. New York: Raven, 1983, p. 205.
32. Melzack, R. The McGill Pain Questionnaire: Major properties and scoring methods. *Pain*, 1975, *1*(3):277.
33. Kruszewski, A.Z., Lang, S.H., & Johnson, J.E. Effect of positioning on discomfort from intramuscular injections in the dorsogluteal site. *Nurs Res*, 1979, *28*(2):103.
34. Heft, M.W., & Parker, S.R. An experimental basis for revising the graphic rating scale for pain. *Pain*, 1984, *19*(2):153.
35. Maxwell, C. Sensitivity and accuracy of the visual analogue scale: A psycho-physical classroom experiment. *Br J Clin Pharmacol*, 1978, *6*(1):15.
36. Clarke, P.R.F., & Spear, F.G. Reliability and sensitivity in the self-assessment of well-being. *Bull Br Psychol Soc*, 1964, *17*(55):18A.
37. Huskisson, E.C. Measurement of pain. *Lancet*, 1974, *2*(7889):1127.
38. Price, D.D., McGrath, D.A., Rafii, A., et al. The validation of visual analogue scales as ratio scale measures for chronic and experimental pain. *Pain*, 1983, *17*(1):45.
39. Revill, S.I., Robinson, J.O., Rosen, M., et al. The reliability of a linear analogue for evaluating pain. *Anaesthesia*, 1976, *31*(9):1191.
40. Dixon, J.S., & Bird, H.A. Reproducibility along a 10 cm vertical visual analogue scale. *Ann Rheumat Dis*, 1981, *40*:87.

41. Carlsson, A.M. Assessment of chronic pain. 1. Aspects of the reliability and validity of the visual analogue scale. *Pain,* 1983, *16:*87.
42. Bond, M.R., & Pilowsky, I. Subjective assessment of pain and its relationship to the administration of analgesics in patients with advanced cancer. *J Psychosom Res,* 1966, *10*(2):203.
43. Scott, J., & Huskisson, E.C. Vertical or horizontal visual analogue scales. *Ann Rheumat Dis,* 1979, *38:*560.
44. Scott, J., & Huskisson, E.C. Accuracy of subjective measurements made with or without previous scores: An important source of error in serial measurement of subjective states. *Ann Rheumat Dis,* 1979, *38:*558.
45. Ohnhaus, E.E., & Adler, R. Methodological problems in the measurement of pain: A comparison between the verbal rating scale and the visual analogue scale. *Pain,* 1975, *1*(4):379.
46. Scott, J., & Huskisson, E.C. Graphic representation of pain. *Pain,* 1976, *2*(2):175.
47. Wallenstein, S.L. Scaling clinical pain and pain relief. In B. Bromm (Ed.), *Pain measurement in man: Neurophysiological correlates of pain.* Amsterdam: Elsevier, 1984, p. 389.
48. Woodforde, J.M., & Merksey, H. Some relationships between subjective measures of pain. *J Psychosom Res,* 1972, *16:*173.
49. Reading, A.E. A comparison of pain rating scales. *J Psychosom Res,* 1980, *24:*119.
50. Downie, W.W., Leatham, P.A., Rhind, V.M., et al. Studies with pain rating scales. *Ann Rheumat Dis,* 1978, *37*(4):378.
51. Kremer, E., Atkinson, J.H., & Ignelzi, R.J. Measurement of pain: Patient preference does not confound pain measurement. *Pain,* 1981, *10:*241.
52. Johnson, J.E. Effects of structuring patients' expectations on their reactions to threatening events. *Nurs Res,* 1972, *21*(6):499.
53. Johnson, J.E. Effects of accurate expectations about sensations on the sensory and distress components of pain. *J Pers Soc Psychol,* 1973, *27*(2):261.
54. Johnson, J.E., & Rice, V.M. Sensory and distress components of pain: Implications for the study of clinical pain. *Nurs Res,* 1974, *23*(3):203.
55. Wells, N. The effect of relaxation on postoperative muscle tension and pain. *Nurs Res,* 1982, *31*(4):236.
56. Tursky, B. The development of a pain perception profile: A psychophysical approach. In M. Weisenberg, & B. Tursky (Eds.), *Pain: New Perspectives in Therapy and Research.* New York: Plenum Press, 1976, p. 171.
57. Tursky, B., Jammer, J.D., & Friedman, R. The pain perception profile: A psychophysical approach to the assessment of pain report. *Behav Ther,* 1982, *13:*376.
58. Andrasik, F., Blanchard, E.B., Ahles, T., et al. Assessing the reactive as well as the sensory component of headache pain. *Headache,* 1981, *21:*218.
59. Urban, B.J., Keefe, F.J., & France, R.D. A study of psychophysical scaling in chronic pain patients. *Pain,* 1984, *20:*157.
60. Bilting, M., Carlsson, C., Menge, B., et al. Estimation of time as a measure of pain magnitude. *J Psychosom Res,* 1983, *27*(6):493.
61. Weeks, D.J. Communication to the Editor (letter). *J Psychosom Res,* 1983, *27*(6):533.
62. Margoles, M.S. The pain chart: Spatial properties of pain. In R. Melzack (Ed.), *Pain measurement and assessment.* New York: Raven, 1983, p. 215.
63. Hanken, A. The measurement of pain. In M. Newton, W. Hunt, W. McDowell, & A. Hanken (Eds.), *A study of nurse action in relief of pain.* Columbus, OH: The Ohio State University School of Nursing, 1964.
64. Hanken, A., & McDowell, W. Development of a rating scale to measure pain. In M. Newton, W. Hunt, W. McDowell, & A. Hanken (Eds.), *A study of nurse action in relief of pain.* Columbus, OH: The Ohio State University School of Nursing, 1964.
65. Chambers, W.G., & Price, G.G. Influence of nurse upon effects of analgesics administered. *Nurs Res,* 1967, *16*(3):228.
66. Bruegel, M.A. Relationship of preoperative anxiety to perception of postoperative pain. *Nurs Res,* 1971, *20*(1):26.
67. Hagle, M.E. *Diurnal variation in pain intensity of cancer patients.* Unpublished master's thesis, University of Illinois at the Medical Center, Chicago, IL, 1980.

68. Bonnel, A.M., & Boureau, F. Labor pain assessment: Validity of a behavioral index. *Pain*, 1985, *22*(1):81.
69. Fordyce, W.E., Lansky, S., Calsyn, D.A., et al. Pain measurement and pain behavior. *Pain*, 1984, *18*(1):53.
70. Follick, M.J., Ahern, D.K., & Laser-Wolston, W. Evaluation of a daily activity diary for chronic pain patients. *Pain*, 1984, *19:*373.
71. Kremer, E.F., Block, A., & Gaylor, M.S. Behavioral approaches to treatment of chronic pain: The inaccuracy of patient self-report measures. *Arch Phys Med Rehab*, 1981, *62*(4): 188.
72. Keefe, F.J., Wilkins, R.H. & Cook, W.A. Direct observation of pain behavior in low back pain patients during physical examination. *Pain*, 1984, *20:*59.
73. Richards, J.S., Nepomuceno, C., Riles, M., et al. Assessing pain behavior: The UAB pain behavior scale. *Pain*, 1982, *14*(4):393.
74. Keefe, F.J., Brantley, A., Manuel, G., et al. Behavioral assessment of head and neck cancer pain. *Pain*, 1985, *23*(4):327.
75. Melzack, R., & Torgerson, W.S. On the language of pain. *Anesthesiology*, 1971, *34*(1):50.
76. Melzack, R., Katz, J., & Jeans, M.E. The role of compensation in chronic pain: Analysis using a new method of scoring the McGill Pain Questionnaire. *Pain*, 1985, *23*(2):101.
77. Graham, C., Bond, S.S., Gerkovich, M.M., et al. Use of the McGill Pain Questionnaire in the assessment of cancer pain: Replicability and consistency. *Pain*, 1980, *8*(3):377.
78. McGuire, D.B. Assessment of pain in cancer inpatients using the McGill Pain Questionnaire. *Oncol Nurs Forum*, 1984, *11*(6):32.
79. Klepac, R.K., Dowling, J., Rokke, P., et al. Interview vs. paper and pencil administration of the McGill Pain Questionnaire. *Pain*, 1981, *11:*241.
80. Byrne, M., Troy, A., Bradley, L.A., et al. Cross-validation of the factor structure of the McGill pain questionnaire. *Pain*, 1982, *13:*193.
81. Prieto, E.J., Hopson, L., Bradley, L.A., et al. The language of low back pain: Factor structure of the McGill pain questionnaire. *Pain*, 1980, *8*(1):11.
82. Reading, A.E. The internal structure of the McGill pain questionnaire in dysmenorrhoea patients. *Pain*, 1979, *7*(3):353.
83. Kremer, E., & Atkinson, J.H. Pain measurement: Construct validity of the affective dimension of the McGill pain questionnaire with chronic benign pain patients. *Pain*, 1981, *11*(1):93.
84. Burckhardt, C.S. The use of the McGill Pain Questionnaire in assessing arthritis pain. *Pain*, 1984, *19*(3):305.
85. Prieto, E.J., & Geisinger, K.F. Factor-analytic studies of the McGill Pain Questionnaire. In R. Melzack (Ed.), *Pain measurement and assessment.* New York: Raven, 1983, p. 63.
86. Buren, J.V., & Kleinknecht, R.A. An evaluation of the McGill Pain Questionnaire for use in dental pain assessment. *Pain*, 1979, *6:*23.
87. Klepac, R.K., Dowling, J., & Hauge, G. et al. Sensitivity of the McGill Pain Questionnaire to intensity and quality of laboratory pain. *Pain*, 1981, *10:*199.
88. Hunter, M., & Philips, C. The experience of headache—An assessment of the qualities of tension headache pain. *Pain*, 1981, *10:*209.
89. Reading, A.E. The McGill Pain Questionnaire: An appraisal. In R. Melzack (Ed.), *Pain measurement and assessment.* New York: Raven, 1983, p. 55.
90. Reading, A.E. A comparison of the McGill Pain Questionnaire in chronic and acute pain. *Pain*, 1982, *13:*185.
91. Grushka, M., & Sessle, B.J. Applicability of the McGill Pain Questionnaire to the differentiation of "toothache" pain. *Pain*, 1984, *19*(1):49.
92. Dubuisson, D., & Melzack, R. Classification of clinical pain descriptions by multiple group discriminant analysis. *Exp Neurol*, 1976, *51*(2):480.
93. Nehemkis, A.M., & Charter, R.A. Comparison of arthritis and cancer pain patients: Are distinct clinical pain syndromes definable using the McGill Pain Questionnaire? *Percept Mot Skills*, 1984, *58*(1):126.
94. Nehemkis, A.M., & Charter, R.A. The limits of verbal pain descriptors. *Percept Mot Skills*, 1984, *59*(1):251.

95. Reading, A.E., Everitt, B.S., & Sledmere, C.M. The McGill Pain Questionnaire: A replication of its construction. *Br J. Clin Psychol,* 1982, *21:*339.
96. Turk, D.C., Rudy, T.E., & Salovey, P. The McGill Pain Questionnaire reconsidered: Confirming the factor structure and examining appropriate uses. *Pain,* 1985, *21*(4):385.
97. Corson, J.A., & Schneider, M.J. The Dartmouth Pain Questionnaire: An adjunct to the McGill Pain Questionnaire. *Pain,* 1984, *19*(1):59.
98. Reading, A.E., & Newton, J.R. A card sort method of pain assessment. *J Psychosom Res,* 1978, *22*(6):503.
99. Carroll, S.L. *A comparison of four methods of assessing acute pain in hospitalized, post-surgical adults.* Unpublished master's thesis, University of Illinois at the Medical Center, Chicago, IL, 1981.
100. Daut, R.L., Cleeland, C.S., & Flanery, R.C. Development of the Wisconsin Brief Pain Questionnaire to assess pain in cancer and other diseases. *Pain,* 1983, *17:*197.
101. Cleeland, C.S. Measurement and prevalence of pain in cancer. *Semin Oncol Nurs,* 1985, *1*(2):87.
102. Ahles, T.A., Ruckdeschel, J.C., & Blanchard, E.B. Cancer-related pain. II. Assessment with Visual Analogue Scales. *J Psychosom Res,* 1984, *28*(2):121.
103. Fishman, B., Pasternak, S., Wallenstein, S.L., et al. The Memorial Pain Assessment Card; A valid instrument for the evaluation of cancer pain. Submitted for publication, 1986.
104. Hunter, M. The Headache Scale: A new approach to the assessment of headache pain based on pain descriptors. *Pain,* 1983, *16*(4):361.
105. Kerns, R.D., Turk, D.C., & Rudy, T.E. The West Haven-Yale Multidimensional Pain Inventory (WHYMPI). *Pain,* 1985, *23*(4):345.

CHAPTER 21

Measuring Alterations in Taste and Smell

Roberta A. Strohl, R.N., M.N.

It has been estimated that over 2 million Americans suffer from some impairment in taste and/or smell. The study and measurements of these disorders have not reflected the frequency of their occurrence. Disturbances in these senses are difficult to measure, and easily used reliable and valid tools do not exist. This factor coupled with their nonlife-threatening nature has led them to be called "the neglected senses."[1] Although not as debilitating as alterations in sight or hearing, taste and smell abnormalities can contribute to nutritional compromise. People who are unable or unwilling to eat because of the unpleasant tastes of foods may not tolerate the treatment they require. Nutritional compromise may contribute to increased side effects and decreased response to therapy.

In order to discuss the alterations of taste and smell and their measurements, it is necessary to describe the normal taste and smell responses.

NORMAL TASTE SENSATION

Adults have approximately 10,000 taste buds, which are located on the tongue, palate, pharynx, tonsils, epiglottis, and in some people in the mucosa of the cheek and lips. Taste buds respond to four primary sensations: sweet, sour, salty, and bitter. Sweet receptors are found on the anterior surface and tip of the tongue, sour and salty on the two lateral sides, and bitter on the circumvillate papillae on the posterior surface. The sour and bitter tastes are perceived most acutely on the palate, whereas salty and sweet tastes are most sensitive on the tongue. Each taste bud is not exclusively sensitive to a single sensation, and all respond to sweet, sour, salty, and bitter but in varying proportions. It is thought that a center in the brain detects all the ratios of tastes, and the summary of these stimuli produces the distinguishable taste.[2]

Sweet taste is caused by a group of substances, mostly organic chemicals, including sugars, alcohols, glycol, ketones, amides, sulfonic acids, and inorganic salts of beryllium and lead. Sour taste results from acids, and salty taste results from ionized salts. Bitter taste is caused by organic substances, such as alkaloids and long-chain acids. Intense bitter taste is objectionable, and this can be seen as a protective mechanism, since many poisons have a bitter taste.[2]

Taste buds consist of a combination of gustatory receptor cells and supporting cells. Each taste bud consists of approximately 50 cells. The life span of a taste cell is about 10 days. Renewal of the cells is made possible by mitotic division in the surrounding epithelium. At the center of each taste bud is a taste pore. Microvilli or taste hairs protrude from the surface of the taste cells and are believed to form the receptor surface for taste. The containerlike structure of the taste bud provides a minute cup for solutions to be tasted, since substances must be mixed in saliva in order to be tasted. Taste nerve fibers that are stimulated by the taste buds are located within the taste cells.[1-3]

When a substance in solution comes in contact with the taste bud, the taste response begins. The taste bud serves as a chemical sieve, which allows the substance to stimulate the taste nerve. A variety of physiologic mechanisms cause changes in the diameter of the taste pore that alter its permeability. These changes in the protein molecules that line the taste bud may be controlled by the equilibrium of metals and thiols. When the taste nerve is stimulated, a change in membrane potential occurs that transmits the stimulus along the nerve fibers.[2,4]

Depending on the location of the taste buds, the stimulus is transmitted by different nerves. Taste buds on the anterior two thirds of the tongue and the palate are innervated by the seventh cranial nerve. The circumvallate papillae are innervated by the ninth nerve, as is the posterior two thirds of the tongue. The tenth nerve innervates the laryngeal and epiglottal taste buds. Those taste buds in the pharynx are mediated by the ninth and tenth nerve. The information is sent to the nucleus of the solitary tract in the medulla, to the pons, thalamus, and finally to the cortical taste area, where the taste response is perceived. There are also neurons that go from the pons into the lateral hypothalamus and free endings of the trigeminal nerve in the oral cavity and tongue that participate in the taste response.[3]

NORMAL SMELL SENSATION

The sense of smell is less well understood. The olfactory membrane is located in the superior part of each nostril, with a surface area of approximately 2.4 cm^2. Olfactory cells are derived from the central nervous system and are specialized bipolar neurons. The olfactory receptor cells have renewal system with a turnover rate of about 30 days. Each person has about 100 million olfactory cells. The cells form an olfactory bulb, which terminates in olfactory hairs or cilia that line the mucus coating the nasal cavity.[1-3]

The chemical process that results in the stimulation of the olfactory sense is unknown, and there is no general agreement about the basic qualities and classifications of smell. Attempts to classify smell have been numerous, starting with Plato, who used only two groups, pleasant and unpleasant. Linneaus, in 1752, reported seven classifications: aromatic, fragrant, ambrosial, alliaceous (garlicy), hircine (goaty), repulsive, and nauseous. Currently, it is postulated that separate olfactory cells may respond to seven primary smells: camphoraceous, musky, floral, pepperminty, etheral, pungent, and putrid. That this list actually reflects all the primary sensations of smell is unlikely, and it is viewed as only another attempt at classification. It may be that there are as many as 50 primary smell sensations.[1-3]

The means of stimulation of olfactory cells also is unclear. The substance must be volatile so that it can reach the cells. It must be somewhat water soluble to pass through the mucus and lipid soluble, since the olfactory cilia and tips of the olfactory cells are composed of lipids. Smell occurs in cycles with inspiration. It is believed that the olfactory cells respond with a change in membrane potential, much like taste cells, which then stimulates the olfactory nerve. The wave theory proposes that the response is triggered by stimulation from direct radiation from the odorous source. Steric theories suggest that chemical reactivity occurs when particles of the odorant react with receptor cells.[1,2]

The nerve fibers when stimulated propagate the response as they converge into larger bundles and leave the epithelium through perforations in the cribiform plate and send axons into the olfactory bulb. These end in dendrites from mitral cells in a structure known as the "glomerulus," located near the bulb's surface. Some of the axons of mitral cells form the olfactory tract, whereas others lead back to tufted cells that send axons back to the glomerulus. This forms a circular pathway that amplifies the message.[1]

The fibers terminate in two areas of the brain called the "medial olfactory area" and "lateral olfactory area." The medial area is located in the midportion of the brain superiorly and anteriorly to the hypothalamus. The lateral olfactory area consists of the uncus, prepyriform area, the lateral portion of the anterior perforated substance, and part of the amygaloid nuclei. The lateral area, which contains parts of the cerebral cortex, is believed to be responsible for the complex association of smell with other sensations. Although taste and smell are separate sensations, it is clear that they are closely related. Loss of the ability to smell during a cold has taught us that the sense of taste is also diminished.[2]

DISORDERS OF TASTE AND SMELL

Noting the complexity of these sensations, it should not be surprising that there are a myriad of situations in which taste and smell may be altered. It is beyond the scope of this chapter to discuss them all. The terminology used to describe taste and smell abnormalities is as follows:[3]

Ageusia	Absence of taste
Dysgeusia	Distortion of normal taste
Hypergeusia	Increased sensitivity of taste
Hypogeusia	Lessened sensitivity of taste
Anosmia	Absence of smell
Dysosmia	Distortion of normal smell
Hyperosmia	Increased sensitivity of smell
Hyposmia	Lessened sensitivity of smell

Schiffman classifies taste and smell disorders into four categories based on cause. Disorders may result from local atrophy of receptor sites, damage to neural projections, surgery or trauma disturbances of cell renewal by factors including disease, drugs, or radiation, and change in receptor cell environment resulting from alterations in saliva or olfactory mucosa (from such substances as drugs or environmental pollutants, such as benzene, carbon disulfide, or ethyl acetate).[3] For purposes of this discussion, changes as a result of disease are emphasized.

Changes in Taste and Smell Resulting from Disease States
A number of diseases have been associated with alterations in taste and smell. More work has been done in the area of taste abnormalities than smell abnormalities, partly because of the difficulty in measurement and lack of understanding of the sense of smell.

TABLE 21–1. CHANGES IN TASTE AND SMELL RELATED TO CANCER

Nature of Change	Explanation	Reference
Lowered bitter threshold	Tumor may secrete substance that stimulates bitter taste buds	5–12
Increase in threshold for sucrose	Depression of cell renewal by tumor; decrease in taste cells; decrease in stimulus received by taste receptor	5–9, 13–16
Weight loss	Correlation with extent of tumor; taste abnormalities improved as tumor regressed; without response, abnormalities increased	6,7
Increase in threshold for salt	Unknown	15
Studies in which no abnormalitis found		10
Alteration in smell	Unknown; patients reported unusual smell in chemotherapy and/or radiation clinic	17

Patients with cancer have been found to report alterations in taste and smell as a result of the disease and its treatment. A study of the literature reveals that there is a need for more research in this area and that there is not a single, simple explanation for the changes in taste and smell reported in people with cancer. The changes related to the disease are presented in Table 21–1. Treatment-related factors in cancer are presented in Tables 21–2, 21–3, and 21–4, and Tables 21–5 and 21–6 show changes related to other diseases and to aging, respectively.

Although there is still significant research to be done in both the measurement and etiology of disturbances of taste and smell, the complexity of these senses and the numerous ways in which response may be altered make it a difficult area to research. The complexity of some of the currently available testing methods makes this an area where collaborative research between nurses, who identify and document changes clinically, and other researchers familiar with testing methods is appropriate. With practice some of the testing methods are within the realm of nursing research.

MEASUREMENT OF TASTE

To evaluate the nature of the changes in taste, the following questions can be asked:

Have you noticed a change in the way food tastes?

TABLE 21–2. CHANGES IN TASTE AND SMELL RELATED TO CANCER SURGERY

Procedure	Alteration	Reference
Removal of tongue	Loss of sweet and salty receptors	18
Removal of palate	Loss of sour and bitter receptors	18
Laryngectomy	Loss of olfactory component of taste	19

TABLE 21–3. CHANGES IN TASTE AND SMELL RELATED TO CANCER CHEMOTHERAPY

Alteration	Explanation	Reference
Loss of taste	Stomatitis with infection and coating of tongue alters receptor sites; taste cells with high mitotic index altered by drugs	20
Metallic taste	Associated with such drugs as cytoxan, vincristine, methotrexate	20
Void aversions	Conditioned response related to association of nausea and vomiting with chemotherapy	20,21

When did you notice this change?

Have you changed the way you season food—if so how?

(Looking for relationship to disease and therapy)

Are the tastes of any particular foods changed?

Do any foods taste better than others?

What foods have you stopped eating and why?

Are the changes constant?

Classification of Taste Changes

Markley et al. placed foods in six categories: breads, fruits, vegetables, meats, milk and dairy, and miscellaneous, including coffee, condiments, and carbonated beverages. Dysgeusia was placed into four classifications of alteration in taste as follows[41]:

Type I   One food or beverage in any single group
Type II   More than one food or beverage but not all items in a group
Type II   All common items in one group
Type IV   All foods and beverages

These classifications may help in comparing weight loss related to taste alterations and charting the progression of taste loss such as occurs with head and neck irradiation. In patients with anorexia nervosa, taste changes can be classified using this approach, and recovery as the patient progresses through therapy may be documented. The questions may be repeated on a weekly basis to document the progression of taste changes and the recovery of taste.

TABLE 21–4. FACTORS IN TASTE AND SMELL ALTERATIONS RELATED TO HEAD AND NECK IRRADIATION[22–27]

Damage to microvilli of taste cells
Loss of saliva related to salivary gland damage
Profound taste loss at dose > 3000 rad (sweet taste may persist longer since there are more sweet taste buds)
Loss of smell related to irradiation of nasal passage and damage to olfactory receptor site
Taste may be partially restored 20–60 days posttreatment and return to normal 60–120 days after treatment
Some hypogeusia may be permanent

TABLE 21–5. TASTE AND SMELL ALTERATIONS IN SOME DISEASE STATES

Disease	Alterations Reported and Rationale	Reference
Diabetes	Higher thresholds for all sensations except sour; degree of alteration correlates with peripheral neuropathy; Most severe taste loss with autonomic neuropathy related to alteration in taste nerves	28,29
Renal disease	Hypogeusia and low zinc levels Persistent unpleasant taste Alteration in cranial nerves related to renal failure Decrease in salivary flow Change in calcium and phosphorus content in saliva	30–33 30–33
Anorexia	Taste loss related to altered zinc and copper levels	34
Head trauma	Smell alteration related to fracture of cribiform plate, laceration of olfactory nerves, and hemorrhage in frontal lobe; hemorrhage into taste center in brain	35–37

Wall and Gabriel tested taste alterations in children with leukemia and a comparison group of healthy children.[15] The taste testing methods and questionnaires were pretested. Children were given an orientation to the four taste qualities using posters showing foods that were sweet, sour, salty, and bitter. A checklist of 62 foods commonly eaten by children was used to determine taste preferences. Parents identified what foods the child preferred before the illness and how the choices had changed since diagnosis. Parents of children without leukemia were given the same checklist of foods. This checklist was pretested in the community. Reliability was determined for the list of preferred foods (87.8 percent agreement first to second test, appetite rating 94 percent agreement, food checklist 98.2 percent agreement). Children were asked three questions:

Do you like to eat?

What are your favorite foods?

What foods do you not like:

The foods were divided into the four basic food groups. A scale was used consisting of 0 = dislike, 1 = tolerate, and 2 = like. Scores were summed for each group by adding the scores and dividing by the number of foods in the group. Significant differences existed only in the meat group ($+47 = 2.69$, $p < 0.0125$).

This study is the best-controlled investigation of taste changes found in this review of the nursing literature.[15] The methods used could be adapted to the adult population to help determine the pattern of food likes and dislikes. Repeating the study during the course of the treatment process should further elucidate the pattern of taste changes and their relationships to treatment.

TABLE 21–6. CHANGES IN TASTE RELATED TO AGING[38–40]

Thinning in epithelium of taste bud
Decrease in vascular supply to taste cells
Decrease in number of taste buds
Decrease in all taste sensations (in edentulous patients may improve if dentures removed)
Decrease in sense of smell related to changes in olfactory receptors

Interviewing patients to determine the nature of any taste changes is a logical first step. Although this is subjective, it will identify changes that may be significant in their influence on eating behaviors. Listing foods from all groups may help cue patients and determine if there is a pattern to taste alterations.

Documenting Taste Response—Taste Thresholds

The most commonly used technique for documenting taste is the measurement of detection and recognition thresholds. Subjects are presented with two bottes, one of which is water and the other is the substance being tested. Three drops of varying concentrations of the test substance are placed on the subject's tongue (usually approximately ten concentrations), with the subject rinsing between tests. The point at which the substance is detected as being different from water is the detection threshold. The point at which the substance is recognized as being sweet, sour, salty, or bitter is the recognition threshold, which is usually a slightly higher concentration than the detection threshold. A group of normal subjects frequently is used as a comparison group. Subjects are matched by age and should be matched for other factors, such as smoking history.[42] Loss of the ability to distinguish tastes in the suprathreshold range is difficult to detect using this method. This is believed to occur in the elderly in both taste and smell, where enough receptors exist to detect a stimulus but not enough to make subtle distinctions.

Schechter et al. used a single-blind study to investigate the effects of zinc sulfate on taste and smell dysfunction.[42] In this trial, subjects were initially given placebo. If no change in taste or smell occurred, the subject was given zinc sulfate, with each subject serving as his or her own control. Subjects who improved on placebo were not given zinc. In this study, patients who did not improve with placebo improved with zinc.[42] Reliability and validity information was not presented.

▪ TASTE SCALE

Henkin et al. have developed a scale to document taste acuity.[43] Using the forced-choice three-drop technique, the detection and recoginition thresholds are determined. The measurements were transformed to a scale, with each concentration designated as a bottle-unit and the change from one concentration to the next a bottle-unit change. This permits a logarithmic transformation, since the tastant concentrations used are approximately log-linear. This method is the most frequently used measure of taste in the studies presented in this chapter. Taste testing kits are commercially available to investigators. This technique was used by Wall and Gabriel, and statistically significant differences were found in detection thresholds for sweet ($+47 = -2.36$, $p < 0.05$) and salt ($+47 = -3.01$, $p < 0.05$) and in recognition thresholds for all modalities, sweet ($+34 = -2.56$, $p < 0.05$), salt ($+47 = -2.99$, $p < 0.05$), sour ($+37 = -2.74$, $p < 0.05$), and bitter ($+33 = -2.26$, $p < 0.05$).[15] Taste testing by this method has been criticized as revealing only certain forms of sensory loss and not controlling the area tested and the number of taste buds stimulated.

▪ MAGNITUDE ESTIMATION

In this method of taste scaling, the subject is asked to assign a number to a perceived intensity of taste. The subject chooses any number to start and assigns subsequent numbers according to the intensity of the stimulus. Magnitude estimation functions describe the growth of perceived intensity with concentration across the whole dynamic range, from threshold to concentrations pereceived to be very strong. This method allows the plotting of a scale with controls compared to the population being tested. Subjects cannot be adequately compared, since the intensity of a substance may be rated the same by two subjects but the absolute intensities of the experience may not be equivalent. What one individual believes is a strong stimulus may not be the same to another subject.[44]

▪ MODALITY MATCHING

In an attempt to remedy this situation, Modality Matching is being used more frequently. In this procedure, a subject is asked to prescribe the same intensity scale to two sensory continua. Patients are asked to match half-log concentrations of sweet, sour, salty, and bitter with five intensities of sound. Matches for normal subjects have been determined. Subjects with loss of taste will match taste concentrations with abnormally weak tones.[44] Reliability and validity information was not presented.

▪ SPATIAL TESTING

Drop techniques have been criticized for testing only specific areas of the tongue and not addressing the spatial summation characteristics of taste; that is, with a given concentration, the taste is more intense if a larger area is stimulated. In this method, arc-shaped pieces of filter paper are soaked in concentrated solutions and placed on the left or right front of the tongue or left or right rear portions. Subjects identify the substance and assign concentrations. This method can identify specific areas of taste change, such as those seen with cranial nerve involvement.[3,44]

A combination of interview and taste testing seems the most reasonable method of assessing taste alterations. Investigations that determine the reliability of tools are needed. If the taste-testing techniques are a limiting factor, collaborative research between nurses who can identify clinical parameters and other investigators should yield significant results.

MEASUREMENT OF SMELL

Interview may help to clarify the nature of smell disorders. Questions to determine alterations include:

Have you noticed a change in smell?

What is the nature of the change?

When did it occur?

Are there certain odors that have become unpleasant?

Does the area in which you are being treated have an odor?

Are there smells that have become more pleasant?

Have you noticed a loss of smell?

Determining Smell Thresholds

Thresholds for smell are determined in the same manner as those for taste. A simple test to obtain a quick idea of the status of smell is to place such substances as coffee, peanut butter, or chocolate in the bottom of a small jar covered with gauze. The patient is given both an empty jar and the one containing the stimulus to smell. If the jar containing the stimulus is chosen, the subject is given a list of possibilities from which to identify the odor. Each nostril must be tested separately. Some investigators have added placing the subject's head into a box containing a volatilized agent for testing in order to exclude odors from the person's body.[2,3]

▪ FORCED CHOICE THREE-SNIFF TECHNIQUE

The Forced Choice Three-Sniff Technique has been used by Henkin[43] and other investigators. Stimuli are pyridine (onion or garliclike), nitrobenzene (bitter almond), and thiophene (burnt rubber). Measurements are transformed to the same bottle-unit logarithmic scale used for taste testing. Hyposmia is defined as thresholds one bottle-unit above normal.

▪ UNIVERSITY OF PENNSYLVANIA SMELL IDENTIFICATION TEST (UPSIT)

A standardized recently developed test is the University of Pennsylvania Smell Identification Test (UPSIT). Subjects are asked to identify microencapsulated odors in a scratch-and-sniff form. Tests that can help identify alterations in smell are still being developed. Schiffman presents an analogy to the type of test that is needed[3]: in assessing color perception one can show a subject red, green, and orange cards and ask them which two are most alike. Subjects choosing red and green have altered color perception. Tests such as this are necessary in the evaluation of both taste and smell.[3,43]

SUMMARY

Alterations in taste and smell may occur for a myriad of reasons. The complexity of the chemosenses has hampered investigation. The sensations are difficult to measure in an objective manner. The stimulus–response cycle is still unclear. Patients may be told that they simply must live with the abnormalities, since they are not life-threatening. However, these alterations need further research. Nurses in a clinical setting may identify the changes and initiate investigation. Collaborative research is required to develop reliable, valid, and usable tools.

REFERENCES

1. Ziporyn, T. Taste and smell: The neglected senses. *JAMA*, 1982, *247*(3):277, 282.
2. Guyton, A. *Textbook of medical physiology*. Philadelphia: Saunders, 1976.
3. Schiffman, S. Taste and smell in disease. Part I. *N Engl J Med*, 1983, *308*(21):1275.
4. Murray, R.G. Ultrastructure of taste receptors. In L.M. Beidler (Ed.), *Handbook of sensory physiology*. New York: Springer-Verlag, 1971, p 31.
5. DeWys, W.D. Abnormalities of taste as a remote effect of a neoplasm. *Ann NY Acad Sci*, 1974, *230:*427.
6. DeWys, W.D., & Walters, K. Abnormalities of taste sensation in cancer patients. *Cancer*, 1975, *36:*1888.
7. DeWys, W.D. Changes in taste sensation in cancer patients: Correlation with caloric intake. In *The chemical senses and nutrition*. New York: Academic Press, 1977, p. 381.

8. DeWys, W.D. Nutritional care of the cancer patient. *JAMA,* 1980, *244*(4):374.
9. Vickers, Z., Nielsen, S., & Theologides, A. Food preferences of patients with cancer. *J Am Diet Assoc,* 1981, *79*(4):441.
10. Trant, A.S., Serin, J., & Douglass, H. Is taste related to anorexia in cancer patients? *Am J Clin Nutr,* 1982, *36*(1):45.
11. Brewin, T. Can a tumor cause the same appetite perversion or taste change as a pregnancy? *Lancet,* 1980, *2:*907.
12. Hall, J.C., Staniland, J.R., & Giles, G.R. Altered taste thresholds in gastrointestinal cancer. *Clin Oncol,* 1980, *6*(2):137.
13. Bruera, E., Carraro, S., Roca, E., et al. Association between malnutrition and caloric intake, emesis, psychological depression, glucose taste and tumor mass. *Cancer Treat Rep,* 1984, *68*(6):873.
14. Barale, K., Aker, S.N., & Martinsen, C.S. Primary taste thresholds in children with leukemia undergoing marrow transplantation. *J Parenter Enter Nutr,* 1982, *6*(4):287.
15. Wall, D.W., & Gabriel, L. Alterations of taste in children with leukemia. *Cancer Nurs,* 1983, *6*(6):447.
16. DeWys, W., Costa, A.G., & Henkin, R. Clinical parameters related to anorexia. *Cancer Treat Rep,* 1981, *65:*49.
17. Hogan, C. Nausea and vomiting. In *Guidelines for cancer care: Symptom management.* Reston, VA: Reston Publishing, 1983.
18. Kashima, H., & Kalinowski, B. Taste impairment following laryngectomy *Ear Nose Throat,* 1979, *58:*88.
19. Donovan, M.I., & Pierce, S.G. *Cancer care nursing.* New York: Appleton-Century Crofts, 1976.
20. Bernstein, I.L., & Bernstein, I.D. Learned food aversions and cancer anorexia. *Cancer Treat Rep,* 1981, *5:*43.
21. Aker, F. The role of taste and taste dysfunction in oral diagnosis. *Quintessence Internat,* 1980, *11*(11):81.
22. Donaldson, S.F. Nutritional consequences of radiotherapy. *Cancer Res,* 1977, *37:*2407.
23. Shatzman, A.R., & Mossman, K.L. Radiation effects on bovine taste bud membranes. *Radiat Res,* 1982, *92*(2):353.
24. Mossman, K.L., & Henkin, R.I. Radiation-induced changes in taste acuity. *Int J Radiat Oncol Biol Phys,* 1978, *4:*633.
25. Johnson, C.A., Keane, T.S., & Prudo, S.M. Weight loss in patients receiving radical radiation therapy for head and neck cancer: A prospective study. *J Parenter Enter Nutr,* 1982, *6*(5):399.
26. Bolze, M.S., Fosmire, G.J., Stryker, J.A., et al. Taste acuity, plasma zinc levels and weight loss during radiotherapy: A study of relationships. *Radiology,* 1982, *144*(1):163.
27. Mossman, K. Long-term effects of radiotherapy on taste and salivary function in man. *Int J Radiat Oncol Biol Phys,* 1982, *8*(2):991.
28. Hardy, S.L., Brennand, C.P., Wyse, B.W. Taste thresholds of individuals with diabetes mellitus and of control subjects. *J Am Dietet Assoc,* 1981, *79*(3):286.
29. Abbasi, A. Diabetes: Diagnostic and therapeutic significance of taste impairment. *Geriatrics,* 1981, *36*(12):73.
30. Russell, R.M., Cox, M.E., & Solomons, W. Zinc and the special senses. *Ann Intern Med,* 1983, *99*(2):227.
31. Mahajan, S.K., Prasad, A.S., Lambuian, J., et al. Improvement of uremic hypogeusia by zinc: A double-blind study. *Am J Clin Nutr,* 1980, *33*(7):1517.
32. Zetin, M., & Stone, R.A. Effects of zinc in chronic hemodialysis. *Clin Nephrol,* 1980, *13*(1):20.
33. Ciechanover, M., Peresecenschi, G., Aviram, A., et al. Malrecognition of taste in uremia. *Nephron,* 1980, *26*(1):20.
34. Casper, R.C., Kirschner, B., Sandstead, H.H., et al. An evaluation of taste function in anorexia nervosa. *Am J Clin Nutr,* 1980, *33*(8):1801.
35. Nakajima, Y., Utsumi, H., & Takahashi, H. Ipsilateral disturbance of taste due to pontine hemorrhage. *J Neurol,* 1983, *229*(2):133.
36. Goto, W., Yakamoto, T., & Kaneko, M. Primary pontine hemorrhage and gustatory disturbance: Clinicoanatomic study. *Stroke,* 1983, *14*(4):507.

37. Schellinger, D., Henkin, R., & Smirniotopoulos, J. CT of the brain in taste and smell dysfunction. *Am J NR,* 1983, *4*(3):752.
38. Koopman, C.F., & Coulthard, S.W. The oral cavity and aging. *Otolaryngol Clin North Am,* 1982, *15*(2):293.
39. NIH. Variation in taste thresholds with human aging. *JAMA,* 1982, *247*(6):775.
40. Schiffman, S. Taste and smell in disease. Part II. *N Engl J Med,* 1983, *308*(22):1337.
41. Markley, E.J., Mattes-Kulig, D.A., & Henkin, R. A classification of dysgeusia. *J Am Dietet Assoc,* 1983, *83*(5):578.
42. Schecter, P.J., Friedewald, W.T., Bancert, D.A., et al. Idiopathic hypogeusia: A description of the syndrome and a single blind study with zinc sulfate. *Int Rev Neurobiol* [Supplement 1], 1972, 125.
43. Henkin, R., Schecter, P., & Friedewald, W. A double blind study of the effects of zinc sulfate on taste and smell dysfunction. *Am J Med Sci,* 1976, *272*(3):285.
44. Bartoshuk, L., Gent, J., Catalanotto, F., et al. Clinical evaluation of taste. *Am J Otolaryngol,* 1983, *4*(4):257.

CHAPTER 22

Measuring Dyspnea

Mary L. Brown, R.N., M.S., C.A.N.P., O.C.N.

Dyspnea, or shortness of breath, is a common symptom of cardiopulmonary pathologic conditions. It may be present during exercise or at rest in acute or chronic diseases requiring nursing assessment and intervention.

Dyspnea is observed most frequently in primary pulmonary disease, heart disease, and neuromuscular disorders affecting respiratory muscles. The symptom can occur in conditions that result in increased ventilation, alteration of physical properties of the lung, or increased respiratory work. It may be present with pregnancy, obesity, and in particular psychologic conditions characterized by anxiety.[1] Dyspnea denotes the patient's awareness of an effort to breathe, which may be excessive for the level of physical activity experienced. Neural pathways involved in the development of dyspnea are not clearly understood, and no single mechanism has been proposed that accounts for all clinical situations in which dyspnea may occur.

Dyspnea may be defined as difficult, labored, and uncomfortable breathing.[2,3] The sensation is subjective and involves the patient's perception and reaction to the sensation. It is sensory, totally perceived, interpreted, and rated by the individual experiencing it.[4] The degree of physical alteration may or may not reflect the subjective interpretation, and objective measurement may not correlate with the subjective feeling. On one end of the continuum are patients who may describe severe dyspnea and demonstrate minor pathophysiologic alterations. At the other extreme are patients describing minimal dyspnea and demonstrating marked change in pulmonary function. This statement has been supported by investigators who have observed and attempted to quantify dyspnea in a wide variety of disease states.[4,5] These investigators agree that pulmonary function disturbances differ according to disease, and no one measurement of lung function can be accepted as an exact definition of respiratory capacity.

In patients with primary pulmonary disease, dyspnea is related to abnormal breathing mechanics.[6] Pulmonary fibrosis, asthma, and emphysema are diseases that demonstrate a relationship between inspiratory work and dyspnea. In pulmonary fibrosis, where lungs and thorax are stiffer than normal, inspiratory muscles must develop greater tension to produce the same tidal volume. A similar situation exists in emphysema and acute asthma when the thoracic volume is abnormally large. In these clinical situations, it is necessary for the patient to breathe near maximum inspiratory level and use accessory inspiratory muscles to overcome high resistance to airflow at normal lung volumes. In acute asthma, dyspnea is correlated with sternocleidomastoid muscle retraction. In emphysema, a large lung volume is created by the loss of elastic recoil at rest. Dyspnea in these patients is related to the decreased capacity to respond to the ventilatory stimulus. Improving mechanical function (using bronchodilators) and decreasing ventilatory stimulus (improved oxygenation levels) are methods used to decrease dyspnea in patients with asthma and emphysema.

In cancer patients, dyspnea may be the result of disease or treatment.[7] It may be present before the diagnosis of malignancy is made, or it may develop at any point during the illness. Patients with primary lung or mediastinal tumors or those with neck or central nervous system tumors involving the respiratory centers have been identified as being at high risk for developing altered ventilatory patterns. Other cancer patients who may develop dyspnea are those who have received radiation to the chest or neck or those who have received antineoplastic agents that may cause pulmonary toxicities. Complications of disease, such as pleural effusion, ascites, pneumonia, or pulmonary emboli, may produce the dyspneic sensation. Patients with concurrent histories of pulmonary disease, congestive heart failure, smoking, environmental/occupational exposures, or anemia may exhibit dyspnea, as may those who have had surgery of the head, neck, chest, or lung.

PHYSICAL AND PSYCHOSOCIAL VARIABLES CORRELATED TO DYSPNEA PERCEPTION

The patient's description of the dyspnea sensation may aid in the diagnostic process. Patients with obstructive disease (e.g., emphysema, chronic bronchitis) recognize that they have great difficulty moving air in and out of their lungs. In contrast, patients with restrictive disease (e.g., pulmonary fibrosis or infiltrative disease) complain of hard breathing with little exertion and appear to experience sensations that would be normal for a higher level of exercise. However, some of these patients and those with pulmonary vascular disease, heart disease, or respiratory muscle weakness may describe a feeling or sense of suffocation, which is different than the shortness of breath sensation described previously.

Efforts have been made to correlate physiologic parameters with the sensation of difficult breathing. Blood gas levels and static lung volumes do not appear to be related directly to the development and production of dyspnea.[8-10] Blood gases are important, however, since they affect the level of ventilation. Although respiratory work and the oxygen cost of breathing are elevated in pulmonary disease, investigators have discovered that they do not correlate with reported dyspnea or cause perceived dyspnea.

Pulmonary function studies have been performed in an effort to correlate specificity of disease, pulmonary dysfunction, and severity of dyspnea. Since restrictive disease decreases vital capacity and limits perfusion, the reduced forced vital capacity ($r = -0.41$) and diffusing capacity ($r = -0.50$) have been shown to correlate moderately with dyspnea severity in these processes. In obstructive diseases, the maximal voluntary ventilation (MVV)—the largest liter volume that can be breathed per minute voluntarily—has the highest reported correlation with dyspnea ($r = 0.78$).[8]

The dyspnea index is a percentage of the MVV and expresses the minute ventilation at a specific level of exercise.[11] For a normal person walking 2 miles per hour on level ground, this measurement is 12 percent ± 4 percent. Studies have shown that if the dyspnea index is less than 30 percent, shortness of breath does not usually occur. Subjects with an index greater than 50 percent are likely to be short of breath at abnormally low exercise levels. However, Fishman and Ledlie demonstrated that patients with obstructive lung disease may not complain of dyspnea even though they may demonstrate a dyspnea index greater than 50 percent.[12]

Since the MVV is tiring and difficult to reproduce, the 1-second forced expiratory volume (FEV_1) is the most convenient and useful measurement for evaluating prolonged expiration and the degree of airway obstruction. It has a slightly lower correlation with dyspnea than the MVV ($r = -0.71$) and depends on individual effort and cooperation. Although incremental exercise tests have provided some investigators with statistically significant correlations, the exact degree of dyspnea that an individual patient will experience remains unpredictable.[10]

As previously described, the severity of dyspnea varies with the degree of pulmonary dysfunction. To determine the threshold at which the dyspnea is perceived, resistive and elastic loads have been added to aid in understanding how some patients can have airflow obstruction and no complaints of breathlessness. Recent studies have shown that for patients with chronically high airway resistance, increased changes in resistance are needed for the detection of dyspnea.[13] Asthmatics have high thresholds and decreased perception of dyspnea, probably due to more frequent episodes of bronchospasm and greater responsiveness to histamine.[5]

Since people can become short of breath when experiencing emotional situations, asthmatics have been studied extensively to try to determine correlations between breathlessness and various psychosocial phenomena. Investigators have demonstrated, however, that dyspnea experienced by patients with asthma is generally acute in nature. These dyspneic events are not generalizable to patients whose dyspnea is chronic and present at rest or during minimal exercise.[14]

EXPERIMENTS TO PRODUCE THE SENSATION OF DYSPNEA

Efforts to study the sensation of dyspnea and gain understanding into ventilatory regulation have focused on producing unpleasant respiratory sensations resembling breathlessness. Examples of these early investigations are breathholding and studies on perceptions of added respiratory loads.[15] Transcutaneous vagal nerve and chest wall blocks also have been performed.[8] Asthmatics, as a special group, have been studied to determine if a relationship exists between the psychology and physiology of dyspnea.[5] These studies have added to the basic understanding of neural, chemical, and muscular functions of the respiratory sensation, but their relationship to dyspnea continues to be vague.

Treadmill and standardized walking tests (2, 6, and 12 minutes) have been used to produce and evaluate dyspnea as it related to exercise.[8,15–17] Butland et al. demonstrated high correlation coefficients between 2-minute, 6-minute, and 12-minute walking tests, indicating that they are similar measures of exercise tolerance (6 minute versus 12 minute, $r = 0.955$; 2 minute versus 12 minute, $r = 0.864$; 2 minute versus 6 minute, $r = 0.892$).[18] Clinically easy to perform and tested for validity, standardized walking tests may be used by nurses to relate pulmonary function and disability in patients over long periods of time.

More sophisticated laboratory investigations have been performed to produce dyspnea. One approach pharmacologically induces bronchoconstriction with histamine or methacholine.[5,19] The threshold at which the patient perceives breathlessness is then determined. Other investigators have used elastic and resistive loads to breathing to determine when subjects detect the loads and are rendered breathless.[20]

INSTRUMENTS TO MEASURE DYSPNEA

Verbal reports of breathlessness and psychophysiologic magnitude estimation techniques have been used to measure dyspnea.[21] Studies have measured dyspnea from a time perspective, that is, the amount of dyspnea perceived daily and the amount of dyspnea produced at a specific time in the experimental setting.

Retrospective determination of daily activity at which breathing difficulty occurs currently is the most common method of evaluating dyspnea. Scales equating dyspnea with activity have been proven to be reliable and correlate with measures of pulmonary function. Figure 22–1 illustrates two dyspnea activity scales.

▪ FIVE-LEVEL SCALE OF BREATHLESSNESS AND MORGAN DYSPNEA DISABILITY SCALE

The first scale, developed by the American Thoracic Society and included in the Standardized Respiratory Disease Questionnaire, contains a Five-Level Scale of Breathlessness that relates dyspnea to activity.[22] Morgan et al. used a similar scale (Morgan Dyspnea Disability Scale), but four grades of dyspnea were used to evaluate disability in patients with chronic lung disease.[23] Both of these scales are retrospective and designed to be used with patients experiencing chronic shortness of breath. They can aid nurses in all settings in determining baseline dyspnea levels during initial nursing assessment and in ongoing evaluation of the dyspneic patient.

A. American Thoracic Society Five-Level Scale of Breathlessness Graded 1 to 5

Grade	Description
1	Are you troubled by shortness of breath hurrying on the level or walking up a slight hill? Yes ___ No ___
2	Do you have to walk slower than people of your age on the level because of breathlessness? Yes ___ No ___
3	Do you ever have to stop for breath when walking at your own pace on the level? Yes ___ No ___
4	Do you ever have to stop for breath after walking about 100 yards (or after a few minutes on the level)? Yes ___ No ___
5	Are you too breathless to leave the house or breathless on dressing or undressing? Yes ___ No ___

Grade of breathlessness _____

B. Degree of shortness of breath graded from 0 to 3 by using the Morgan Dyspnea Disability Scale

Grade	Description
0	No unusual shortness of breath compared to other persons of the same age, height, and sex
1	More shortness of breath than a person of the same age when walking up hills or hurrying on ground level
2	Shortness of breath while walking on level ground
3	Shortness of breath at rest or while dressing

Figure 22–1. Instruments to measure dyspnea and activity.

▪ MODIFIED BORG SCALE

Other quantifiable rating scales have been developed to assess dyspnea perception produced at one specific time point by a particular stimulus. In a study of breathlessness perception in asthmatics, Burdon et al. used an adaptation of a scale developed by Borg (Modified Borg Scale).[5] This scale uses words describing increasing degrees of breathlessness rated by numbers between 0 and 10. The 12-item scale has been used to determine perceived breathlessness in relation to changes in specific pulmonary function studies. Breathlessness increased as the FEV_1 decreased, indicating a close linear relationship between the two indices (mean $r = 0.88 \pm 0.15$ SD). There was, however, a considerable variation in the severity of breathlessness for any degree of airflow obstruction (mean intercept 0.50 ± 0.89 SD). A significant relationship ($p < 0.01$) between bronchial responsiveness and magnitude of respiratory distress was indicated.

▪ VISUAL ANALOG SCALES (VAS)

As in measuring other sensations, Visual Analog Scales (VAS) have been used to measure dyspnea (Fig. 22–2).[3,24] The VAS is a measured line with descriptive phrases at each end. The line is marked by the subjects at a point that corresponds with symptom severity. Investigators have related these scales to standardized exercise tests and pulmonary function studies to aid in determining relationships between exercise and breathlessness. Harries et al. studied relationships between standardized walking tests, lung function, and the VAS.[16] Subjects were divided into groups according to pulmonary diagnosis: 70 were bronchitic and 33 were emphysematous. In those patients with emphysema, a significant correlation existed between the walking test and VAS ($r = 0.7$, $p < 0.0001$), whereas bronchitic patients demonstrated correlations between the walking test and FEV_1 ($r = 0.62$, $p < 0.0001$).

A. Visual Analog Scale

0		10
No difficulty breathing		Unable to breathe

B. Modified Borg Scale

0	Nothing at all
0.5	Very, very slight (just noticeable)
1	Very slight
2	Slight
3	Moderate
4	Somewhat severe
5	Severe
6	
7	Very severe
8	
9	Very, very severe (almost maximal)
10	Maximal

Figure 22–2. A Visual Analog Scale to measure dyspnea and the Modified Borg Scale.

▪ OXYGEN COST DIAGRAM

The Oxygen Cost Diagram is a variation of the VAS. It determines the point at which a specific activity level corresponds to the subject's perception of dyspnea. A 100 mm vertical line is used, with everyday activities placed in proportion to their oxygen cost. The point where shortness of breath limits exercise is marked by the subjects.[15]

▪ MAGNITUDE ESTIMATION

Magnitude Estimation is a psychophysiologic technique that measures the subjective magnitude of a sensation. A range of physical stimulus intensities has been used to measure dyspnea.[25-28] The proportional increase in dyspnea is estimated from the subject's own reference point as loads are added. Since learning is required by the patient, this testing is performed most easily on the ambulatory patient.

▪ BASELINE DYSPNEA INDEX AND TRANSITION DYSPNEA INDEX

Two newly developed indices have been used to correlate lung function and exercise capacity.[29] Tested for reliability on 21 patients with COPD the Baseline Dyspnea Index grades the severity of dyspnea at a single point in time. The Transition Dyspnea Index indicates changes in dyspnea from the baseline assessment. Each index scale contains three classification axes: functional impairment, magnitude of task in exertional capacity, and magnitude of subject effort. Each main axis contains five categories, numerically rated 0 to 4. The grades are added to form a baseline score ranging from 0 to 12. Each main axis in the Transition Index contains seven grades, ranging from −3 (major deterioration) to +3 (major impairment). These grades are added to form a Transition Score (−9 to +9). These indices, along with spirometry and 12-minute walking distance, were used to measure dyspnea, lung function, and exercise capacity in patients with obstructive pulmonary disease. The investigators concluded that the indices can be used to quantify dyspnea severity and identify changes. Using Jaspen's multiserial correlation coefficient (m), the study demonstrated statistically significant relationships between the mean Baseline Dyspnea Score and the 12-minute walking test ($m = 0.54$) and forced vital capacity ($m = 0.63$). In addition, agreement between paired observers was nearly perfect.

In another study, these same indices were used to assess the effects of theophylline on dyspnea, lung function, and exercise performance on 12 male ambulatory patients with non-reversible airway obstruction.[30] Arterial gas tensions, steady-state, and maximal exercise performance and the 12-minute walking distance also were measured. Results demonstrated that theophylline reduced dyspnea but did not improve lung function, gas exchange, or exercise performance.

▪ STANDARDIZED RESPIRATORY DISEASE QUESTIONNAIRE

In addition to the previously mentioned instruments, two questionnaires are available to aid in evaluating the behavioral manifestations of dyspnea.[22,31] The Standardized Respiratory Disease Questionnaire developed by the American Thoracic Society provides extensive demographic data as well as specific information on pulmonary symptomatology (cough, mucus production, and wheezing) that may occur with dyspnea. Historical information on related pulmonary disease, occupational exposures, medication use, and smoking can also be obtained. Examples of questions are:

A. Does your chest ever sound wheezy or whistling:
   1. When you have a cold: 1. Yes ___   2. No ___
   2. Occasionally apart from colds?   1. Yes ___   2. No ___
   3. Most days or nights?   1. Yes ___   2. No ___

B. For how many years has this been   _____
   present?   Number of years

C. Have you ever had an attack of wheezing   1. Yes ___   2. No ___
   that made you feel short of breath?

D. How old were you when you had your   ___ Age in years
   first attack?

E. Have you had 2 or more such episodes? 1. Yes ___   2. No ___

F. Have you ever required medicine for   1. Yes ___   2. No ___
   treatment of the(se) attacks?

• DYSPNEA INTERVIEW SCHEDULE

The Dyspnea Interview Schedule developed by Carrieri and Janson-Bjerklie is a semistructured interview that asks questions related to the patient's dyspnea perception, aggravating and alleviating factors, prodromal indicators, and physiologic, psychologic, and behavioral correlates.[31] Information about adaptive mechanisms, social support, and effects of dyspnea on activities of daily living is obtained from this Interview Schedule. Typical questions are:

1. When were you first aware of having shortness of breath?
   a. What did you do about it?
   b. Did you talk to someone about it?
   c. How long did you have shortness of breath before you sought medical advice?
   d. What were you told was the cause of your shortness of breath?

2. Do your present eating habits differ from what was normal for you before your illness?
   a. Do people bring food to you?
   b. Are you able to cut your own food?
   c. Is pouring milk or coffee a problem for you?

This instrument illustrates how investigators have begun to focus on behavioral manifestations that are demonstrated by patients experiencing dyspnea. These behavioral manifestations, along with careful descriptions of feelings during dyspneic episodes, have given additional insight into the sensation of dyspnea. Efforts have been made to describe differences and commonalities among patients with chronic dyspnea (i.e., those having lung cancer, emphysema, chronic bronchitis, COPD) and those who experience dyspnea more acutely (those patients with asthma).

SUMMARY

A recent study of 30 lung cancer patients and their perceptions of their dyspnea points out the need for careful and thoughtful consideration of this sensation.[32] The purposes of this study were to describe and determine patterns in the sensation of dyspnea, identify coping and adaptive strategies used by lung cancer patients, and determine the relationship between activity and dyspnea in this patient population. A convenience sample was interviewed twice over a 2-month interval. At Time 1, the American Thoracic Society Questionnaire (including the Grade of Breathlessness Scale, or GBS), the Dyspnea Interview Schedule, the Dyspnea Visual Analog Scale (DVAS), and the Karnofsky Performance Scale (KPS) were used. At Time 2, the GBS, KPS, and DVAS were administered.

Data were analyzed using parametric and nonparametric statistics. The semistructured interview provided thematic descriptions of physical and emotional sensations experienced during episodes of dyspnea. Precipitants and patterns of dyspnea also were identified. Patients reported significant dyspnea, felt extreme fatigue, and experienced loss of concetration, memory, and appetite when short of breath. Many patients in the sample had preexisting obstructive and restrictive pulmonary disease that had been present for some time. This may have added to the high average number of self-taught strategies identified by study patients. Of concern was the fact that no patient identified any useful strategies that had been taught by nurses.

Severity of dyspnea was measured quantitatively by the GBS and DVAS. Moderate correlations were seen between these two instruments. Although slightly lower at Time 2, the degree of breathlessness did not change significantly over the 8-week period (Time 1, worst dyspnea $p = 0.001$, usual dyspnea $p = 0.001$; Time 2, worst dyspnea $p = 0.002$, usual dyspnea $p = 0.002$).

The KPS scores were predictably lower at Time 2, but a statistically significant correlation between KPS and GBS occurred (Time 1, $p = 0.001$, and Time 2, $p = 0.002$). A moderate correlation between KPS and perceived level of dyspnea (measured by the DVAS) was also evident when usual and worst dyspnea were evaluated and related to activity.

This study demonstrated that dyspnea is a significant problem for patients with lung cancer. It also points out the need for careful evaluation of dyspnea using multiple instruments that will measure the sensation qualitatively and quantitatively. The DVAS, GBS, and KPS can easily be administered clinically to aid in detecting the level of dyspnea a patient may be experiencing. The information obtained can then lead to appropriate planning for change, with nursing interventions based on reliable measurement of the subjective symptom of dyspnea. The patients themselves provided a wealth of information on how to manage dyspnea. Future patients would benefit from this information rather than having to rely on trial and error in isolation.

Further investigations with dyspneic patients experiencing other pulmonary diagnoses has been started.[33] The importance of these studies is underscored by the need for ongoing research in symptom management for patients with chronic illness. The use of multiple instruments to investigate these complex phenomena can assist in providing a solid base for the science of clinical therapeutics in nursing.

REFERENCES

1. Carrieri, V., Janson-Bjerklie, S., & Jacobs, S. The sensation of dyspnea: A review. *Heart Lung,* 1984, *13*(4):436.

2. Comroe, J. Some theories in the mechanism of dyspnea. In J. Howell & E. Campbell (Eds.), *Breathlessness*. Oxford: Blackwell Scientific Publications, 1966, p. 1.
3. Comroe, J. *Physiology of respiration* (2nd ed.). Chicago: Year Book, 1974.
4. Widimsky, J. Dyspnea. 1979, *Cor Vasa, 21*(2):128.
5. Burdon, J., Juniper, E., Killian, K., et al. The perception of dyspnea in asthma. *Am Rev Respir Dis,* 1982, *126*(5):825.
6. Ball, W., & Summer, W. Clinical manifestations and diagnosis of pulmonary disease. In A. Harvey, R. Johns, V. McKusick, et al. (Eds.), *The principles and practice of medicine.* New York: Appleton-Century-Crofts, 1980, p. 353.
7. Krzysko, A., Erdel, S., Greiner, M., & Lawrance, A. Guidelines for nursing care of patients with altered ventilation. *Oncol Nurs Forum,* 1983, *10*(2):113.
8. Epler, G., Sabec, F., & Gaensler, E. Determination of severe impairment (disability) in intersitial lung disease, *Am Rev Respir Dis,* 1980, *121*(4):647.
9. McDadden, E., Kiser, R., & DeGroot, W. Acute bronchial asthma. *N Engl J Med,* 1973, *288*(5):221.
10. Morgan, W. Pulmonary disability and impairment. *Am Thorac Soc News Basis RD,* 1982, *10:*1.
11. Carrieri, V., & Janson-Bjerklie, S. Dyspnea. In V. Carrieri, A. Lindsey, & C. West (Eds.), *Pathophysiological phenomena in nursing.* Philadelphia: Saunders, 1986, p. 191.
12. Fishman, A.P., & Ledlie, J.F. Dyspnea. *Bull Eur Physiol Respir,* 1979, *15*(5):789.
13. Gottfried, S., Altose, M., Kelson, S., & Cherniak, N. Perception of changes in airflow resistance in obstructive pulmonary disorders. *Am Rev Respir Dis,* 1981, *124*(5):566.
14. Burki, N. Dyspnea. *Clin Chest Med,* 1980, *1*(1):47.
15. McGavin, C., Artivinli, M., Nave, H., & McHardy, G. Dyspnoea, disability, and distance walked: Comparison of estimates of exercise performance in respiratory disease. *Br Med J,* 1978, *2:*241.
16. Harries, D., Booker, H., Rehaln, M., & Collins, J. Measurement and perception of disability in chronic airways obstruction (Abstr.). *Am Rev Respir Dis,* 1983, *127*(Suppl):119.
17. Bilman, M., Rambhatla, K., Blair, G., & Sieck, G. Breathlessness index, a simple and repeatable exercise test for patients with chronic obstructive pulmonary disease/(Abstr.). *Am Rev Respir Dis,* 1983, *127*(Suppl):109.
18. Butland, R., Pand, J., Gross, E., et al. Two-, six-, and 12-minute walking rests in respiratory disease. *Br Med J,* 1982, *284*(6329):1607.
19. Rubinfeld, A., & Pain, M. Conscious perception of bronchospasm as a protective phenomenon in asthma. *Chest,* 1977, *72*(2):154.
20. Burki, N., Mitchell, K., & Chaudhary, B. The ability of asthmatics to detect added resistive loads. *Am Rev Respir Dis,* 1978, *117*(1):71.
21. Gottfried, S., Altose, M., Kelson, G., & Cherniack, N. Perception of changes in airflow resistance in obstructive pulmonary disorders. *Am Rev Respir Dis,* 1981, *124*(5):566.
22. American Thoracic Society. Recommended respiratory disease questionnaire for use with adults and children in epidemiological research. *Am Rev Respir Dis,* 1978, *118*(1):7.
23. Morgan, W., Lapp, N., & Seaton, D. Respiratory disability in coal miners. *JAMA,* 1980, *243*(23):2402.
24. Joyce, C., Zutshi, D., Hrubes, V., & Mason, R. Comparison of fixed interval and visual analogue scales for rating chronic pain. *Eur J Clin Pharmacol,* 1975, *8*(6):415.
25. Killian, K., Mahutte, C., Howell, J., & Campbell, E. Effect of timing, flow, lung volume and threshold pressure on resistive load detection. *J Appl Physiol,* 1980, *49*(6):958.
26. Killian, K., Burens, D., & Campbell, E. Effect of breathing patterns on the perceived magnitude of added loads to breathing. *J Appl Physiol,* 1982, *52*(3):578.
27. Killian, K., Campbell, E., & Howell, J. The effect of increased ventilation on resistive load discrimination. *Am Rev Respir Dis,* 1979, *120*(6):1233.
28. Burki, N., Davenport, P., Safdar, R., & Zechman, F. The effects of airway anesthesia on magnitude estimation of added inspiratory resistive and elastic loads. *Am Rev Respir Dis,* 1983, *127*(1):2.
29. Mahler. D., Weinberg, D., Wells, C., & Feinstein, A. Measurement of dyspnea: Description of two new indexes, interobserver agreement, and physiologic correlations (Abstr.). *Am Rev Respir Dis,* 1982, *125*(Suppl):138.

30. Mahler, D., Matthay, R., Berger, H., et al. Sustained-release theophylline reduces dyspnea in non-reversible obstructive airway disease. *Am Rev Respir Dis,* 1983, *127*(Suppl):87.
31. Carrieri, V., & Janson-Bjerklie, S. *Dyspnea Interview Schedule.* Unpublished paper. University of California, San Francisco, 1983.
32. Brown, M., Carrieri, V., Janson-Bjerklie, S., & Dodd, M. Lung cancer and dyspnea: The patient's perception, *Oncol Nurs Forum,* 1986, *13*(5):19.
33. Carrieri, V., & Janson-Bjerklie, S. Strategies patients use to manage the sensation of dyspnea. *West J Nurs Res,* 1986, *8*(3):284.

CHAPTER 23

Measuring Skin Integrity

Barbara J. Braden, R.N.,M.S.

The primary problem in skin integrity for the nurse is that of pressure sore development. Because other skin lesions and problems are more appropriately described than measured, this chapter is devoted almost exclusively to measurement involving pressure sores.

The critical factors in pressure sore development are the intensity and duration of the pressure and the skin tolerance for pressure.[1] Contributing factors identified in the literature are those that predispose to intense and prolonged pressure or to poor tolerance of the skin for pressure. Some of these contributing factors are advanced age, depression, prolonged immobility, paralysis, loss of sensation, poor nutritional status, cachexia, anemia, exposure of the skin to moisture, exposure of the skin to friction and shear, low cardiac output, and infection. It is outside the scope of this chapter to discuss measurement of all of these contributing factors.

Many instruments are available to the clinical researcher concerned with skin integrity. Selection of an instrument or instruments will depend on the purpose of the inquiry. The common purposes of inquiry in this area are to identify patients who are at risk for skin breakdown, to predict the effectiveness of clinical modalities in preventing pressure sores, and to determine the effectiveness of treatment modalities in healing pressure sores. Instruments available for these purposes can be divided into four categories: (1) instruments that measure an etiologic factor directly, that is, a direct measure of pressure over a bony prominence, (2) instruments designed to provide a direct measurement of a secondary effect of an etiologic factor, such as changes in skin oxygen tension resulting from pressure, (3) instruments that assess etiologic factors indirectly and summatively in an attempt to determine the patient's overall risk for developing pressure sores, and (4) instruments that describe the stage of development of the pressure sore or measure the size of the pressure sore on one or more dimensions.

It is important to note that many factors contribute to the development and healing of pressure sores, and some probably remain to be discovered or adequately delineated. Certainly, many of these factors interact in ways that are not fully understood. Although it is expedient and wise to use instruments currently available, the clinical researcher should collect as much additional data as possible in an effort to uncover new relationships. Furthermore, ancedotal data on a per case basis may be as enlightening as aggregate data and should be collected systematically throughout the process of inquiry. The clinicians providing direct care are important sources of this type of information, and their intuitive judgments about why pressure sores develop or heal in one patient and not in others should be solicited and evaluated.

DIRECT MEASUREMENT OF ETIOLOGIC FACTORS

Instruments to measure the etiologic factors of pressure, shear, and loss of sensation are reported in the literature. Many of these are complex devices that are not always commercially available, and some require a special design suited to the phenomena of interest. In addition, the instruments may have little or no clinical use after the conclusion of the research. Nevertheless, a clinical researcher may be able to acquire these instruments through collaboration with the biomedical engineering department of a hospital, university, or medical supplies company. In discussing these instruments, greater emphasis is placed on those with the simplest designs and widest applicability.

Instruments to Measure Pressure and Shear

▪ CONTINUOUS PRESSURE MONITOR

Measurements of pressure have been important aspects of studies concerned with the effect of positioning on pressure points, the effectiveness of therapeutic mattress surfaces or wheelchair pads in reducing skin surface pressure, and comparison of the effects of identical skin surface pressures on varying patient populations. Recent studies have used relatively simple devices to measure pressure. The simplest of these devices, a Continuous Pressure Monitor, was used to study skin pressure measurements in cancer patients on various mattress surfaces.[2,3] This device has three components, all connected by tubing: (1) a pressure-sensing inflatable bladder with a 1 square inch surface area, (2) a pump that inflates the bladder in response to internal pressures, and (3) a mercury manometer to measure the pressure inside the bladder. The bladder is placed between the patient and the mattress at various points at which pressure sores commonly occur. Internally, both walls of the inflatable bladder have electrically conductive strips that are connected to the pump. When the bladder is flat, the conductive strips make contact and activate the pump. The pump inflates the bladder until the conductive strips separate. The separation occurs at a pressure that is equal to or slightly greater than the surface pressure between the patient and the mattress; this pressure is reflected on the mercury manometer. When the conductive strips separate, the pump is switched off and the bladder deflates until contact is reestablished. One group of researchers report the accuracy of this device to be ± 2 mm Hg at a pressure of 50 mm Hg and below and ± 4 mm Hg from 50 to 80 mm Hg.[3]

▪ PRESSURE EVALUATION PAD (PEP)

The Pressure Evaluation Pad (PEP) is reported in a study of the effects of various side-lying positions on trochanteric pressure.[4] It is more complex than the Continuous Pressure

Monitor and possibly more accurate in establishing the point of maximal pressure. The PEP, like the Continuous Pressure Monitor, uses an inflatable pad with internal contact switches attached to a pneumatic pump. Whereas the Continuous Pressure Monitor is small and has one internal contact switch, the PEP is larger and has a 12 × 12 matrix of contact switches connected to a readout board. The readout board contains 144 light-emitting diodes that become illuminated with pressure on the corresponding switches. Similar to the Continuous Pressure Monitor, the standard error using the PEP ranged from 2.83 mm Hg to 4.49 mm Hg. However, multiple repositionings of the pad to determine the point of maximal pressure were not necessary using the PEP, and this appears to render it less vulnerable to human error. This device is commercially available and has been used to evaluate wheelchair pressure-relief cushions.[5]

• MONITOR FOR PRESSURE, SHEAR, AND PULSATILE BLOOD FLOW

An instrument has been reported that allows for measurement of pressure, shear, and pulsatile blood flow.[6] This device consists of a hard, clear plastic seat containing flush-mounted sensors capable of monitoring all three variables. It has been used to determine differences in pressure, shear, and pulsatile blood flow among paraplegic, geriatric, and normal subjects in a sitting position.[7] This device has limited applications in clinical research because it cannot be used within soft pressure-relief mattresses or cushions and is prone to certain types of quantification errors in untrained hands. Nevertheless, it has several unique qualities for researchers with special interest in this area.

Instruments to Measure Loss of Sensation
Instruments that measure sensation or loss of sensation are simple, inexpensive, and commercially available. The clinical researcher may use these instruments for any study in which a determination of cutaneous sensory function in any part of the body is important. Furthermore, these instruments may be useful for clinical assessments as well as scientific inquiry.

• COMPASS-TYPE CALIPER

The instrument most commonly used is a Compass-Type Caliper to determine two-point discrimination ability. Two-point discrimination is defined as the ability to differentiate two, non-noxious, light-touch stimuli applied separately but simultaneously to the skin.[8] Nolan suggests that an ECG caliper is easily adapted for this purpose by gentle sanding of the points until they become blunt, thus insuring that light touch will not produce noxious stimuli.[9] The instrument measures the distance between the two points in millimeters and is not inherently prone to error other than slippage. The clinical researcher who wishes to use two-point discrimination should be aware of intrinsic and extrinsic factors that influence two-point discrimination and the range of possibilities for interindividual and intraindividual variations.[9] Although the test of two-point discrimination seems relatively easy to perform, considerable skill is required to elicit and interpret patient responses. An excellent discussion of the procedure for evaluating cutaneous sensibility quantitatively and qualitatively is reported by Werner and Omer.[10]

▪ WEINSTEIN-SEMMES PRESSURE AESTHESIOMETER

Also reported by Werner and Omer is an additional instrument for evaluating cutaneous sensibility, the Weinstein-Semmes Pressure Aesthesiometer, which is used to establish the threshold of light touch to deep pressure.[10] This instrument allows the investigator to use a series of 20 calibrated nylon monofilaments that exert pressure ranging from 1.65 to 6.65 mg of pressure. Because the filament bends when pressed against the skin, the pressure exerted is a function of the length and diameter of each monofilament and is not attributable to the investigator. The calibration of the monofilaments allows for a quantification of cutaneous sensibility that is not possible with older, more commonly used techniques, such as dragging cotton wool across the skin. The instrument is relatively impervious to error when used to obtain quantifiable results. However, like two-point discrimination testing, the investigator's skill in eliciting and interpreting patient responses is important if qualitative determinations are to be made.

DIRECT MEASUREMENT OF SECONDARY EFFECTS OF ETIOLOGIC FACTORS

For every known etiologic factor in pressure sore development, there are several secondary effects. Many of these effects are internal and involve changes in the dynamics and architecture of the vascular bed, lymphatic channels, and soft tissue. Measurement of most effects requires complex, invasive techniques that are not discussed here, since they are not of general interest to clinical researchers working with human subjects. Readers with further interest in this area are referred to a review article by Krouskop.[11] However, some secondary effects of pressure, such as skin oxygen tension and skin temperature, can be measured noninvasively.

▪ SKIN OXYGEN SENSOR

Skin oxygen tension is particularly easy to study in that the necessary equipment is available commercially. The Skin Oxygen Sensor was developed for monitoring the arterial oxygen partial pressure in the newborn and was subsequently used by Seiler and Stahelin in adult subjects to measure the effects of pressure on skin.[12] To standardize conditions for all subjects, these researchers heated the skin sensor to a constant temperature of 44°C to achieve maximal vasodilation in the cutaneous tissues underneath the sensor. They then tested the skin oxygen tension over a hard site (greater trochanter) and a soft site (quadriceps muscle) before, during, and after applying varying amounts of pressure to these areas. In this manner, they were able to demonstrate a "high sensitivity of skin oxygen availability to any imposed pressure at hard sites" (p. 1301).[12] This instrument would seem to have many further applications in studies of positioning and pressure relief devices and possibly in areas of inquiry unrelated to pressure.

▪ ELECTRIC THERMOMETER AND THERMOGRAPHY

Another secondary effect of pressure that can be measured with relative ease is the increase in skin temperature that occurs with reactive hyperemia following the release of pressure. A number of instruments ranging from simple to complex have been used to measure skin temperature. Howell[13] used an Electric Thermometer, accurate to within ± 0.2°. This type of instrument has the advantage of being simple to use, commonly available, and inexpensive. Other researchers[14,15] have used thermisters and thermocouplers but offer no explanation of methods to determine instrument accuracy. Thermography also has been used to document changes in skin temperature resulting from pressure.[15] This technique requires complex and expensive equipment, including a cathode ray tube (CRT) with a CRT display. However, this equipment is available in the radiology department of most acute care facilities.

When using any of these instruments, the clinical researcher must be careful to control for ambient temperature, time of day, and activity level. Sufficient time must be allowed for the subject to adjust to the temperature of the test room (usually 1 hour), and baseline temperatures should be obtained. Depending on the purpose of the inquiry, temperature may be monitored during exposure to pressure as well as at 1- to 2-minute intervals after exposure. If areas of the skin are to be tested with repeated applications of pressure, a rest period of at least 20 minutes should be provided to allow the skin temperature to equilibrate. In addition, duration and intensity of pressure must be controlled, since these variables affect the peak skin temperature rise.

Skin temperature can be a valuable measure in a variety of studies. It may be useful in evaluating pressure-relief devices.[14] It has possibilities for testing patient tissue tolerance[13,14] and may, therefore, be of value in predicting risk of pressure sore development. The use of hypothermia to reduce the metabolic demands of a region has been explored.[15]

MEASUREMENT OF RISK OF SKIN BREAKDOWN

Several instruments designed to predict the risk of skin breakdown have been reported in the literature.[16–19] These instruments use summative rating scales based on observations of factors contributing to skin breakdown and specify critical scores for identifying patients at risk. Researchers or clinicians considering the use of these instruments should be reminded that they are designed to measure risk for skin breakdown rather than to predict with absolute accuracy the occurrence of skin breakdown. It is important also to note that these instruments were tested using almost exclusively hospitalized and institutionalized elderly subjects. It would, therefore, be unwise to expect predictive values to be similar to those previously reported when these instruments are used to study younger subjects.

▪ NORTON SCALE

The instrument developed by Norton et al.[16] and first reported in 1962 has been studied most extensively.[20–22] This tool consists of five parameters: physical condition, mental state, activity, mobility, and incontinence, each of which is rated on a scale of 1 to 4, with one- or two-word descriptors for each rating (Fig. 23–1). The sum of the ratings for all five param-

E Incontinence	
Not	4
Occasionally	3
Usually of urine	2
Doubly	1

Figure 23–1. Example from the Norton Scale.

eters yields a score that can range from 4 to 20. Norton found an almost linear relationship between the scores of the elderly patients and the incidence of pressure sores, with a score of 14 indicating the "onset of risk" and a score of 12 or below indicating a high risk for pressure sores.

Roberts and Goldstone, using the Norton tool in a study of 64 patients over age 60 admitted to an orthopedic ward, found that 32 patients received scores below 14 and that 12 of these at-risk patients developed pressure sores more serious than erythema.[20] A predictive value for positive results of 37.5 percent can be calculated from these data. Only 1 patient with a score above 14 developed a pressure sore. These investigators trained a team of nurses to rate the patients but give no indication of studying the interrater reliability of this tool. They do indicate that the patient with a score above 14 who broke down was probably scored improperly. In a later study, Goldstone and Goldstone used only one rater in an apparent attempt to control the reliability of the scores.[22] Among patients over age 50 admitted to an orthopedic ward, 30 of 40 were judged to be at risk (Norton score 14 or below); 16 of the at-risk patients developed pressure lesions, and 2 of the patients with Norton scores above 14 developed pressure lesions. A predictive value for positive results of 53 percent can be calculated from these data. In both studies, the difference in the mean Norton scores between patients who developed pressure sores and those who did not was statistically significant ($p = <0.001$). Goldstone and Goldstone do not define pressure lesions, but it is likely that they classified skin erythema as a pressure lesion, which may account for the improvement in the predictive value.

Roberts and Goldstone included a report of a pilot study in which patients were not excluded on the basis of age.[20] Of 125 patients in this age-heterogeneous sample, only 29 received scales of 14 or below, and only 1 of these 29 developed pressure sore (a predictive value of only 3.4 percent. Goldstone and Goldstone found the sums of physical conditions rating and the incontinence rating to be as predictive as the total Norton score.[22]

▪ GOSNELL SCALE

A second tool for assessing patient risk for skin breakdown was reported in 1973 by Gosnell.[17] It consists of five parameters (or subscales): mental status, continence, mobility, activity, and nutrition. This tool is an adaptation of Norton's instrument. In a major departure, Gosnell substituted a 3-point nutrition rating scale (good, fair, poor) for Norton's 4-point physical condition rating scale. In addition, she altered the descriptors slightly in Norton's incontinence rating scale (Fig. 23–2) and added a fifth rating, confusion, to Norton's Mental Status Scale.

The range of possible scores remained 4 to 20, but Gosnell changed the cutoff score for risk to 16. Gosnell also developed two- or three-sentence descriptive statements for each

CONTINENCE control of urination and defecation	1. No control: incontinent of urine and feces	2. Minimally controlled: often incontinent of urine; occasionally incontinent of feces	3. Usually controlled: incontinent occasionally or has catheter and is occasionally incontinent of feces	4. Fully controlled: total control of urine and feces

Figure 23–2. Example from scale developed by Gosnell.

rating on each scale. The use of the descriptive statements appears to be aimed at increasing the reliability of the instrument when used by multiple raters. However, the investigator performed all ratings in this study and did not report any study of interrater reliability.

Gosnell used her instrument to study 30 patients over age 65 admitted to extended care facilities.[17] On admission, 21 patients received scores of 16 or above, and 9 patients received scores below 16. At the conclusion of the study, 4 patients had experienced skin breakdown, 2 with admission scores of 16 or better and 2 with admission scores below 16. However, 3 of the 4 patients had scores below 16 at the time of skin breakdown.

Gosnell's instrument did not appear to predict as well as Norton's, with a predictive value for positive results of only 33 percent when used to evaluate elderly patients. Although the inclusion of a nutrition rating scale is logically supported in studies of etiologic factors of pressure sores,[23,24] difficulties exist in the accuracy with which staff estimate intake on a traditional "good," "fair," "poor" rating scale.[25]

Gosnell studied a number of additional variables, such as body temperature, blood pressure, skin tone and sensation, medications, and medical diagnosis. These factors were given no weight in the score, and development of a scheme for including some of these factors in an assessment tool may be of interest to other clinical researchers.

▪ BRADEN SCALE

A third instrument, the Braden Scale, has been developed to predict the risk for skin breakdown.* The Braden Scale is composed of six subscales that conceptually reflect degrees of sensory perception, skin moisture, physical activity, nutritional intake, friction and shear, and ability to change and control body position. All subscales are rated from 1 to 4, with the exception of the friction and shear subscale (Fig. 23–3), which is rated from 1 to 3. Each rating is accompanied by a brief description of criteria for assigning the rating. Potential scores range from 4 to 23, and a patient with a score of 16 or below is considered at risk.

This instrument is being used at present in a 3-year study of factors related to pressure sore development among elderly patients. Some preliminary testing of this instrument has been completed. Content validity has been established by expert opinion. Two studies of

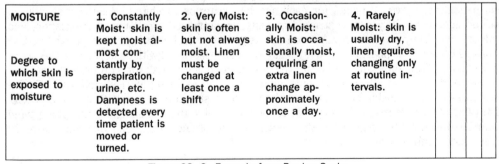

MOISTURE	1. Constantly Moist: skin is kept moist almost constantly by perspiration, urine, etc. Dampness is detected every time patient is moved or turned.	2. Very Moist: skin is often but not always moist. Linen must be changed at least once a shift	3. Occasionally Moist: skin is occasionally moist, requiring an extra linen change approximately once a day.	4. Rarely Moist: skin is usually dry, linen requires changing only at routine intervals.			
Degree to which skin is exposed to moisture							

Figure 23–3. Example from Braden Scale.

---

*The Braden Scale. Copyright © 1985. Available through Barbara J. Braden, Associate Professor, Creighton University School of Nursing, Omaha, NB 68178.

reliability have been carried out in two extended care facilities.[26] The purpose of the first study was to estimate interrater reliability between a graduate student research assistant and registered nurses trained in the use of the tool. The Pearson product moment correlation among 84 pairs of observations scores was $r = 0.99$ ($p<0.001$). The purpose of the second study was to determine the reliability of the scale when used by Licensed Practical Nurses (LPNs) and nurse aides (NAs) who were not trained in the use of the tool. Pearson product moment correlations among 53 pairs of scores ranged from $r = 0.83$ to $r = 0.87$ ($p<0.001$).

Studies of predictive validity have been conducted using patient populations in a skilled nursing facility, a general nursing unit, and a critical care stepdown unit in an acute care setting.[26] Preliminary results in the study using subjects over age 65 admitted to a skilled nursing facility indicate that, using a score of 17 as the critical cutoff score, the predictive value of positive results is about 75 percent ($n = 150$). In the two studies conducted in acute care settings ($n = 99$, $n = 100$) where adult-subjects were heterogeneous with regard to age, the tool demonstrated 100 percent sensitivity and, respectively, 90 percent and 64 percent specificity at a cutoff score of 16. However, the predictive value of positive results diminished to 44 percent and 20 percent, respectively, in these two studies. The differences in predictive validity when using the tool in different settings probably occur as a result of variances in age among subjects as well as the variance in caregiver/patient ratios in all three settings.

These data indicate that the Braden Scale is highly reliable when used by registered nurses trained in its use and that untrained nursing personnel achieve satisfactory reliability when using this instrument. In certain clinical situations, a score of 17 is an efficient predictor of pressure sore formation, whereas in other situations, a score of 16 will tend to overpredict in varying degrees. It is recommended that pilot studies be conducted to determine a cutoff point appropriate to the purposes of the investigator or clinician. For those patients with scores of 16 or below, measurements should be repeated at intervals (perhaps weekly), since patients who eventually break down show a downward trend in their scores and those who do not break down show an upward trend.

▪ ANDERSON ET AL. SCALE

Other tools reported in the literature appear to be either less predictive or less practical than the instruments described previously. Anderson et al. prepared a simple tool consisting of eight risk criteria divided into two categories, those of absolute risk criteria and relative risk criteria.[19] Unconsciousness, dehydration, and paralysis are classified as absolute risk criteria, and patients are given 2 points for each absolute criterion exhibited. Relative risk criteria include age above 70 years, restricted mobility, incontinence, pronounced emaciation, and redness over bony prominence. A score of 1 is given for each relative criterion exhibited. A total of 11 points was possible, with highest risk being associated with highest scores. A score of 2 is considered sufficient to classify the patient as being at risk for skin breakdown.

In Anderson's study, 600 patients were classified as being at risk, and only 35 (5.8 percent) experienced skin breakdown. Although this instrument is simple to use, the predictive value of positive results is very low. It should be noted that the sample in this study came from 2916 hospitalized patients without exclusion according to age and that age above 70 years added only 1 point to the score.

▪ TAYLOR SCALE

Taylor describes a tool developed after a small exploratory study of physiologic problems commonly associated with pressure sores.[18] The tool is described as consisting of four preliminary questions, followed by a ten-item scoring system. If two or more of the preliminary questions are answered in the affirmative, the ten-item assessment is completed. The scale is reported to take only 2 minutes to complete. No specific examples of items or preliminary questions are given, but this tool has the apparent advantage of quickly excluding patients who are not at risk. However, no studies of reliability and validity were performed, and considerable testing would be necessary before this tool could be used confidently for making either research or clinical decisions.

Selection of a Risk Predictor Scale

Predictive value is, of course, the critical consideration for selection of a risk prediction instrument. The clinical researcher is concerned almost equally with the reliability of the instrument. The interrater reliability should be important to the clinician if the intent is to use ratings completed by a number of staff members as a basis for making clinical decisions. The time involved in completing a rating is important, and all of the instruments reported here take less than 2 minutes to complete. Research and clinical protocols should include repeated measurements at specified intervals in consideration of possible changes in patient condition.

MEASUREMENT OF PRESSURE SORES

Staging or Grading Pressure Sores

• CLINICAL GRADING SYSTEM

Most systems for staging or grading pressure sores include four or five categories. The Clinical Grading System reported by Reddy[27] is used commonly but should be compared to the five stages of pressure sore development reported by Tepperman et al.[28] (Table 23–1). It should be noted that although neither of these authors appears to be the primary inventor of the classification systems, a review of the literature did not uncover a single primary source. No studies of interrater reliability could be found, probably because either classification system is used as a simple heuristic device.

TABLE 23–1. FIVE STAGES OF SORE DEVELOPMENT

Clinical Grading System[26]	Stages of Development[27]

Grade I
  Reactive hyperemia lasting more than 24 hours
	Stage I
	  Branching hyperemia—redness that blanches with light finger pressure

Grade II
  Blister and eschar formation
	Stage II
	  Nonblanching hyperemia

Grade III
  Superficial ulceration involving skin and subcutaneous tissue
	Stage III
	  Blister and eschar formation

Grade IV
  Ulceration extending down to muscle
	Stage IV
	  Clean ulcer

Grade V
  Deep ulceration to bone joint structure
	Stage V
	  Infected ulcer

Certainly, the clinical researcher using any grading or staging system should use clear and descriptive terminology in operationally defining the terms of the system. It is common in clinical usage to see Grades IV and V in the clinical grading system collapsed, since differentiation can be difficult without intrusive exploration of the wound.[29,30]

Measuring Pressure Sore Surface Area

Meticulous and accurate measurement of pressure sore surface area is probably most important in studies related to the effectiveness of therapeutic modalities in enhancing healing. Several methods are reported in the literature, some requiring less sophisticated equipment than others. Bohannon and Pfaller compared three common methods, all of which require the investigator to trace the sore surface.[31] The materials for tracing are sterilized transparency film and a fine-tip transparency marker. To obtain the tracing, the investigator places the sterilized transparency film over the sore and traces the perimeter with the transparency marker. The tracing then is cut from the transparency film and quantified by one of three methods. The first method used by Bohannan and Pfaller involved placing the tracing over metric graph paper and counting the square millimeters within the perimeter, the second method consisted of weighing the tracing on a gram balance scale, and the third method required the edges of the tracing to be retraced with an electronic planimeter.

To determine the accuracy of each method in their study, Bohannon and Pfaller used multiple tracings of the same sore obtained by two different clinicians, resulting in ten pairs of tracings. Mean differences in the area mass identified by each of the three methods were then calculated in the ten pairs. The mean difference with the weighing technique was 4.4 percent, with the counting technique was 3.9 percent, and with the planimetry was 3.6 percent. According to these investigators, the greatest percentage differences were found in the tracings of smaller wounds but were of no greater magnitude than the difference between larger tracings. They reported that the greatest difference found in the calculated areas of tracings of the same wound by two different clinicians was 8.8 percent, or 0.81 cm^2.

Although the small number of pressure sores studied makes absolute judgments of reliability and validity difficult, it appears that any of the three methods would provide measurements sufficiently accurate for most studies of pressure sore healing. In clinical research, the measurements obtained using a given method are compared to subsequent measurements of the same pressure sore at specified time intervals.

A fourth method of measurement is reported by Anthony and Barnes and requires complex and expensive equipment.[32] Using this method, a transparent polyester film, framed with a highly accurate grid and sized slightly larger than the pressure sore, is taped over the area of the sore. The pressure sore is photographed using slide film, and, after development, the slide is projected by a photographic enlarger onto a digitizer. The digitizer is described by Anthony and Barnes as consisting of a probe attached by simple electronic circuitry to a computer. The probe is used to trace sore perimeters on the enlarged photograph, and the computer is calibrated to measure the area of the sore. The computer used by Anthony and Barnes is programmed to correct for errors resulting from distortion. These authors report procedures for minimizing error but do not report any investigations related to accuracy. They specify that the program is written in BBC Basic and that copies of the program are available.[32]

Abbey,[33] in a commentary on a study of Kurzuk-Howard et al.,[29] suggests some possible methods to establish the depth of a pressure sore through use of two small light beams or serial photographs taken with several adjustments in focus. In the context of the commentary, Abbey does not give further details or indicate that she has tested these methods. Nevertheless, Abbey is experienced in instrumentation techniques, and a researcher who needs a method to measure pressure sore depth should explore her suggestions.

It is obvious that decisions about the use of any of these instruments will depend on the purposes and resources of the individual investigator. Where time and precision are of concern, the method of transposing a tracing on graph paper and counting the squares may be burdensome. Conversely, when monetary resources are in short supply, the purchase of equipment from a computer to a gram scale—may be impractical. Investigators may be able to justify purchase of equipment if they can find alternate uses after the conclusion of their study.

SUMMARY

This chapter is devoted almost solely to instruments that would be useful in research related to pressure sores and their prevention and treatment. Literature found on the other types of skin lesions primarily describes the lesions and implications for care rather than actual measurement.[34,35] The last section of this chapter deals with methods to measure surface area of pressure sores, and these methods may be useful also to the researcher interested in measuring other types of skin lesions.

REFERENCES

1. Braden, B., & Bergstrom, N. A conceptual schema for the study of the etiology of pressure sores. *Rehabil Nurs,* 1987, *12*(1):8.
2. Shaw, B. Continuous pressure monitor. *Engl Med,* 1979, *8*(2):105.
3. Berjian, D., Douglass, H., Holyoke, E., et al. Skin pressure measurements on various mattress surfaces in cancer patients. *Am J Phys Med,* 1983, *62*(5):217.
4. Garber, S., Campion, L., & Krouskop, T. Trochanteric pressure in spinal cord injury. *Arch Phys Med Rehabil,* 1982, *63*(11):549.
5. Garber, S., Krouskop, T., & Carter, R. System for clinically evaluating wheelchair pressure-relief cushions. *Am J Occup Ther,* 1978, *32*(9):565.
6. Bennett, L. Transferring load to flesh. Part III. Analysis of shear stress. *Bull Prosthetics Res,* 1979, (10–31):38.
7. Bennett, L., Kavnern, D., Lee, B., et al. *Arch Phys Med Rehabil,* 1984, *65*(4):186.
8. Moberg, E. Nerve repair in hand surgery: An analysis. *Surg Clin North Am,* 1968, *48*(5):985.
9. Nolan, M. Limits of two-point discrimination ability in the lower limb in young adult men and women. *Phys Ther,* 1983, *24*(5):347.
10. Werner, J., & Omer, G. Evaluating cutaneous pressure sensation of the hand. *Am J Occup Ther,* 1970, *24*(5):347.
11. Krouskop, T. A synthesis of the factors that contribute to pressure sore formation. *Med Hypotheses,* 1983, *11*(2):255.
12. Seiler, W., & Stahelin, H. Skin oxygen tension as a function of imposed skin pressure: Implication for decubitus ulcer formation. *J Am Geriatr Soc,* 1979, *27*(7):298.
13. Howell, T. Skin temperature in bedsore areas in the aged. *Exp Gerontol,* 1981, *16*(2):137.
14. Mahanty, S., Roemer, R., & Meisel, H. Thermal response of paraplegic skin to the application of localized pressure. *Arch Phys Med Rehabil,* 1981, *62*(12)608.
15. Verhonick, P., Lewis, D., & Goller, H. Thermography in the study of decubitus ulcers. *Nurs Res,* 1972, *21*(3):233.
16. Norton, D., McLaren, F., & Exton-Smith, A. *An investigation of geriatric nursing problems in hospital.* Edinburgh: Churchill Livingston, 1975.

17. Gosnell, D. An assessment tool to identify pressure sores. *Nurs Res,* 1973, *22*(1):55.
18. Taylor, V. Decubitus prevention through early assessment. *J Gerontol Nurs,* 1980, *6*(7):389.
19. Anderson, K., Jensen, O., Kvorning, S., & Bach, E. Prevention of pressure sores by identifying patients at risk. *Br Med J,* 1982, *284*(6326):1370.
20. Roberts, B., & Goldstone, L. A survey of pressure sores in the over sixties on two orthopaedic wards. *Int J Nurs Stud,* 1979, *16:*355.
21. Goldstone, L., & Roberts, B. A preliminary discriminant function analysis of elderly orthopaedic patients who will or will not contract a pressure sore. *Int J Nurs Stud,* 1980, *17:*17.
22. Goldstone, L., & Goldstone, J. The Norton score: An early warning of pressure sores? *J Adv Nurs,* 1982, *7*(5):419.
23. Moolten, S. Bedsores in the chronically ill patient. *Arch Phys Med Rehabil,* 1972, *53*(9):430.
24. Hunter, T., & Rajan, J. The role of ascorbic acid in the pathogenesis and treatment of pressure sores. *Paraplegia,* 1971, *8:*211.
25. Braden, B., Bergstrom, N., Brandt, J., & Krall, K. Adequacy of descriptive scales for reporting diet intake in institutionalized elderly. *J Nutr Elderly,* 1986, *6*(1):3.
26. Bergstrum, N., Braden, B., Laguzza, A., & Holman, V. The Braden Scale for predicting pressure sore risk. *Nur Res,* 1987, *36*(4):205.
27. Reddy, M. Decubitus ulcers: Principles of prevention and management *Geriatrics,* 1983, *38*(7):55.
28. Tepperman, P., DeZwirek, S., Chiarcossi, A., & Jimenez, J. Pressure sores: Prevention and step-up management. *Postgrad Med,* 1977, *62*(3):83.
29. Kruzuk-Howard, G., Simpson, L., & Palmieri, A. Decubitus ulcer care: A comparable study. *West J Nurs Res,* 1985, *7*(1):58.
30. Cameron, G. Presure sores: What to do when prevention fails. *Nursing '79,* 1979, *9*(1):42.
31. Bohannan, R., & Pfaller, B. Documentation of wound surface area from tracings of wound perimeters. *Phys Ther,* 1983, *63*(10):1622.
32. Anthony, D., & Barnes, E. Measuring pressure sores accurately. *Nurs Times,* 1984, *80*(36):33.
33. Abbey, J. Commentary. *West J Nurs Res,* 1985, *7*(1):75.
34. Miaskowski, C. Potential and actual impairments in skin integrity related to cancer and cancer treatment. *Top Clin Nurs,* 1983, *2:*64.
35. Verhonick, P. Decubitus ulcer observations measured objectively. *Nurs Res,* 1961, *10*(4):211.

CHAPTER 24

Assessment of the Oral Cavity

Sharon Rothenberger, R.N., M.S.

Current cancer treatment with chemotherapy or radiation therapy is designed to effect cure, produce long-term remissions, or provide palliation.[1] Unfortunately, there are side effects associated with these therapies, and stomatitis is one of these treatment-associated side effects.[2] Nurses must be especially interested in altering this side effect because, although not related to the disease itself, stomatitis can have a significant impact on the patient's quality of life.

Stomatitis is a known, potential side effect of selected chemotherapy agents and of radiation to the head and neck region.[3,4] It results from either a direct cytotoxic action of the chemotherapy agent on the replicating basal cells, from radiation damage to these cells, or as a result of the overall impaired host response. The mucosal lining of the oral cavity is a very delicate and rapidly proliferating tissue, thus making it very sensitive to the effects of chemotherapy and radiation.[5-7] Table 24–1 lists those chemotherapy agents commonly associated with mucositis.[8]

Stomatitis is an inflammatory reaction of the oral mucosa caused by local or systemic factors involving the buccal and labial mucosa, palate, tongue, floor of the mouth, and gingiva.[9] The initial complaint is a sore dry mouth with mild erythema and edema of the gums. Areas of inflammation may progress from small patches to large, painful ulcers. These ulcerations develop most commonly on the ventral surface and along the sides of the tongue, soft palate, posterior buccal mucosa, and floor of the mouth and often extend down the esophagus. The number and size of the ulcerations vary. Chewing and swallowing can become quite painful, with patients complaining of pain to such a degree that they are reluctant to eat or even open their mouths. If the ulcerations persist and involve a major portion of the mouth, parenteral pain medication may be necessary.

The timing and duration of stomatitis generally follow a predictable course. Oral erythematous stomatitis may appear as early as 3 days after chemotherapy, depending on the dose of drug and the treatment schedule (e.g., 24-hour infusions of bleomycin can result in early development of stomatitis).[10] The ulcerative form of stomatitis in general develops 5 to

**TABLE 24–1. CHEMOTHERAPY AGENTS ASSOCIATED
WITH A HIGH INCIDENCE OF STOMATITIS**

Dactinomycin
Bleomycin
Cytarbine (ARA-C)
Daunorubicin
Doxorubicin
Floxuridine (FUDR)
Fluorouracil (Maypasine)
6-Mercaptopurine
Methotrexate
Methyl-GAG[a]
Mitomycin-C
Mithramycin
PALA disodium[a]
Tegafur[a]
6-Thioguanine
Triazinate[a]
Vinblastine
Vinvesine

[a]Investigational agent.
*From Brager, Yasko. Care of the patient receiving chemother-
apy, 1984, p. 275. Courtesy of Reston Publishing Company.*

14 days after therapy, with symptoms persisting for 7 to 10 days. If secondary infection occurs, the healing process can take up to 3 to 4 weeks.

Infection of the oral cavity can alter significantly the course of the cancer patient's treatment. The oral cavity, the first line of defense against infection, can serve as the first site of infection and lead to further systemic infections. Bacteriemia associated with the oral cavity is well documented.[3,11]

There are a variety of factors that may encourage a persistent oral infection, such as preexisting oral/dental status, the integrity of the mucosal lining, the immunologic status of the patient, impaired host defense mechanisms, and a variety of physical factors that irritate or perpetuate the oral infection.[10] For example, prior injury to the oral mucosa by radiation therapy to the head and neck can increase the risk factors of infection. A variety of infections are common, for example, candidiasis (thrush), herpes simplex, gram-negative bacterial infections, and gram-positive bacterial infections.[3]

Oral pain associated with stomatitis begins as a burning sensation or general discomfort of the oral cavity. As the severity of the stomatitis increases with the appearance of ulcers, patients will begin to complain of sensitivity to cold or warm food and fluids, although they will continue to be able to eat and drink with minimal discomfort. When stomatitis is most severe, patients can experience severe, diffuse, debilitating pain. The patient usually refuses any oral intake because of the intensity of the pain.

The resulting oral pain and consequent nutritional compromise can affect the dose of chemotherapy that may be administered, resulting in dose modifications or delay of treatment. This may affect the patient's long-term prognosis or alter the response to chemotherapy treatment. Stomatitis may require the patient to be hospitalized, increase the number of days as an inpatient, affect compliance to the regimen, and increase the cost of treatment.

Stomatitis can have a significant impact on the patient's quality of life. The mild form of stomatitis simply may alter oral intake. The more severe the stomatitis, the greater the

TABLE 24—2. CHEMOTHERAPEUTIC AGENTS COMMONLY ASSOCIATED WITH MUCOSITIS

Drug	Related Factors
Methotrexate	May be quite severe with prolonged infusions or compromised renal function; severity is enhanced by radiation; may be prevented with adequate citrovorum rescue factor
5-Fluorouracil	More severe with higher doses, frequent schedule, and arterial infusions
Dactinomycin	Very common and may prevent oral alimentation; severity enhanced by radiation
Doxorubicin	May be severe and ulcerative; increased with liver disease; severity enhanced by radiation
Bleomycin	May be severe and ulcerative
Vinblastine	Frequently ulcerative

From Mitchell, Schein. Semin Oncol, 1982, 9(1):56.

impact on the overall nutritional status of an already compromised patient. Table 24–2 lists the chemotherapy agents most likely to cause severe stomatitis.[12]

Knowledge of the chemotherapeutic regimen or radiation field should alert the clinician to the potential for developing mucositis. All investigators suggest pretreatment assessment of the mouth to determine the patient's oral/dental status and the presence of preexisting periodontal infection or tissue breakdown. Assessing the status of the oral mucosa requires adequate lighting, removal of dentures or appliances, and examination of soft tissues to determine areas of irritation.

INSTRUMENTS TO EVALUATE STOMATITIS

The following literature review describes the various instruments that have been developed to evaluate degrees of stomatitis and the efficacy of nursing interventions for the care of the oral cavity. Adequate clinical assessment tools to assess the oral contents are important to evaluate consistently the effectiveness of a particular nursing intervention.

▪ GINSBURG STANDARDS OF ORAL HYGIENE

In 1961, Ginsburg identified the need for standards of oral hygiene, stating that oral care has always been an integral part of nursing care.[13] She observed that a particular nursing intervention was chosen more by subjective feelings of the nurse than by objective assessment because there was no valid method of comparing one nursing intervention with another. An attempt was made to identify the principles underlying the oral hygiene nursing care given to patients for the prevention or alleviation of stomatitis. All the patients in this study were diagnosed as being in acute renal failure. Using a flashlight and tongue blade the investigator inspected the oral cavity and recorded her observations. No attempts at objective standards of evaluation were made. The data-collection instruments included (1) a line drawing of the mouth, lips, and nose with a word description, (2) use of photographs, and (3) a condition checklist to determine the general condition of the patient. Data included intake and output, weight, orientation (time, person, and place), and other symptoms (dyspnea, nausea and vomiting, cough, sputum production). Standards of oral care were identified but not validated, and the evaluation tool was not validated. Success of therapy was determined by whether or not the patient showed evidence of stomatitis. Ginsberg concluded that the frequency and regularity of oral hygiene nursing care was the most important factor in preventing stomatitis.

▪ PASSOS AND BRAND NUMERICAL RATING GUIDE

Passos and Brand noted that there was no body of knowledge about oral hygiene to validate a nurse's judgment about who should receive oral hygiene and what techniques worked.[14] The purpose of their study was to evaluate and compare the effectiveness of three agents for oral hygiene care of the acutely ill, hospitalized surgical patient. None of their 66 patients could perform his or her own oral care. A pretreatment evaluation was made of the condition of the mouth using a numerical rating guide developed by Greene and Vermillion.[15] Figure 24–1 is an example of the guide used by Passos and Brand. The numerical ratings of eight categories (saliva, tongue, palates, membranes and gums, teeth, odor, lips, and nares) are added together. A rating of 8 would represent normal characteristics; a rating of 24 would indicate the worst possible condition of the oral contents.

▪ VANDRIMMELSEN AND ROLLINS TOOL

VanDrimmelsen and Rollins adapted the guide from Passos and Brand to evaluate the effectiveness of lemon juice and glycerine as an oral agent.[16] The adapted tool was tested for reliability, and the instrument was refined after use on 23 patients. The reliability coefficient was 0.96. Both the oral care and the numerical evaluations were performed by the investigators. The results showed that it was the process of giving oral care rather than the specific agent used that appeared to influence the general condition of the mouth.

▪ DEWALT TOOL

DeWalt extensively reviewed studies of oral hygiene. The first study (1969) was of recorded observations made on the subject's saliva, oral mucosa, tongue, lips, and teeth while receiving continuous nasal oxygen.[17] The subjects' reactions were noted at 15-minute intervals for 5 hours. Another study identified and compared the effects of using a toothbrush or toothette

Category	Numerical and Descriptive Ratings		
	1	2	3
Saliva	Cavity moist	Scanty, with or without debris	Viscid or ropy, with or without debris
Tongue	Wet or moist, coating absent to small amount of coating	Dry, slight or moderate coating	Dry or moist, with abundant coating
Palates	Wet or moist, debris absent to small amount, soft	Dry, with or without small amount of soft debris	Dry or moist, moderate to large amount of soft or hard debris

Figure 24–1. Passos and Brand Guide for Numerical Rating of the Condition of the Mouth.

Dependent Variable	Tools for Data Collection	Methods of Measurement	Numerical and Descriptive Ratings		
			1	2	3
Salivation	Tongue blade	Insert blade into mouth, touching gums, palates, and floor of mouth; slowly remove and observe	Ropy or viscid	Dry or scanty	Moist
Tongue moisture	Visual and palpitory assessment	Feel and observe appearance of tissue	Coated	Dry	Moist

Figure 24–2. DeWalt adaptation of Passos and Brand Numerical Rating Guide.

on the oral mucosa, performing oral care at varying time intervals.[18] An adaptation of the Passos and Brand Numerical Guide was used (Fig. 24–2).

The tool not only provides the numerical scale for rating the appearance of a particular aspect of the oral cavity but also lists how the assessment is to be made and by what method of measurement. Use of the guide resulted in a 0.92 interrater reliability. Data from this study supported the conclusion that a nursing intervention can produce observable improvement of oral tissues.

• BRUYA AND MADEIRA GUIDE FOR ASSESSMENT OF THE MOUTH

Bruya and Madiera devised a guide for assessment of the mouth from an adaptation of all the previously noted assessment tools (DeWalt, Passos and Brand, VanDrimmelsen and Rollins).[19] They recommended using this guide to assess stomatitis after chemotherapy (Fig. 24–3); no reliability or validity testing was reported.

The guide provides a standard for future studies of nursing care because it is an extensive review of observations of both normal and abnormal oral cavities. The authors encourage nurses not only to study the need for frequent mouth care but also to determine the relationship between the therapeutic interventions and observable results.

• BECK ORAL GUIDES

Beck initiated a descriptive study to assess the effects on stomatitis from chemotherapy after teaching staff nurses about stomatitis, oral assessment, and nursing interventions before their implementing a systematic oral care protocol.[20] The control group consisted of 25 inpatients over a 25-day period. The experimental group, which received the teaching and implementation of the oral care protocol, consisted of 22 patients during a second 25-day period. The nursing interventions outlined in the protocol depended on whether the patient had mild or severe stomatitis. The data collection began with visual observation and assessment of the mouth before chemotherapy to establish a baseline measurement. Three assessment instruments were developed. The tools were:

1. Oral Exam Guide. This is an adaptation of previous tools from nursing, dental, and medical literature that numerically assessed the patient's mouth condition. Categories

		Numerical and Descriptive Rating		
Variables		3	2	1
Oral cavity				
Lips				
	Texture	Cracked, bleeding	Rough	Smooth, soft
	Color	Red, inflamed, some bleeding	Some reddened areas	Pink
	Moisture	Dry, cracked	Blistered	Moist
Tongue				
	Texture	Coated at base, engorged, deeply grooved, thicker than normal	Vallate papillae and lingual groove prominent	Firm, without fissures or prominent papillae
	Color	Very red tip, sides blistered	Pink with reddened areas	Pink
	Moisture	Dry with indentations; patient complains of burning	"Tongue sticks to roof of mouth," dry	Moist
	Mucous membranes of the palate, uvula, and tonsillar fossa	Red with general inflammation, blisters, and pinpoint brown spots on pallate	Dry, pale palate	Moist, pink

Figure 24–3. Bruya and Madiera Guide for Assessment of the Mouth.

of 16 descriptors with a numerical rating of 1 to 4 were included in the Oral Exam Guide.

2. Oral Perception Guide. This guide was developed by Beck. It asked the nurse to rate the patient's sensory perceptions of the mouth, teeth, taste, voice changes, and ability to eat.

3. Physical Condition Tool. This guide asked the nurse to measure the overall physical condition of the patient (level of consciousness, breathing habits, diet, and self-care ability).

A Basic Information Sheet listed the specific chemotherapy drugs, dose, and prior treatment (both chemotherapy and radiation therapy). There is no validity or reliability reported for these various instruments.

Results of the study indicated a significant difference in improved Oral Exam scores before and after implementation of the oral care protocol. Several limitations can be noted with this study that are important for further investigation of cancer patient's oral care status. Patients received a variety of chemotherapeutic agents at varying doses. The effect of a nursing intervention could be better assessed if all patients received the same chemotherapy regimen. Also, a randomized study between normal oral nursing care measures and various nursing approaches would more adequately assess a difference. The various instruments need to be tested for reliability and validity. The definition of various degrees of stomatitis should be clearly delineated. Rating the degree of stomatitis over the total time it is present would provide valuable information for the nurse about the usual course of the stomatitis and if the nursing intervention made any difference in prevention or treatment of stomatitis symptoms.

· LINDQUIST ET AL. STOMATITIS GRADING SYSTEM

Lindquist et al. followed a stomatitis grading system of Grade 0 (no stomatitis) to Grade III (severe intraoral pain with inability to eat).[21] They studied the relationship between the amount of dental plaque present and the development of stomatitis during chemotherapy. All 20 patients received 5-fluorouracil, doxorubicin, and cytoxan according to a specified dosage (mg/m^2) and schedule. They recommended that stomatitis could be reduced if patients had dental scaling and prophylaxis performed before chemotherapy.

· HICKEY ET AL. GRADING SCALE

Hickey et al. recognized that severe stomatitis is a known complication of patients with testicular cancer receiving velban and bleomycin.[9] They noted that treatment schedules often need to be altered because of the length of time the stomatitis is present. Studying patients with a particular cancer diagnosis and treatment regimen eliminates some intervening variables that could affect the frequency, severity, and duration of stomatitis. In this case, all patients had testicular cancer, were 18 to 34 years old, and had no other medical problems. The subjects were randomized regardless of dental status. The Hickey et al. Grading Scale used in this study is shown in Table 24–3. Assessment of effect was determined by the average number of days stomatitis lasted with each course of chemotherapy.

Results showed that water lavage made no significant difference in the severity and duration of stomatitis. Those patients who received prechemotherapy oral care with reinforced teaching of oral hygiene and necessary dental treatment by a dentist or dental hygienist had less severe stomatitis for a shorter duration of time. Study results assessed the occurrence and course of stomatitis in relation to the leukocyte count. Mucositis started 3 to 5 days before the drop in leukocytes and was most severe just before the leukocyte nadir. Resolution of the mucositis occurred before the leukocytes reached normal limits. A difficulty noted with assessing mucositis was that the presence of clinical signs of inflammation could be altered by the degree of immunosuppression.

SUMMARY

Further research is necessary to assess both general oral care nursing measures and specific nursing interventions that can prevent, palliate, or decrease the duration and severity of

TABLE 24–3. HICKEY et al. GRADING SCALE

Grade	Status
0	No stomatitis
I	Whitish gingival area observable, or patient mentions slight burning sensation or discomfort in oral cavity
II	Moderate erythema and ulcerations or white patches present; patient complains of pain but can eat, drink, and swallow
III	Severe erythema and ulcerations or white patches present; patient complains of severe pain and cannot eat, drink, or swallow

From Hickey, Toth, Lindquist. Prosthet Dent, 1982, 47: 190.

stomatitis due to chemotherapy or radiation therapy.[22–26] The benefits of research that would lead to improved nursing care measures are (1) decreasing the occurrence of secondary infection, (2) improving patient comfort and decreasing oral pain, (3) maintaining adequate nutrition, (4) decreasing the need for alterations in treatment schedules and affecting patient compliance, and (5) decreasing medical costs to the patient.[27]

Research is needed to further define and anticipate those conditions that make the patient susceptible to stomatitis. Identification of drug and drug combinations known to cause stomatitis is important as a means of determining susceptibility to the development of stomatitis and, ideally, how stomatitis can be prevented. Baseline assessment of the patient's oral and dental status must become an established nursing responsibility. A classification system for oral complications that is concise and easy to implement in actual clinical settings must be devised.[28–30] The present instruments could be adapted to provide a standard assessment tool, so that data can be compared from one setting to another. Evaluation of stomatitis should include exact location and size of ulcers over the period of time the patient experiences this side effect. Intervening variables to be considered include status of immunocompetence, previous radiation therapy, prior oral/dental status and practices, secondary infection, leukocyte count, blood chemistries, platelet and coagulation studies. Nurses are encouraged to continue to improve interventions that can improve significantly the patient's quality of life.

REFERENCES

1. DeVita, V., Hellman, S., & Rosenberg, S. *Cancer: Principles and practice of oncology.* Philadelphia: Lippincott, 1982.
2. Bodey, G.P. Oral complications of the myeloproliferative diseases. *Postgrad Med,* 1971, *49:*115.
3. Dreizen, S., Bodey, G.P., & Rodriquez, V. Oral complications of cancer chemotherapy. *Postgrad Med,* 1975, *58*(2):75.
4. Trowbridge, J., & Carl, W. Oral care of the patient having head and neck irradiation. *Am J Nurs,* 1975, *75*(12):2146.
5. Guggenheimer, J., Verbin, R.S., Appel, V., et al. Clinicopathologic effects of cancer chemotherapeutic agents on human buccal mucousa. *Oral Surg,* 1977, *44:*58.
6. Dreizen, S. Stomatotoxic manifestations of cancer chemotherapy. *J Prosthet Dent,* 1978, *40*(5):650.
7. Dreizen, S., McCredie, K.B., & Keating, M.J. Chemotherapy induced oral mucositis in adult leukemia. *Postgrad Med,* 1981, *69:*103.
8. Brager, B., & Yasko, J. *Care of the client receiving chemotherapy.* Reston VA: Reston, 1984.
9. Hickey, A.J., Toth, B.B., & Lindquist, S.B. Effect of intravenous hyperalimentation and oral care on the development of oral stomatitis during cancer chemotherapy. *J Prosthet Dent,* 1982, *47:*188.
10. Toth, B.B., & Frame, R.T. Dental oncology: The management of disease and treatment-related oral/dental complications associated with chemotherapy. *Curr Prob Cancer,* 1983, *7*(10):7.
11. Williams, L.T., Peterson, D.E., & Overholser, C.D. Acute periodontal infection in myelosuppressed oncology patients: Evaluation and nursing care. *Cancer Nurs,* 1982, *5*(6):465.
12. Mitchell, R., & Schein, D. Gastrointestinal toxicity of chemotherapeutic agents. *Semin Oncol,* 1982, *9*(1):56.
13. Ginsberg, M. A study of oral hygiene nursing care. *Am J Nurs,* 1961, *61*(10):67.
14. Passos, J.Y., & Brand, L.M. Effects of agents used for oral hygiene. *Nurs Res,* 1966, *15*(3):196.
15. Greene, J.C., & Vermillion, J.R. The oral hygiene index: A method for classifying oral hygiene status. *J Dent Assistant,* 1960, *61:*172.
16. VanDrimmelsen, J., & Rollins, H. Evaluation of a commonly used oral hygiene agent. *Nurs Res,* 1969, *18*(4):327.
17. DeWalt, E., & Haines, A. The effects of specified stressors on healthy oral mucousa. *Nurs Res,* 1969, *18*(1):22.

18. DeWalt, E. Effect of timed hygienic measures on oral mucosa in a group of elderly subjects. *Nurs Res,* 1975, *24*(2):104.
19. Bruya, M., & Madiera, N. Stomatitis after chemotherapy. *Am J Nurs,* 1975, *75*(8):1349.
20. Beck, S. Impact of a systemic oral care protocol on stomatitis after chemotherapy. *Cancer Nurs,* 1979, *2*(3):185.
21. Lindquist, S.F., Hickey, A.M., & Drane, J.B. Effect of oral hygiene on stomatitis in patients receiving cancer chemotherapy. *J Prosthet Dent,* 1978, *40:*312.
22. Hart, C.N., & Rasmussen, D. Patient care evaluation: A comparison of current practice and nursing literature for oral care of persons receiving chemotherapy. *Oncol Nurs Forum,* 1982, *9*(2):22.
23. Daeffler, R. Oral hygiene measures for patients with cancer. I. *Cancer Nurs,* 1980, *3*(5):347.
24. Daeffler, R. Oral hygiene measures for patients with cancer. II. *Cancer Nurs,* 1980, *3*(6):427.
25. Daeffler, R. Oral hygiene measures for patients with cancer. III. *Cancer Nurs,* 1981, *4*(1):29.
26. Bersani, G., & Carl, W. Oral care of the cancer patient. *Am J Nurs,* 1983, *83*(4):533.
27. Ostchega, Y. Preventing and treating cancer chemotherapy's oral complications. *Nursing '80,* 1980, *10*(8):47.
28. Meissner, J. A simple guide for assessing oral health. *Nursing '80,* 1980, *10*(4):84.
29. Peterson, D.E., & Sonis, S. Oral complications of cancer chemotherapy: Present status and future studies. *Cancer Treat Rep,* 1982, *66*(6):1251.
30. Schweiger, J.L., Lang, J.W., & Scheiger, J.W. Oral assessment: How to do it. *Am J Nurs,* 1980, *80*(4):654.

CHAPTER 25

Assessment of Vaginitis

Marcia M. Grant, R.N., D.N.Sc. and Sue B. Davidson, R.N., M.S.

Unlike stomatitis, altered skin integrity, and vein problems, which are secondary to a specific medical condition or treatment, vaginitis is encountered most frequently as a primary medical diagnosis. Three perspectives to vaginitis are pertinent: that of the office or clinical nurse, that of the practitioner, be it a nurse or a physician, and that of the researcher. Nurses are interested in helping patients with vaginitis manage distressing symptoms and instructing patients on when to seek additional medical care. Practitioners are interested in the accuracy of the diagnosis and the effectiveness of the specific treatment prescribed. A researcher, on the other hand, selects specific and reliable data pertinent to the study being conducted. For example, in studying the incidence of *Trichomonas* infection, the researcher may select only those variables specific to a *Trichomonas* infection. The authors' perspective is primarily that of researchers of a problem firmly embedded in the clinical nursing care of patients with diabetes mellitus. The authors became interested in vaginitis as a recurrent and distressing clinical problem for these women and were interested in testing the effectiveness of a noninvasive and nonpharmacologic approach to symptom management.[1]

Because of our combined clinical and research perspectives, our approach is from the practice setting and includes aspects pertinent to nurses as well as to practitioners and researchers.

DEFINITION AND OCCURRENCE

Vaginitis is one of the most common problems causing women to seek medical care. In one review of reasons for outpatient gynecologic clinic referrals, vaginal discharge or irritation comprised 37 percent of the complaints.[2] Vaginitis is described frequently as the most common reason for women to be seen in a physician's office.[3,4]

Vaginitis is an inflammation of the vulvar and vaginal tissues, usually associated with changes in the vaginal environment, changes in the usual distribution of microbes, or the presence of abnormal pathogenic organisms. Four factors are associated with maintenance of the noninfected vagina[5]: secretion of normal estrogen levels in order to maintain a normal vaginal epithelial lining, availability of glycogen in vaginal tissue, presence of sufficient numbers of lactobacilli (Döderlein's bacilli) to produce lactic acid, and sufficient lactic acid to maintain the vaginal acidity at a pH of 4.0 to 4.5. Changes in one or more of these factors predispose the woman to vaginitis.

The two organisms most commonly associated with vaginitis are *Candida albicans,* which is a fungus previously referred to as *Monilia,*[6] and *Trichomonas vaginalis,* which is a flagellated protozoa.[7] In the past, cases in which neither of these pathogens has been identified have been referred to as "nonspecific vaginitis" and associated with *Corynebacterium vaginale (Haemophilus vaginalis).*[8] This organism has recently been renamed *Gardnerella vaginalis* and is a gram-negative bacillus.[9-12]

Infections with the herpes virus are much less frequent and generally involve the vulvar tissues only, causing blisters that become shallow painful ulcerations.[10] Herpes occasionally infects both the vagina and the cervix. Vaginitis also may be associated with other sexually transmitted diseases. Approximately 1 million cases of gonorrhea were reported in 1983, and it is estimated that only 1 in 5 actual cases are reported.[13] However, 70 to 80 percent of these infections in women are asymptomatic.[14] Another very common sexually transmitted pathogen that causes cervicitis is *Chlamydia trachomatis;* an estimated 3 million cases occurred in the United States in 1983.[15] In women, *Chlamydia* may cause cervicitis, salpingitis, and acute urethral syndrome, but it is common for symptoms to be nonspecific, mild, or not present at all.[16,17] Venereal warts, *condylomata acuminata,* may occur on the vulva, vagina, or cervix of infected patients.[18] Although these warts have slow growth cycles, they spread if not treated early. They are identified here because they constitute a common infection, with over 1 million cases occurring each year,[16] although they frequently do not produce symptoms other than a mild pruritis of the vulva.

Besides positive identification of the presence of a causative organism, objective signs and subjective symptoms specific to each type of infection have been described for classic cases. However, exceptions to these patterns of signs and symptoms are not uncommon, and controversies occur about whether or not vaginitis of a specific type is present when either positive organism identification without other typical signs and symptoms is present or typical signs and symptoms without a positive organism identification are present (Fig. 25–1). Some physicians treat patients only if both a positive organism identification and positive signs and symptoms are present, whereas others treat patients if either a positive organism identification or typical signs and symptoms are present.[4,5,19] Therefore, practitioners differ over what parameters are needed for the diagnosis of vaginitis. Part of this controversy is related to the cost of cultures, especially if the organism has already been identified on immediate wet mount examination of secretions or the Pap report indicates a vaginal infection and no abnormalities are noted on examination or history.

Another aspect of this controversy concerns the methods used to identify the organisms, since different methods may reveal different incidences of positive cultures. In a study by Osborne et al., the difference in prevalence of several organisms that could cause vaginitis was compared in a group of symptomatic and a group of nonsymptomatic women.[20] Findings revealed that although the presence of symptoms was significantly related to positive identification of pathogenic organisms, 9 percent of the women with symptoms had no pathogenic organisms identified, and a significant number of women who did have organisms present did not have symptoms. Thus, in comparing studies on the incidence and treatment of vaginitis, the parameters used to define vaginitis must be specified in order to interpret findings across studies.

Within nursing, the relevant diagnostic label for vaginitis is altered skin integrity related

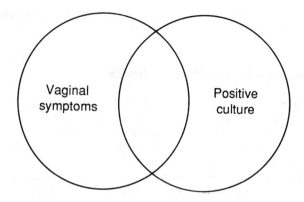

Figure 25–1. Symptoms and cultures in vaginitis.

to pruritis.[21] This diagnosis is not specific for vaginitis but would include the signs and symptoms related to skin irritation and would require nursing interventions aimed at relieving pruritis. In older women, pruritis of the vulvar area is considered an early symptom of vulvar cancer and deserves further evaluation.

Treatment of vaginitis differs according to the type of infection apparently present.[3,5,22] Systemic antibiotic therapy and local agents are available for *Gardnerella* infections. Local antifungal agents are used to treat *Candida* infections, and an antiprotozoon agent is available for *Trichomonas* infections. For genital herpes, oral acyclovir has been proven effective in controlled clinical trials for first-episode cases but does not seem to prevent virus latency or recurrent disease.[23] The usual treatment for gonorrhea is aqueous procaine penicillin or ampicillin, although some strains resistant to these medications are seen.[13] The usual treatment for *Chlamydia* infection is changing as more efficacious drugs are found; tetracycline, a broad-spectrum antibiotic, is the present treatment of choice.[15] Thus, determination of the exact type of vaginitis is critical to the prescription of accurate therapy for both nursing and medical professionals.

Vaginitis occurs primarily in females after puberty. It occurs in both menstruating and postmenopausal women and is characterized by frequent recurrences. Several risk factors for candidiasis have been identified. Diabetic females are particularly prone to develop vaginal infections—as many as half of the women with diabetes mellitus may have it. This increased occurrence may be associated with an increased incidence of *Candida* on the skin surfaces of diabetics and increases in blood glucose, with associated glucosuria.[24–26] Since glucosuria can result in residual glucose on the vulvar tissues following urination, it has been hypothesized that such glucose provides an environment for excessive growth of *Candida*, with resulting vaginitis.[1]

Another risk factor involves atrophic conditions of the vagina in which the squamous epithelium is compromised.[27] A decrease in estrogen has been associated with these epithelial changes and can occur in women taking oral contraceptives, during pregnancy, and after menopause. These epithelial changes lead to a change in the distribution of normal flora, allowing an overgrowth of pathogenic bacteria.[5]

Since vaginal infections are passed between sexual partners, increased exposure to a variety of sexual partners also may be associated with an increase in vaginitis. Even with one partner, vaginitis can recur if the sexual partner is infected and untreated. In multiple vaginal infections, such as *Trichomonas, Gardnerella,* and *Chlamydia* infections, treatment of the sexual partner is essential.[28]

PARAMETERS USED TO DESCRIBE VAGINITIS

Most studies on vaginitis have had as their purpose an examination of the incidence of the problem in the population in general or a test of specific approaches to prevention and treatment. Development of an instrument to measure vaginitis has been the focus of few publications. Some studies, however, have compared incidence rates using different methods for identification of organisms and different sets of signs and symptoms.

The parameters used in the assessment of vaginitis can be classified into three groups: identification of pathogenic organisms, complaints of subjective symptoms, and observation of objective signs. For each group, clinicians and investigators may select different methods and different parameters dependent on sensitivity and reliability as well as cost and availability.

Identification of Pathogenic Organisms

Two major approaches are used to identify pathogenic organisms associated with vaginitis. The wet mount, or immediate microscopic examination, is done right after the vaginal examination and collection of vaginal secretions. A slide is prepared and examined under the microscope for characteristics of suspected pathogens. In the second method, secretions obtained during the vaginal examination are transferred onto various culture media. They are incubated for at least 48 hours, after which pathogenic organisms are identified.

Since the organism associated with vaginitis may be a yeast, a bacterium, or a protozoon, different methods must be used in identification. A typical procedure involves both wet mount and culture.[7] Performing the vaginal examination to obtain exudate and conducting the wet mount examination are technologies done generally by the health practitioner, either medical or nursing. If nurses in more traditional roles are responsible for these procedures, advanced training is needed.

A swab of exudate from the vagina is used to prepare two slides for immediate wet mount or microscopic examination, one with potassium hydroxide and one with saline.[7,20,29] The presence of a fishy odor on the slide with potassium hydroxide indicates that *Gardnerella* is present.[30] This is generally called the "whiff" test.[5] Yeasts are identified by the presence of budding cells, pseudohyphae, and spores during microscopic examination of the potassium hydroxide slide.[7,22,29] These characteristics of the yeast are seen most easily on the potassium hydroxide slide, since the medium destroys leukocytes, epithelial cells, and bacteria. On the normal saline slide, *Gardnerella* is identified by the presence of clue cells, which have a typical stipled or granulated appearance.[11,22] *Trichomonas* is identified by its flagella, a typical pear shape, and a corkscrew movement.[7,20,22]

Exudate from the vaginal walls and/or the cervix for cervicitis is obtained on cotton swabs and transported to the laboratory for preparation of cultures. Rapid transportation for fragile organisms, such as *Neisseria gonorrhoeae,* is critical. Typical media used include trypticase, soy blood agar, Nickerson medium, and chocolate agar.[7,8,29] Several kinds are used, since each fosters the growth of different organisms (Table 25–1). After incubation, the presence of specific microbes is determined by the characteristics of the colonies and by carrying out various tests, such as a gram stain of the organisms that have grown.

Validity and reliability of the various methods of identifying the microbes associated with the occurrence of vaginitis involve comparing results of microbe identification across the various methods and various preparations and comparing results obtained among different

TABLE 25–1. CULTURE MEDIA USED FOR DETECTION OF VAGINAL PATHOGENS

Organism	Media
Candida albicans	Nickerson's medium Sabouraud's medium
Chlamydia trachomatis	Tissue culture McCoy cells
Gardnerella vaginalis	Casman broth medium CNAF modified medium Chocolate agar
Genital herpes	Viral culture
Neisseria gonorrhoeae	Thayer-Martin medium Transgrow medium Martin-Lewis medium New York City medium
Trichomonas vaginalis	Feinberg-Whittington medium Trichosal broth

investigators. A number of studies have been performed comparing immediate wet mount and microscopic examination versus culture and subsequent examination.[7,31–33] In general, these results show that additional identification of organisms occurs when culture data are added to data obtained from immediate microscopic examination only. In practical terms, the approach of treating patients without culture confirmation of pathogenic organisms is usually based on expediency; that is, the patient has acute symptoms that are typical, and treatment is not held up for 3 days to await culture results. In addition, costs (cultures using various media and requiring laboratory identification procedures) can be prohibitively expensive.[4,22]

A number of studies have compared different methods for identifying organisms. O'Brien reported on a study of 1034 patients for whom the incidence of positive vaginal candidiasis was compared using wet smear techniques, culture with Nickerson's medium, and clinical impressions.[34] Nickerson's medium contains bismuth hydroxysulfite and facilitates the growth of *Candida* while inhibiting bacterial growth. Clinical impressions included the character of the vaginal discharge and the state of the vulva and vaginal tissues. The wet smear was prepared with normal saline and examined immediately for characteristics of *Candida* and *Trichomonas*. Findings indicated that only 40 percent of the Nickerson-positive cases were also identified clinically, and in only 40 percent of these was the wet smear positive. Thus, the potential for diagnostic error was 60 percent if information from the culture results had not been available. Using only microscopic information resulted in a large number of false negatives.

Another study that compared traditional *Candida* culture methods with a new culture slide and wet mount microscopy was conducted by Pattman et al.[35] Growth results on the two different culture media were comparable, achieving 96 percent agreement. The wet smear technique alone, however, would have missed 10 (29 percent) cases. It appears that the incidence of positive organism identification using culture techniques exceeds the incidence with wet mount microscopy and clinical signs and symptoms only. These studies illustrate the validity of using culture methods to confirm and add to the results of immediate microscopic examination for identifying *Candida*.

For recurrent vaginal candidiasis, additional cultures may be helpful. Concern for the source of reinfection has led to the hypothesis that the intestine serves as a reservoir.[36] In a series of 98 young women who complained of recurrent vaginal candidiasis, results showed that if the vaginal culture was positive for *Candida,* the stool culture was positive as well, and if the vaginal culture was negative for *Candida,* the stool culture was negative as well. Thus, for recurrent vaginal candidiasis, assessment of the stool is an important variable. Treatment approaches for recurrent candidiasis include decreasing contributing causes as much as possible.[14]

Another study involved comparing practices currently in use for diagnosing *Trichomonas* infection in various English clinics.[19] The most common approach (54 percent, $n = 93$) was a combination of immediate microscopic examination and a culture of vaginal secretions using a variety of growth media (e.g., Feinberg-Whittington's medium for *Trichomonas* and Sabouraud's agar for *Candida*). The second most common method of identification was immediate microscopic examination alone (45 percent of the cases). Diagnosis by culture only was done in only three clinics. These results illustrate the usual clinical approaches and the potential difficulty of comparing incidence rates among settings without a clear definition of methods used in organism identification.

Immediate microscopic examination for clue cells in identification of *Gardnerella* has a reported accuracy rate of 90 percent.[11] The relationship of clue cells to positive cultures of *Gardnerella,* however, has not been established. In one study, positive identification of clue cells was associated with the presence of positive cultures in 4 of 17 patients (24 percent); clue cells were found in the absence of positive cultures in an additional 3 of 10 patients (30 percent).[8] These results replicate those of an earlier study.[37]

In a review of the diagnostic criteria to be used in identifying nonspecific vaginitis, Amsel et al. compared microscopic examination with culture and with other clinical criteria.[9] A total of 397 consecutive unselected female students were studied at a university health clinic. Results illustrated the value of a variety of laboratory and clinical parameters to obtain the most accurate rate of diagnosis. More than 90 percent of the patients with nonspecific vaginitis had clue cells on microscopic examination, and less than 10 percent of the normal patients had clue cells. This indicates that identification of clue cells is valuable, but some false positives are likely to occur in almost 10 percent of the patients. Positive growth of *Gardnerella* cultures was obtained in 77 percent of the women with clue cells versus 13 percent of women who did not have clue cells. These rates contrast with those reported previously.[8]

Because of the fragility of the organism, producing a culture of *N. gonorrhoeae* presents a greater challenge than exists with the other vaginal pathogens. Both temperature and transit delays can decrease gonococcal viability, and up to 10 percent of all isolates are inhibited by the concentration of vancomycin found in all the culture media.[38] The use of New York City medium, which has a decreased concentration of vancomycin, has improved the positive rate of recovery of *N. gonorrhoeae* by 13 percent.[39] A new enzyme immunoassay approach was developed in response to the need for quicker, more accurate results. This approach works well on specimens from males but produces a large percentage of false positives among women.[38,39]

In summary, reliability of organism identification appears to be related primarily to concern for identification of organisms via immediate microscopic examination. With adequate training, an appropriate level of reliability appears to be achievable. Validity of organism identification, in terms of which is the best method and the best medium, is less clear. *Candida* grows easily in specialized media, such as Nickerson's medium, and to exhibit individual characteristics on microscopy. *Trichomonas,* too, seems readily identifiable. What is less clear is the identification of *Gardnerella,* since the need for clinical symptoms to confirm the diagnosis has been recommended. Studies containing statistical analyses for tool reliability and validity are scarce or nonexistent. Combinations of both laboratory and clinical data appear to be most valid.

Subjective Symptoms

The second group of parameters used to assess vaginitis is the subjective symptoms obtained during patient interview. They generally include pruritis, discharge, odor, dyspareunia, dysuria, and vaginal pressure, soreness, or burning.[4,22,40] These symptoms may be continuous or intermittent. Symptom patterns can be used to differentiate specific vaginal infections (Table 25–2). For *Candida* infection, typical symptoms include intense pruritis, dysuria, and a white, curdlike discharge.[22,41] *Trichomonas* infection produces a large amount of frothy, yellowish green, foul-smelling vaginal discharge, which may or may not be accompanied by pruritis.[41] *Gardnerella* does not generally precipitate an inflammatory response and thus is not accompanied by soreness, itching, or burning. Rather, it is associated with a copious and odorous yellow or gray discharge with a fishlike odor.[11,41]

Genital herpes is characterized by intense vulvar pain associated with rupture of vulvar vesicles. If the lesions enter the urethra, dysuria may occur, and catheterization may be required.[42] Secondary infection of ruptured lesions occurs. Most patients with gonorrhea are asymptomatic, and those who have symptoms complain of vaginal discharge that is cervical in origin, dysuria, menstrual irregularity, and right upper quadrant pain.[13] The majority of patients with positive *Chlamydia* infections also are asymptomatic. Those who have symptoms complain of vaginal discharge and urethral symptoms[18] (Table 25–2).

Validity of these symptoms has been explored in several studies. In a study of 821 patients attending an ambulatory clinic, McCue et al. analyzed which symptoms aided in the differential diagnosis of a specific type of vaginitis.[4] Data were collected during an interview by a nurse practitioner. All patients were able to distinguish internal dysuria felt inside the body from external dysuria, which involved pain felt on the external genitalia when urine passed over it. A total of 578 of the patients had had diagnosed episodes of a pure vaginitis, which were defined as having diagnostic clinical and laboratory findings specific to one kind of vaginitis and no evidence of a concomitant second illness that could produce similar findings. A

TABLE 25–2. SYMPTOM PATTERNS IN SPECIFIC VULVOVAGINAL INFECTIONS

Symptom	Candida	Trichomonas	Gardnerella	Herpes	Gonococcus	Chlamydia
Pruritis	Intense Painful	Sometimes	Seldom	Sometimes		
Lesions				Vesicles	Abscess of Bartholin glands	
Pain				Tender groin nodes	Right upper quadrant pain	
Discharge	White, curdlike	Yellowish green	Grayish yellow		Mucopurulent from cervix	Mucopurulent from cervix
Odor		Foul	Fishlike			
Dyspareunia	Present					
Dysuria	Present			Present	Present	Present
Fever				Moderate		
Asymptomatic		25%	50%		70–80%	50%

total of 285 cases of *Candida,* 70 cases of *Trichomonas,* and 210 cases of nonspecific vaginitis were found. In these cases, vaginal discharge was reported by at least 90 percent in each group, and vulvar irritation occurred in the vast majority of those with *Candida* infections (93 percent) but in only 83 percent of those with *Trichomonas* and 74 percent of those with nonspecific vaginitis. External dysuria occurred in 31 percent of those with *Candida* infections, 29 percent of those with *Trichomonas,* and 23 percent of those with nonspecific vaginitis. Internal dysuria occurred far less frequently: in 4 percent of those with *Candida,* 11 percent of those with *Trichomonas,* and 3 percent of those with nonspecific vaginitis. From these results, it appears that history of vaginal discharge and complaints of vulvar irritation are sensitive symptoms for assessment of vaginitis in general but that they do not differentiate between types of vaginitis.

In a study by Daus and Hafez, 92 randomly selected pregnant and nonpregnant women were examined for incidence of vaginal candidiasis in an attempt to identify factors contributing to this diagnosis.[29] A positive diagnosis of vaginal candidiasis was defined as either positive characteristics of yeasts on immediate wet mount microscopic examination or, if that was negative, positive yeast culture on Nickerson's medium. A positive diagnosis was made in 45 percent of the women. Of these positive cases, there were no complaints of burning on urination, no complaints of dysuria, and no complaints of dyspareunia. However, pruritis vulvae was a common symptom, indicating its value in the assessment of vaginitis.

As well as the traditional symptoms of vaginitis, other historical data have been associated with its occurrence. Areas of concern include personal hygiene factors that may foster pathogenic growth. For example, excessive douching may irritate the vaginal mucosa, change the pH, and lead to growth of one or more pathogens.[30] Tightly fitting clothing, nylons, and lingerie may add to the warmth and moisture in the labial area, enhancing the growth of microorganisms. If the rectum is the source for vaginal contamination, inappropriate techniques for wiping and cleansing the perineum after urination and elimination, as well as poor handwashing technique, may facilitate the transfer of organisms from the rectum to the vagina. Other data that may be of value include changes in laundry detergents, use of scented deodorants, emotional upheaval, sexual practices, contraception practices, and the use of drugs, such as broad-spectrum antibiotics, that alter the vaginal environment.[22,43] These factors are untested but appear theoretically relevant and are of concern to many practitioners.[30]

Observation of Objective Signs

The third group of parameters used to assess vaginitis includes the objective signs obtained during patient examination. The external genitalia may be examined for erythema, lesions, and edema. During the internal examination using a vaginal speculum, erythema, secretions, and lesions are examined. Secretions can be tested for pH and glucose. Typical signs for each type of vaginitis have been described. For *Candida,* typical signs include white, cheesy or curdlike discharge with a yeasty odor, excoriation of the vulva, and small lesions appearing like open sores.[4,5,22,29,44] For *Trichomonas,* clinical signs include vulvar inflammation, green to yellowish foul discharge, and hemorrhagic lesions on the vaginal wall.[30] However, as many as 25 percent of the patients with positive identification of *Trichomonas* do not exhibit any clinical signs. For *Gardnerella,* the predominant sign is a very malodorous gray-white homogeneous discharge that does not reveal an inflamed mucosa when it is wiped away.[5,22] In addition, the normal acid pH of 4.0 to 4.5 is changed to 5.0 to 5.5.[5]

Herpes lesions are vesicles 2 to 4 mm in size that may occur on the vulva or the urethra. When they rupture, the base becomes pale yellow and the edges remain reddened.[42] Signs seen in gonorrhea include a mucopurulent discharge from the cervix and occasional abscess formation in Skene's or Bartholin's glands.[13] However, signs are not present in 70 to 80 percent of the women who have cultures positive for gonorrhea. Because it is predominantly a cervicitis rather than a vaginitis, the major sign seen in *Chlamydia* infection is a mucopurulent drainage from the cervix.[16] Another sign typical of *Chlamydia* infection occurs when swabbing the cervical area for culture leaves a bleeding, patchy area.

Sensitivity and validity of these objective symptoms have been explored in a number of studies. In the study by McCue et al., objective data were collected and compared for frequency of occurrence during pure *Candida, Trichomonas,* or nonspecific vaginitis.[4] A curdlike appearance of vaginal secretion, growth of *C. albicans* on a culture plate, presence of *Candida* on microscopic examination, and presence of *Trichomonas* on microscopic examination of the saline suspension were the four objective indicators examined. There was no correlation between a positive *Trichomonas* infection and the three *Candida* symptoms, indicating good differentiation and validity of the indicators. In addition, positive and significant correlations were present among the three *Candida* indicators, giving some evidence of reliability of these three factors. Both the sensitivity and specificity of three of the indicators for *Candida* infections were calculated. Sensitivity was calculated by how often an indicator was positive when both of the other two indicators were also positive. The specificity was calculated by determining how often the indicator was negative when both of the other two indicators were also negative. Microscopic examination was both most sensitive (0.91) and most specific (0.96), followed by curdlike discharge (0.77 and 0.86, respectively), and *Candida* on culture (0.82 and 0.80, respectively).

Probably because the incidence of clinical signs varies in *Trichomonas* infection, emphasis on valid criteria has focused on identification of the organism on wet mount microscopic examination and culture rather than on the occurrence of other subjective symptoms and objective signs. The incidence of pruritis has been reported at 50 percent.[41]

Signs of *Gardnerella* infection have been studied in more detail. Amsel et al. studied 397 consecutive female university students for the purpose of evaluating criteria with microbiologic and epidemiologic characteristics.[9] Criteria included vaginal pH, thin homogeneous vaginal discharge, release of a fish odor from a potassium hydroxide wet mount slide of vaginal discharge, the presence of abnormal amines in vaginal fluid, and the presence of clue cells in wet mount microscopic examination. The validity of pH was determined by examining it against cases diagnosed with at least two of the following three criteria: clue cells, potassium hydroxide odor, or thin homogeneous discharge. The most discriminating pH value for differentiating infected women from those with nonspecific vaginitis was 4.5. That is, 14 women with nonspecific vaginitis had a pH of 4.5 or less, and 158 women had a vaginal pH above 4.5. Correlations were done with the three criteria plus pH above 4.5, evidence of *Gardnerella* by the usual culture techniques, and a positive culture using medium highly selective for small amounts of bacteria. Results indicated that although the presence of the four signs occurred almost exclusively with patients who had positive cultures, about 18 percent of the patients with positive cultures did not have other objective signs. These results give validity to the clinical signs recommended but leave room for symptomatic patients to be missed if culture information is not included in the assessment.

PROTOCOLS FOR ASSESSING VAGINITIS

Management Tools
With the development of the extended role of the nurse and the physician's assistant, protocols have been developed to assist in the diagnosis and differentiation of the various kinds of vaginitis. These protocols include assessment tools to differentiate types of vaginitis clinically.

• SCHODDE PROTOCOL

One protocol, developed by Schodde, includes subjective symptoms (e.g., odor, burning after urination), laboratory tests (e.g., wet mount, culture), objective signs (e.g., vulvar inflammation, vaginal discharge), and an area for interpreting the assessment data and planning the follow-up treatment.[44] Schodde did not report on the validity of the assessment parameters selected or any statistical analysis for the reliability of the parameters.

• GREENFIELD ET AL. PROTOCOL

Greenfield et al. developed a protocol to be used by nurses in the management of dysuria, urinary frequency, and vaginal discharge.[45] The branching logic format includes historicy, physical examination, and laboratory criteria, which were validated by a group of medical consultants. The effectiveness of the protocol was tested on 146 patients. One group of patients was seen by the nurse using the protocol form and then by a physician who used the usual medical approach. The other group of patients was seen by tbe physician first and then by the nurse using the protocol form. Agreement between medical history factors was 139/146. Six of the seven discrepancies were physician error. For physical examination parameters, 137 of 146 were essentially the same. Similar results were obtained for laboratory data. The criteria were validated by demonstrating that patients receiving the protocol-directed treatment obtained the same high degree of symptom relief as those patients treated by the physician. Reliability of nurse identification of *Candida* under microscopic examination was determined by comparing nurse results with laboratory technician results. This comparison revealed that the laboratory failed to identify *Candida* in 9 cases of the 39 positive cases identified. The criteria in this protocol appear to have initial reliability and validity and include parameters relevant to dysuria and frequent urination as well as vaginitis.

Assessment Tools

• VAGINITIS ASSESSMENT FORM

An assessment form was developed and used in a study of vaginitis in female diabetics.[1] The purpose of the study was to test the effectiveness of a perineal care technique on the prevention and management of vaginitis. Subjects were followed weekly for 1 month. The Vaginitis Assessment Form included subjective symptoms, objective signs, and laboratory findings. In the development of the form, a panel of expert nurse practitioners familiar with assessing vaginitis in clinical practice was used to provide content validity for the variables selected and to test the format (Fig. 25–2). Patient interview was used to identify subjective symptoms, which included pruritis, discharge, odor, dyspareunia, dysuria, and burning. Objective signs were obtained during vaginal examination. The external genitalia were examined for erythema, lesions, and edema. Using a vaginal speculum, the vagina was examined for mucosal color, edema, discharge, odor, and lesions. Laboratory procedures included wet mount examination of vaginal saline and potassium hydroxide smears for the presence of hyphae or spores (*Candida*) and flagella or corkscrew movement (*Trichomonas*). Vaginal secretions were tested for pH, glucose, and ketones.

On the first 31 subjects, simultaneous cultures were made of the vagina and the labia to determine which site would reveal the greatest variety of data and the greatest number of

INTERVIEW

A. Menstrual cycle
1. LMPs _____
2. Length
3. Due date

B. Self-care practices
1. Douching
   a. No. of times/week _____
   b. Solution
2. Lingerie
3. Clothing
4. Urination/defecation practices

C. Sexual activity
1. Frequency
2. Types
   a. Heterosexual
   b. Homosexual
   c. Bisexual
3. Partner/s
4. Dyspareunia
5. Other _____
   a. Masturbation

D. Contraception practices:
1. IUD
2. Condom
3. Diaphragm
4. Pill – Name _____
5. Jelly/foam _____
6. Other _____

E. Drugs
1. Birth control pills
2. Antibiotics
3. Steroids
4. Tranquilizers
5. Barbiturates
6. Alcohol
7. Antihypertensives

F. Vaginitis history
1. Pruritis
   a. Labia
   b. Anterior perineum
   c. Perianal
2. Discharge
   a. Amount
   b. Color
3. Odor
4. Vaginal burning
5. Vaginal pressure
6. Vaginal soreness
7. Dysuria
8. Other _____

G. Psychosocial responses
1. Depression
2. Anxiety
3. Anger
4. Sadness
5. Fear
6. Other _____

PHYSICAL EXAMINATION

External Examination	Yes	No	Internal Examination	Yes	No
Erythema			Color		
Labia			Abnormal		
Anterior perineum			Erythema		
Perianal			Beefyred		
Pustules			Cyanotic, pale		
Labia majora			Edema (congested)		
Labia minora			Secretions		
Anterior perineum			Small		
Perianal			Moderate		
Edema			Profuse		
Labia			Odor		
Anterior perineum			Discharge		
Perianal			Clear		
Odor			White		
Discharge			Yellow		
White			Other _____		
Yellow-green			Plaques		
Gray			Cervical os		
Bloody (menses)			Round		
Groin, abdominal folds			Transverse		
Erythema			Excoriated		
Odor			Lesions		
Vesicles					
Discharge					

LABORATORY TESTS

	+	–		Additional information
Wet mount				
Hyphae				
Flagella				
Other _____				Problems/diagnosis
pH				
Vaginal glucose				
Culture				

Figure 25–2. Vaginitis Assessment Form.

411

organisms generally associated with vaginitis. Results showed that differences between the two culture sites were minimal, with positive cultures occurring more frequently from vaginal secretions. Selecting a random weekly examination assessment from each of the 143 subjects, the three sections of the instrument were analyzed for sensitivity and reliability. The history section consisted of those variables collected during patient interview: pruritis, discharge, odor, burning, vaginal pressure, vaginal soreness, dyspareunia, and dysuria. Chronbach coefficient alpha was calculated, and the results were 0.78. The external examination section consisted of those aspects of the examination involving the external genitalia: erythema, pustules, and edema. Chronbach alpha was calculated, and the results were 0.97. The third section consisted of the variables collected during the internal vaginal examination: vaginal wall color, edema, secretions, odor, discharge, and plaques or lesions. Chronbach alpha was calculated, and the results were 0.82. When all the variables were totaled for a grand scale total the Chronbach alpha revealed 0.92. These results indicate that some consistency is occurring within the subscale as well as in the total scale.

The relationship between the occurrence of vulvovaginal symptoms and positive cultures in this study population was illustrated through a comparison of the percentage of subjects having positive vulvovaginal symptoms at the beginning of the study (64 percent) versus the number of subjects who had positive cultures for *Candida, Trichomonas,* and/or *Gardnerella* (13 percent). The high incidence of patients with positive symptoms and negative cultures points to the need for an assessment tool that includes signs and symptoms as well as culture data.

SUMMARY

Assessment of vaginitis may involve three kinds of information: identification of pathogenic organisms, subjective symptoms, and objective signs. Different combinations of information are useful depending on whether the nurse, the practitioner, or the researcher is involved in the assessment. Most studies dealing with the validity and reliability of the variables have focused on methods for organism identification. Continuing issues in assessment of vaginitis include testing predisposing factors, the problem of mixed infections, the recurrence of the problem, and how to manage symptoms. These issues illustrate the need for a more thorough assessment of the patient in order to further explain the problem. For researchers, the variables used in assessment are often most valuable when they are standardized and understood. For the nurse working with patients clinically, management of symptoms is an important focus. One way to enrich this clinical practice would be to supplement the tools already developed for assessing vaginitis with some qualitative information; for example, what relationships occur between vaginitis and sexual function, personal hygiene, and clothing styles. In this way, tools developed via a qualitative methodology could be used to assess, measure, and diagnose the responses of women to vaginitis and begin to identify additional variables to be explored in other research projects.

ACKNOWLEDGMENT

Supported in part by NU00725, Division of Nursing, Bureau of Health Manpower, Health Resources Administration, Department of Health and Human Resources; Oregon Affiliate, American Diabetes Association; Office of Research Development and Utilization, School of

Nursing, Oregon Health Sciences University; and Department of Nursing Research, City of Hope National Medical Center, California.

REFERENCES

1. Grant, M., & Davidson, S. *Effects of perineal care on diabetic vulvovaginitis: Final report of project.* Supported by Grant Number 00725, Division of Nursing, Bureau of Health Manpower, Health Resources Administration, Department of Health and Human Resources, 1984.
2. Fisher, A.M. Clinical aspects, vaginal discharge, vaginitis and pruritus vulvae. *Clin Obstet Gynecol,* 1981, *8*(1):241.
3. Capraro, V.J., Rodgers, D.E., & Rodgers, B.D. Abnormal vaginal discharge. *Med Aspects Human Sexuality,* 1983, *17*(8):84,89,92,93,97,98.
4. McCue, J.D., Komaroff, A.L., Pass, T.M., et al. Strategies for diagnosing vaginitis. *J Fam Pract,* 1979, *9*(3):395.
5. King, J. Vaginitis. *J Obstet Gynecol Nurs,* 1984, *13*(Suppl):41s.
6. Kawada, C.Y. Treatment of vaginitis. *Am J Hosp Pharm,* 1980, *37*(8):1061.
7. Hall, L.F., Shayegani, M., & Hipp, S.S. Genital infections in women. *NY State J Med,* 1982, *82*(9):1317.
8. Levison, M.E., Trestman, I., Quach, R., et al. Quantitative bacteriology of the vaginal flora in vaginitis. *Am J Obstet Gynecol,* 1979, *133*(2):139.
9. Amsel, R., Totten, P.A., Spiegel, C.A., et al. Nonspecific vaginitis: Diagnostic criteria and microbial and epidemiologic associations. *Am J Med,* 1983, *74*(1):14.
10. Hurd, J.K. Vaginitis. *Med Clin North Am,* 1979, *63*(2):423.
11. Gardner, H.L. *Haemophilus vaginalis* vaginitis after twenty-five years. *Am J Obstet Gynecol,* 1980, *137*(3):385.
12. Cibley, L.J. *Trichomonas vaginalis* vaginitis. *Med Aspects Human Sexuality,* 1980, *14*(3):53.
13. Rivlin, M. Gonorrhea. In M. Rivlin, J.C. Morrison, & G.W. Bates (Eds.), *Manual of clinical problems in obstetrics and gynecology.* Boston: Little, Brown, 1983, p. 247.
14. Fiumara, J.N. Diagnosing and treating vaginal infection. *Consultant,* 1981, *21*(2): 281,284, 285,288,289,292.
15. Sanders, L., Harrison, H.R., & Washington, A.E. Treatment of sexually transmitted chlamydial infections. *JAMA,* 1986, *255*(13):1750.
16. Rivlin, M.E. Chlamydia, genital warts, and acquired immune deficiency syndrome. In M. Rivlin, J. Morrison, & G. Bates (Eds.), *Manual of clinical problems in obstetrics and gynecology.* Boston: Little, Brown, 1983, p. 258.
17. Handsfield, H., Jasman, L., Roberts, P., et al. Criteria for selective screening for *Chlamydia trachomatis* infection in women attending family planning clinics. *JAMA,* 1986, *255*(13):1730.
18. Schneider, G. Vaginal infections: How to identify and treat them. *Postgrad Med,* 1983, *73*(2):255.
19. O'Connor, B.H., & Adler, M.W. Current approaches to the diagnosis, treatment, and reporting of trichomoniasis and candidiasis. *Br J Vener Dis,* 1979, *55*(1):52.
20. Osborne, N.G., Grubin, L., & Pratson, L. Vaginitis in sexually active women: Relationship to nine sexually transmitted organisms. *Am J Obstet Gynecol,* 1982, *142*(8):962.
21. Carpenito, L.J. *Nursing diagnosis: Application to clinical practice.* Philadelphia: Lippincott, 1983.
22. Herbert, W.N.P. Recurrent vaginitis: Clues to successful therapy lie in identifying the causes. *Consultant,* 1984, *24*(9):46,53,56.
23. Bryson, Y., Dillon, M., Lovett, M., et al. Treatment of first episodes of genital herpes simplex virus infections with oral acyclovir. *New Engl J Med,* 1983, *308*(16):916.
24. Alteras, I., & Saryt, E. Prevalence of pathogenic fungi in toe webs and toe nails of diabetic patients. *Mycopatholgia,* 1979, *67*(3):157.
25. Knight, L., & Fletcher, J. Growth of candida in saliva: Stimulated by glucose associated with antibiotics, corticosteroids and diabetes mellitus. *J Infect Dis,* 1971, *123*(4):371.

26. Mehnert, B., & Mehnert, H. Yeasts in urine and saliva of diabetic and nondiabetic patients. *Diabetes,* 1958, *7*(4):293.
27. Friedrich, E.G. Vulvovaginitis. In H.G. Conn (Ed.), *Current therapy.* Philadelphia: Saunders, 1980.
28. Crenshaw, T. Vaginitis and epididymitis: When partners reinfect each other. *Med Aspects Human Sexuality,* 1985, *19*(11):74.
29. Daus, A.D., & Hafez, E.S.E. *Candida albicans* in women. *Nurs Res,* 1975, *24*(6):430.
30. Smith, L.S., & Lauver, D. Assessment and management of vaginitis and cervicitis. *Nurse Pract,* 1984, *9*(6):34,39,67.
31. Feinberg, J.G., & Whittington, M.J. A culture medium for *Trichomonas vaginalis* and species of *Candida. J Clin Pathol,* 1957, *10*:327.
32. King, A.J., & Nicol, C.S. In *Veneral Disease.* London: Balliere, Tindall & Cassell, 1975.
33. Oriel, J.D. Clinical overview of candidal vaginitis. Proc R Soc Med, 1977, *70*(Suppl 4):7.
34. O'Brien, J.R. Nickerson's medium in the diagnosis of vaginal moniliasis. *J Can Med Assoc,* 1964, *90*(18):1073.
35. Pattman, R.S., Sprott, M.S., & Moss, T.R. Evaluation of a culture slide in the diagnosis of vaginal candidiasis. *Br J Vener Dis,* 1981, *57*(1):67.
36. Miles, M.R., Olsen, L., & Rogers, A. Recurrent vaginal candidiasis. *JAMA,* 1977, *238*(17):1836.
37. Smith, R.F., Rodgers, H.A., Hines, P.A., & Ray, R.M. Comparisons between direct microscopic and cultural methods for recognition of *Cornebacterium vaginale* in women with vaginitis. *J Clin Microbiol,* 1977, *5*(3):268.
38. Granoto, P., & Rolfaro, M. Comparative evaluation of enzyme immunoassay and culture for the laboratory diagnosis of gonorrhea. *Am J Clin Pathol,* 1985, *83*(5):613.
39. Branato, P., Schneible-Smith, C., & Weiner, L. Use of New York City medium for improved recovery of *Neisseria gonorrhoeae* from clinical specimens. *J Clin Microbiol,* 1981, *13*(5):963.
40. Davidson, S.B., & Grant, M.M. Effects of perineal care on diabetic vulvovaginitis. *West J Nurs Res,* 1983, *5*(3):55.
41. Novotny, T. Vaginal disease: Venereal and nonvenereal types. *Postgrad Med,* 1983, *73*(5):303.
42. Hatch, K. Practical management pointers for an embarrassing problem. *Consultant,* 1982, *22*(3):45.
43. Gorline, L.L., & Stegbauer, C.C. What every nurse should know about vaginitis. *Am J Nurs,* 1982, *82*(12):1851.
44. Schodde, G. A vaginitis protocol that helps teach. *Nurse Pract,* 1975, *1*(2):64.
45. Greenfield, S., Friedland, G., Scifers, S., et al. Protocol management of dysuria, urinary frequency, and vaginal discharge. *Ann Int Med,* 1974, *81*(4):452.

Index

Note: Page numbers followed by an *f* refer to figures; those followed by a *t* refer to tables.

Note: Page numbers followed by an *f* refer to figures; those followed by a *t* refer to tables.

Note: Page numbers followed by an *f* refer to figures; those followed by a *t* refer to tables.

Note: Page numbers followed by an *f* refer to figures; those followed by a *t* refer to tables.

Note: Page numbers followed by an *f* refer to figures; those followed by a *t* refer to tables.

Note: Page numbers followed by an *f* refer to figures; those followed by a *t* refer to tables.

Note: Page numbers followed by an *f* refer to figures; those followed by a *t* refer to tables.